Register Now for Online Access
to Your Book

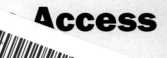

SPRINGER PUBLISHING
C⏻NNECT™

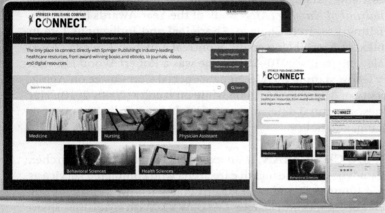

Your print purchase of *Health Equity and Nursing* **includes online access to the contents of your book**—increasing accessibility, portability, and searchability!

Access today at:

http://connect.springerpub.com/content/book/978-0-8261-9507-4
or scan the QR code at the right with your smartphone
and enter the access code below.

PXW5SGSE

Scan here for quick access.

SPRINGER **PUBLISHING COMPANY**
View all our products at springerpub.com

Margaret P. Moss, PhD, JD, RN, FAAN, is a member of the Mandan, Hidatsa, and Arikara Nation, Three Affiliated Tribes of North Dakota. Dr. Moss is the first and only American Indian to hold both nursing and juris doctorates. She is currently director of the University of British Columbia's First Nations House of Learning and a tenured associate professor in the Faculty of Applied Science-Nursing. Formerly, Dr. Moss was assistant dean of diversity and inclusion, and associate professor (tenured) at the University of Buffalo, School of Nursing. She published the first nursing textbook on American Indian health and nursing (Springer Publishing Company, 2015). This text won two *American Journal of Nursing (AJN)* Book of the Year Awards (2016). Dr. Moss was a Fulbright Visiting Research Chair in Aboriginal and Indigenous Life in the North American Context at McGill University, Montreal, Quebec, Canada (2014) while on the faculty at Yale University (2010–2015). She was a Robert Wood Johnson Foundation Health Policy fellow staffing the U.S. Senate Special Committee on Aging. She tenured at the University of Minnesota in 2006 while on faculty (2000–2010). Her focus is in health disparities, structural determinants of health especially in American Indian/Alaska Natives, aging, and policy.

Janice M. Phillips, PhD, RN, CENP, FAAN, is an experienced clinician, researcher, educator, and public policy advocate in the health care arena who completed service as a 2010–2011 Robert Wood Johnson Foundation Health Policy fellow, working in the congressional office of Senator John D. Rockefeller IV (D-WV). With specialties spanning oncology, public health, women's health, minority health, nursing regulation, and research administration, she is passionate about eliminating health disparities and achieving health equity. Dr. Phillips holds a BSN from North Park College and an MS in community health from St. Xavier College, both in Chicago, and a PhD in nursing from the University of Illinois, College of Nursing. She is the director of nursing research and health equity at Rush University Medical Center in Chicago and an associate professor at the Rush University College of Nursing. Dr. Phillips was appointed by the Secretary of Health and Human Services in October 2019 to serve a 4-year term on the National Advisory Council of Nurse Education and Practice (NACNEP or "Council") of the Health Resources and Services Administration (HRSA). The Council provides advice and recommendations to the secretary and Congress with respect to the administration of Title VIII of the Public Health Service Act.

Health Equity and Nursing

Achieving Equity Through Policy, Population Health, and Interprofessional Collaboration

Margaret P. Moss, PhD, JD, RN, FAAN
Janice M. Phillips, PhD, RN, CENP, FAAN
Editors

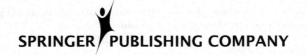

SPRINGER PUBLISHING COMPANY

Copyright © 2021 Springer Publishing Company, LLC

Springer Publishing Company, LLC
11 West 42nd Street, New York, NY 10036
www.springerpub.com
connect.springerpub.com/

Acquisitions Editor: Adrianne Brigido
Compositor: Exeter Premedia Services Private Ltd.

ISBN: 978-0-8261-9506-7
ebook ISBN: 978-0-8261-9507-4
DOI: 10.1891/9780826195074

20 21 22 23 / 5 4 3 2 1

The author and the publisher of this Work have made every effort to use sources believed to be reliable to provide information that is accurate and compatible with the standards generally accepted at the time of publication. The author and publisher shall not be liable for any special, consequential, or exemplary damages resulting, in whole or in part, from the readers' use of, or reliance on, the information contained in this book. The publisher has no responsibility for the persistence or accuracy of URLs for external or third-party Internet websites referred to in this publication and does not guarantee that any content on such websites is, or will remain, accurate or appropriate.

Library of Congress Cataloging-in-Publication Data

Names: Moss, Margaret P., editor. | Phillips, Janice Mitchell, editor.
Title: Health equity and nursing : achieving equity through policy, population
    health, and interprofessional collaboration / Margaret P. Moss, Janice M. Phillips,
    editors.
Description: New York, NY : Springer Publishing Company, LLC, [2021] |
    Includes bibliographical references and index.
Identifiers: LCCN 2019054764 (print) | LCCN 2019054765 (ebook) | ISBN
    9780826195067 (paperback) | ISBN 9780826195074 (ebook)
Subjects: MESH: Nurse's Role | Health Equity | Health Policy | Population
    Health Management | Social Determinants of Health |
    Nursing--organization & administration | United States
Classification: LCC RT51 (print) | LCC RT51 (ebook) | NLM W 76 AA1 | DDC
    610.73--dc23
LC record available at https://lccn.loc.gov/2019054764
LC ebook record available at https://lccn.loc.gov/2019054765

Contact us to receive discount rates on bulk purchases.
We can also customize our books to meet your needs.
For more information please contact: sales@springerpub.com

Publisher's Note: New and used products purchased from third-party sellers are not guaranteed for quality, authenticity, or access to any included digital components.

Printed in the United States of America.

Dedicated to my late parents—a physician and a nurse who propelled me along my professional journey. My father, Dr. Charles P. Henke, was a tireless, lifelong advocate and administrator in the (former) Veterans Administration, and my mother, Norma K. Henke, was nurse to my family and the community. Together, they served as an interprofessional, policy, and provider example for me.

—Margaret P. Moss, PhD, JD, RN, FAAN

Dedicated to the many unsung sheroes and heroes who are committed to ensuring health equity for those most in need.

—Janice M. Phillips, PhD, RN, CENP, FAAN

Contents

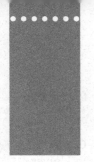

Contributors

Franchesca A. Cifuentes-Andrade, MS, Member of the Board of Directors, Kigezi Women and Children Health Initiative

Margherita Procaccini Clark, MSN, Dean, Health and Human Services, Lansing Community College, Lansing, Michigan; Member of the Board of Directors, Kigezi Women and Children Health Initiative

Daniel E. Dawes, JD, Director, Satcher Health Leadership Institute, Morehouse School of Medicine, Atlanta, Georgia

Myra Michelle DeBose, PhD, MSN, MSEd, RN, Assistant Professor, Graduate Program, Prairie View A & M University College of Nursing, Houston, Texas

Joanne Disch, PhD, RN, FAAN, Professor ad Honorem, University of Minnesota School of Nursing, Minneapolis, Minnesota

Nelson J. Dunlap, JD, Public Policy Manager, Satcher Health Leadership Institute, Morehouse School of Medicine, Atlanta, Georgia

Jacqueline Fawcett, PhD, ScD (hon), RN, FAAN, ANEF, Professor, Department of Nursing, University of Massachusetts Boston, Boston, Massachusetts

Diana Peña Gonzalez, MPH, CHES, Health Education Specialist, Institute for Healthcare Advancement, La Habra, California

Sinsi Hernández-Cancio, JD, Founding Director of the Center on Health Equity Action for System Transformation, Families USA, Washington, District of Columbia

Tonda L. Hughes, PhD, RN, FAAN, Henrik H. Bendixin Professor of International Nursing, Professor of Psychiatry (in Nursing), Director of Global Health Research, Columbia University, New York, New York

Kirby Johnson, MPH, CHES, Health Educator, Emergency Preparedness and Response Division, Los Angeles County Department of Public Health, Los Angeles, California

Debbie Ann Jones, PhD, MS, RN, Clinical Assistant Professor, Prairie View A & M University College of Nursing, Houston, Texas

Wrenetha A. Julion, PhD, MPH, RN, CNL, FAAN, Professor & Department Chair, Women, Children and Family Nursing, Rush University College of Nursing, Chicago, Illinois

Mia Keeys, MA, Director of Health Equity Policy and Advocacy, Center for Health Equity, American Medical Association, Washington, District of Columbia

Sharon Larson, PhD, Professor and Executive Director, Main Line Health Center for Population Health at Lankenau Institute for Medical Research and Jefferson University College of Population Health, Wynnewood, Pennsylvania

Kevin C. Lo, MPH, Public Health Administrator and Advocate, New York, New York

Barry D. Mann, MD, FACS, Chief Academic Officer, Professor of Surgery, Jefferson Medical College, Lankenau Medical Center, Annenberg Conference Center, Wynnewood, Pennsylvania

Heather Miller, BSN, RN, College of Nursing, Rush University Medical Center, Chicago, Illinois

Patricia J. Moreland, PhD, CPNP, RN, FAAN, Assistant Clinical Professor, Lillian Carter Center for Global Health and Social Responsibility, Nell Hodgson Woodruff School of Nursing, Emory University, Atlanta, Georgia

Angela M. Moss, PhD, RN, APRN-BC, Assistant Dean of Faculty Practice & Assistant Professor, Rush University College of Nursing, Chicago, Illinois

Margaret P. Moss, PhD, JD, RN, FAAN, Hidatsa/Dakota, Director-First Nations House of Learning & Associate Professor in the Faculty of Applied Science, School of Nursing, University of British Columbia, Vancouver, British Columbia

Christopher M. Nolan, MPA, System Manager, Community Health and Benefit, Rush University System for Health; Instructor, Department of Health Systems Management, Rush University College of Health Sciences, Chicago, Illinois

Chinwe Onyekere, MPH, System Director, Health Equity and Graduate Medical Education, Designated Institutional Official, Lankenau Medical Center, Annenberg Conference Center, Wynnewood, Pennsylvania

Janice M. Phillips, PhD, RN, CENP, FAAN, Director of Nursing Research and Health Equity, Nursing Administration, Rush University Medical Center, Chicago, Illinois

Monique Reed, PhD, RN, Assistant Dean Generalist Entry Program, Associate Professor Department of Community Systems and Mental Health Nursing, Rush University College of Nursing, Chicago, Illinois

Rachel Roberts, MPH, CHES, Manager, Community Health Engagement and Strategy, Institute for Healthcare Advancement, La Habra, California

Shonalie Roberts, MHA, ARM, Lankenau Medical Center, Program Administrator, Medical Student Advocate Program and Health Equity, Main Line Health, Wynnewood, Pennsylvania

William E. Rosa, PhD, APRN-BC, FCCM, FAANP, FAAN, Robert Wood Johnson Foundation Future of Nursing Scholar, University of Pennsylvania School of Nursing, Philadelphia, Pennsylvania

Sandra Ross, MSW, LSW, Manager, Undergraduate Medical Education, Lankenau Medical Center, Annenberg Conference Center, Wynnewood, Pennsylvania

Sharon L. Ruyak, PhD, CNM, RN, Assistant Professor, College of Nursing, University of New Mexico, Albuquerque, New Mexico

Linda Spoonster Schwartz, DrPH, MSN, RN, FAAN, Senior Advisor, Vietnam Veterans of America, Associate Clinical Professor of Nursing, Yale University, New Haven, Connecticut

Raj C. Shah, MD, Associate Professor, Family Medicine and Rush Alzheimer's Disease Center, Co-Director, Center for Community Health Equity, Rush University Medical Center, Chicago, Illinois

Karen Fitzpatrick Smith, BS, Manager, Workforce Development, Human Resources, Main Line Health, Radnor, Pennsylvania

Ejim Sule, PhD, MSN, RN, Assistant Professor, Prairie View A & M University College of Nursing, Houston, Texas

Noelle Thompson, Former Health Equity Intern, Families USA, Washington, District of Columbia

Justina A. Trott, MD, FACP, Clinical Professor of Medicine, Internal Medicine, University of New Mexico Health Sciences Center, Albuquerque, New Mexico

Thomas Tsang, MD, MPH, CEO and Co-Founder, Valera Health, Brooklyn, New York

Barbara Wadsworth, DNP, RN, FAAN, FNAP, FACHE, Senior Vice President/Chief Nursing Officer, Main Line Health, Bryn Mawr, Pennsylvania

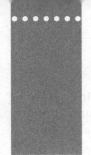

Foreword

At the forefront of the American healthcare system there are concerns about equity and growing disparities. These issues are not new but seem to draw growing concern in the midst of the opioid, behavioral health, obesity, and vaping epidemics. Across the nation we see vast differences in access to health and healthcare services but recognize there are significant challenges in finding cost-effective and sustainable solutions.

There are many factors that impact health and healthcare, some of which will be addressed in this textbook, *Health Equity and Nursing*. The text is presented in three sections that provide the reader with key concepts, principles, pathways, and strategies to achieving health equity. Section I: Policy Issues and Implications for Nursing describes the role of nursing and call to action in achieving health equity. Section II: Population Health provides a discussion on the important change in thinking from eliminating health disparities to achieving health equity through a population lens. Section III: Interprofessional Collaboration captures initiatives, programs, and professionals in and out of the health sciences as examples of how nursing can and must work with other bodies to achieve health equity.

This textbook is timely given the many health-related challenges facing the United States. Disparities in minority health and healthcare will have growing implications for an increasingly diverse nation. Much attention has been focused on health disparities and inequities in recent years. These disparities span the spectrum of health and healthcare services and are reflected in increased incidence and mortality rates across numerous diseases. Disparities are also seen in measures of healthcare access. This can include inadequate access in rural communities, gaps in resources for individuals with disabilities, and lack of access for racial and ethnic minority groups and underserved populations. What is often not addressed is the role the nursing profession can play in reducing inequities and disparities at the community level through leadership, policy development, care delivery, community engagement, and interprofessional education.

Nurses have a powerful voice that can stimulate innovation and change in care delivery, policy development, and health equity. The concepts in this text provide a foundation to understand the policy issues and the implications for nursing in addressing inequities in health. This text also provides a framework for translating data into actions that can change the healthcare landscape, improve access to care for the underserved, close the gap in social determinants of health, and improve the quality of care regardless of where one lives, works, plays, or worships.

In our country there are a number of barriers to achieving full health for many groups. Health should not be dependent upon how much you make or what you look like. These inequities in our country must be fixed, and working together we have the power to change that. We must commit ourselves to the simple and just idea that health equity is everyone's right. This text acquaints the reader with tools and strategies needed to understand the intersection of policy, nursing, and health.

The health of the nation will be best served by nurses who are engaged in creating policy change that improves health equity across the life span. This will require nurses at all levels to obtain and use knowledge, skill, and experience to achieve health equity for all.

Sylvia Trent-Adams, PhD, RN, FAAN

Preface

Health Equity and Nursing: Achieving Equity Through Policy, Population Health, and Interprofessional Collaboration is designed to do the following:

1. Illuminate the role of nursing in achieving health equity
2. Examine current and emerging topics of relevance to achieving health equity
3. Articulate future directions for advancing the health equity agenda through nursing education, practice, research, and policy advocacy

Doctor of Nursing Practice programs are designed around "The Essentials of Doctoral Education for Advanced Nursing Practice" (American Association of Colleges of Nursing, 2006) of which some are explicitly made into sections in this text: Policy, Population Health, and Interprofessional Collaboration. Others such as some of those listed here are found *within* these sections.

    I.   Scientific Underpinnings for Practice
    II.   Organizational and Systems Leadership for Quality Improvement and Systems Thinking
    III.   Clinical Scholarship and Analytical Methods for Evidence-Based Practice
    IV.   Information Systems/Technology and Patient Care Technology for the Improvement and Transformation of Healthcare
    V.   Healthcare Policy for Advocacy in Healthcare
    VI.   Interprofessional Collaboration for Improving Patient and Population Health Outcomes
    VII.   Clinical Prevention and Population Health for Improving the Nation's Health
    VIII.   Advanced Nursing Practice

This textbook consists of 18 chapters divided into three sections. Each chapter includes learning objectives, key terms, key objectives, and related resources. The proposed text expands on existing discussions and resources on health equity by including an in-depth overview on health equity coupled with specific implications for the nursing profession. Although there are many nurse leaders who have contributed to this text, we also included interprofessional examples and contributors. It is through understanding policy and change, the populations that are most affected by inequalities, and the necessity of interprofessional collaboration that we can move the needle on achieving health equality.

    This text, although focused on health equity for all of nursing, speaks to several essentials of the Doctor of Nursing Practice (DNP) and PhD educational requirements.

Section I: Policy Issues and Implications for Nursing describes the role of nursing and call to action in achieving health equity. The book opens with a discussion on the power of nursing to make substantive contributions to improving the health for all populations. Influential nurse leaders describe emerging trends and issues such as creating a culture of health and solidifying the presence of nursing in the health policy arena. Authors issue a clarion call for greater nursing leadership in eliminating health disparities, reversing health inequities, and addressing the social determinants of health; all are critical steps in our journey toward achieving health equity. This section includes genetics as well.

Section II: Population Health provides a timely discussion on the transition from eliminating health disparities to achieving health equity. A reduction in or the elimination of health disparities serves as evidence that we are moving in the right direction toward achieving health equity. This section of the book opens with an overview of key concepts, principles, and pathways related to enhancing health equity. Authors describe population-based and population-specific inequities in health outcomes among diverse populations such as veterans and racial and ethnic minorities. There are chapters on social determinants of health and structural determinants of health.

Section III: Interprofessional Collaboration captures initiatives, programs, and professionals in and out of the health sciences as examples of how nursing can and must work with other bodies to achieve health equity, recognizing that no one discipline/profession can or has been able to make significant strides in "closing the gap."

We hope that this book will serve as a valuable resource for graduate nursing students as well as other audiences with a vested interest in and commitment to achieving health equity. It is our hope that the reader will be intellectually enhanced and empowered to remain front and center in efforts devoted to achieving the best of health for all populations.

Margaret P. Moss, PhD, JD, RN, FAAN

Janice M. Phillips, PhD, RN, FAAN, CENP

■ Reference

American Associaton of Colleges of Nursing. (2006). *The essentials of doctoral education for advanced nursing practice.* Retrieved from https://www.aacnnursing.org/Portals/42/Publications/DNPEssentials.pdf

Policy Issues and Implications for Nursing

I

1

Introduction: Health Equity Does Not Equal Health Equality

Janice M. Phillips and Margaret P. Moss

CHAPTER OBJECTIVES

- ◉ Define health equity and its importance in shaping the health and well-being of populations
- ◉ Elucidate the connection among health equity, health disparities, and the social and structural determinants of health
- ◉ Highlight implications for nursing in achieving health equity

KEY CONCEPTS

Health equity

Health inequities

Social determinants of health

Structural determinants of health

Social justice

◼ Introduction

The goal of achieving health equity has received considerable attention within the past decade and will remain a major concern nationally and internationally well into the 21st century. Although there are several definitions of health equity, for the purposes of this book, we use the definition of health equity as defined by the Robert Wood Johnson Foundation (RWJF). The RWJF defines health equity as follows:

> Health equity means that everyone has a fair and just opportunity to be as healthy as possible. This requires removing obstacles to health such as poverty, discrimination, and their consequences, including powerlessness and lack of access to good jobs with fair pay, quality education and housing, safe environments, and health care. (2017, para. 1)

Noted scholar and health equity professor Paula Braveman (2014) called for greater clarity regarding definitions of health disparities and health equity and underscored that explicit definitions call for the integration of an ethical and a human rights perspective.

To advance the work in this area, *Healthy People 2020* defines health disparities as:

> a particular type of health difference that is closely linked with social, economic, and/ or environmental disadvantage. Health disparities adversely affect groups of people who have systematically experienced greater obstacles to health based on their racial or ethnic group; religion; socioeconomic status; gender; age; mental health; cognitive, sensory, or

> physical disability; sexual orientation or gender identity; geographic location; or
> other characteristics historically linked to discrimination or exclusion. (Office of
> Disease Prevention and Health Promotion [ODPHP], n.d.-b, para. 6)

Explicit definitions of health equity and health disparities are critical to helping ensure that resources are properly allocated to populations in need, particularly economically disadvantaged populations (Braveman, 2014). However, throughout this text, contributors will use the accepted or emerging definitions relevant to their work. Importantly, the terms "health equity" and "health disparities" are interwoven in that any progress toward achieving health equity will be measured by our progress in reducing and ultimately eliminating health disparities. In contrast, the term "health inequality," as defined by UK researcher Margaret Whitehead, refers to health differences that are unavoidable, unjust, and unnecessary (Whitehead, 1991). Social justice principles are the underpinnings for achieving health equity and eliminating inequities that result in poor health outcomes. One cannot achieve health equity until disparities are eliminated, health inequities are successfully addressed, and social justice principles are integrated paving the way for individuals, communities, and populations to experience their fullest health potential.

Equally relevant to achieving health equity are the social determinants of health. There is a growing consensus that addressing the social determinants of health, factors outside of clinical determinants of health, is critical to achieving health equity especially for our most vulnerable populations. The World Health Organization (WHO) provides one of the most frequently cited definitions on the social determinants of health.

> The social determinants of health are the conditions in which people are born,
> grow, live, work and age. These circumstances are shaped by the distribution of
> money, power and resources at global, national and local levels. The social determi-
> nants of health are mostly responsible for health inequities – the unfair and avoid-
> able differences in health status seen within and between countries. (2012, para. 1)

There is ample evidence that shows that health is defined as being more than traditional clinical care, which is believed to account for approximately 20% of health outcomes, with the remaining 80% of health outcomes are attributed to the social, behavioral, and economic factors (University of Wisconsin Population Health Institute, 2019).

Thus initiatives devoted to achieving health equity must include a focus on addressing the social determinants of health, personal, social, structural, economic, and environmental factors that influence health status and health outcomes (ODPHP, n.d.-a). To that end, we also offer a chapter on the less studied structural determinants of health and a model for thinking about how it fits with social determinants of health and health outcomes. These concepts reflect the nursing metaparadigm: person, health, nurse, and environment; as well as the holistic perspective of the person. Collectively, health equity, health disparities, health inequities, and the social determinants of health work together.

The urgency to achieve health equity underscores the need for nurses at all levels and practice settings to develop the necessary acumen, knowledge, expertise, and partnerships that will enable them to be full participants in achieving the highest level of health for all populations. In fact, it is imperative that nurses become active advocates in all arenas surrounding healthcare.

Given that nursing represents the largest sector of the health professions with more than 3.5 million RNs in the United States (American Association of Colleges of Nursing, 2019), nurses are well positioned to play a leadership role in this endeavor and are invited to do so. In the United States, where nursing continues to evolve as one of the most respected, well-recognized, and trusted professions, nurses have increased opportunities to extend their influence in helping all populations experience optimal health, thus moving us toward achieving health equity for the nation. Numerous nurse leaders are calling for more nursing engagement in this arena and have identified a number of implications for nursing practice, education, research, and policy advocacy (Lathrop, 2013; National League for Nursing [NLN], 2019; Persaud, 2018; Schroeder, Kohl Malone, McCabe, & Lipman, 2018; Williams, Phillips, & Koyama, 2018).

■ Discussion Questions

- Does your employing institution, professional organization, or local or state government have a health equity strategic plan? If so, how might you utilize your expertise and influence in helping to achieve the health equity goals outlined in the health equity plan and related initiatives?
- How might you infuse the concepts "health equity," "health inequity," and the "social determinants of health" into clinical practice and nursing research?
- What steps might you as a nurse take to help achieve health equity?

■ Resources

American Association of Colleges of Nursing. (2006). *The essentials of doctoral education for advanced nursing practice*. Retrieved from https://www.aacnnursing.org/Portals/42/Publications/DNPEssentials.pdf

Braveman, P., Arkin, E., Orleans, T., Proctor, D., & Plough, A. (2017). *What is health equity? And what difference does a definition make?* Princeton, NJ: Robert Wood Johnson Foundation.

Haddad, L. M., & Toney-Butler, T. (2019). Nursing shortage. In *StatPearls*. Treasure Island, FL: StatPearls Publishing. Retrieved from https://www.ncbi.nlm.nih.gov/books/NBK493175

■ References

American Association of Colleges of Nursing. (2019). *Nursing fact sheet*. Retrieved from https://www.aacnnursing.org/News-Information/Fact-Sheets/Nursing-Fact-Sheet

Braveman, P. (2014). What are health disparities and health equity? We need to be clear. *Public Health Reports, 129*(Suppl. 2), 5–8.

Lathrop, B. (2013). Nursing leadership in addressing social determinants of health. *Policy, Politics and Nursing Practice, 14*(1), 41–47. doi:10.1177/1527154413489887

National League for Nursing. (2019). *A vision for integration of the social determinants of health into nursing education curricula*. Retrieved from http://www.nln.org/docs/default-source/default-document-library/social-determinants-of-health.pdf?sfvrsn=2

Office of Disease Prevention and Health Promotion. (n.d.-a). *Healthy People 2020: Social determinants of health.* Retrieved from https://www.healthypeople.gov/2020/topics-objectives/topic/social-determinants-of-health

Office of Disease Prevention and Health Promotion. (n.d.-b). *Healthy People 2020: Social disparities.* Retrieved from https://www.healthypeople.gov/2020/about/foundation-health-measures/Disparities

Persaud, S. (2018). Addressing the social determinants of health through advocacy. *Nursing Administration Quarterly, 42*(2), 123–128. doi:10.1097/naq.0000000000000277

Robert Wood Johnson Foundation. (2017). *What is health equity?* Retrieved from https://www.rwjf.org/en/library/research/2017/05/what-is-health-equity-.html

Schroeder, K., Kohl Malone, S., McCabe, E., & Lipman, T. (2018). Addressing the social determinants of health: A call to action for school nurses. *The Journal of School Nursing, 34*(3), 182–191. doi:10.1177/1059840517750733

University of Wisconsin Population Health Institute. (2019). *2019 County Health Rankings Key Findings Report.* Retrieved from https://www.countyhealthrankings.org/reports/2019-county-health-rankings-key-findings-report

Whitehead, M. (1991). The concepts and principles of equity and health. *Health Promotion International, 6*(3), 217–228. doi:10.1093/heapro/6.3.217

Williams, S., Phillips, J., & Koyama, K. (2018). Nurse advocacy: Adopting a health in all policies approach. *The Online Journal of Issues in Nursing, 23*(3), Manuscript 1. Retrieved from http://ojin.nursingworld.org/MainMenuCategories/ANAMarketplace/ANAPeriodicals/OJIN/TableofContents/Vol-23-2018/No3-Sept-2018/Policy-Advocacy.html

World Health Organization. (n.d.). *Social determinants of health.* Retrieved from https://www.who.int/social_determinants/sdh_definition/en

2

Nursing as a Force for Health Equity

Joanne Disch

CHAPTER OBJECTIVES

- ⊙ Examine nursing's historical role in promoting health equity
- ⊙ Explore the impact of the nursing lens
- ⊙ Describe several actionable steps that nurses can take in promoting health equity

KEY CONCEPTS

Health equity

Diversity

The nursing lens

Historical nursing constructs

Nursing *Code of Ethics*

Systems thinking

Person- and family-centered care

Empowering care

The human condition

KEY TERMS

Ethics

Safe, Timely, Effective, Efficient, Equitable, Patient-Centered (STEEEP)

Quality and Safety Education for Nurses (QSEN)

Unique attributes

Advocacy

Action

Clear mandate

Nursing expertise

Nursing curricula

Self-reflection

Political consciousness

Equity

◼ Introduction

"Health equity" is defined as "the absence of disparities or avoidable differences among socioeconomic and demographic groups or geographic areas in health status and health outcomes such as disease, disability, or mortality" (Health Resources and Services Administration [HRSA], 2018, p. 6). In the rest of this book, health equity and inequity, as well as health disparities, are examined from numerous perspectives. The purpose of this chapter is to review some of the historical nursing constructs that position nursing to be especially attuned to promoting health equity and to offer actionable recommendations as to what nurses should be doing, both individually and collectively, in carrying out this special responsibility. To this point, Gloria Smith has argued that nursing is the health profession best suited for leadership in reducing disparities, noting that nursing and health disparities are "inextricably linked by their very natures" since caring is the very essence of nursing and "health disparities are fundamentally the result of lack of caring within society" (2007, p. 285).

■ Health Equity as a Rising Concern

The impetus for the Alma Ata Declaration 40 years ago (World Health Organization [WHO], 1978) was the growing recognition that health is not evenly distributed within and among countries. Since that time, increased attention has been paid by national and world organizations to reduce health disparities, for example, WHO (Commission on Social Determinants of Health, 2008); the U.S. Department of Health and Human Services (HHS, 2011); the HRSA (2017).

Concurrent with these efforts, the Institute of Medicine (now the National Academy of Medicine) published its landmark report *Crossing the Quality Chasm* (2001), declaring that "equity" was one of the six fundamental components of healthcare safety and quality. These six components formed the STEEEP acronym (safe, timely, effective, efficient, equitable, patient-centered) to represent the performance measures that need to be in place if quality care is to be delivered. Two more recent efforts aimed at helping individuals achieve health equity are one by the National Academies of Practice (*Communities in Action: Pathways to Health Equity*; Weinstein, Geller, Negussie, & Baciu, 2017) and the Robert Wood Johnson Foundation (n.d.) modules on its website to help individuals learn about and adopt strategies to achieve health equity.

■ Health Equity as a Fundamental Principle Within Nursing

The nursing profession's *Code of Ethics* expressly states in Provision 1 that "[t]he nurse practices with compassion and respect for the inherent dignity, worth, and unique attributes of every person" (American Nurses Association [ANA], 2015, p. 1) Furthermore, Provision 8 (see Box 2.1) speaks to the specific obligation to advance health and human rights and reduce disparities.

Beyond the *Code of Ethics*, by which every nurse is accountable for his or her practice, other nursing initiatives reinforce the responsibility for working to achieve equity and reduce disparities. Examples include the work of the following:

- The National Advisory Council on Nurse Education and Practice (NACNEP) in its Report to the HHS Secretary and the Congress on Achieving Health Equity Through Nursing Workforce Diversity (NACNEP, 2013)
- The Quality and Safety Education for Nurses (QSEN) Initiative through its work on helping faculty learn—and be better able to teach—the competencies that form the foundation of quality care (STEEEP); and defining patient-/family-centered care as "recognizing the patient or designee as the source of control and full partner in providing compassionate and coordinated care based on patient's preferences, values and needs" (Cronenwett et al., 2007, p. 123)
- The African American Health Engagement Study (AAHES), a collaboration of Pfizer, the National Medical Association (NMA), and the National Black Nurses Association to gain insights to increase health equity in African American communities (NMA, 2018)
- Barnsteiner, Disch, and Walton (2014) in publishing *Person and Family-Centered Care*, which underscores the need to move to *person-* and family-centered care since, increasingly, the recipients of nursing care are not always patients but school

Box 2.1: ANA Code of Ethics, Provision 8.3: Obligation to Advance Health and Human Rights and Reduce Disparities

Advances in technology, genetics, and environmental science require robust responses from nurses working together with other health professionals for creative solutions and innovative approaches that are ethical, respectful of human rights, and equitable in reducing health disparities. Nurses collaborate with others to change unjust structures and processes that affect both individuals and communities. Structural, social, and institutional inequalities and disparities exacerbate the incidence and burden of illness, trauma, suffering, and premature death. Through community organizations and groups, nurses educate the public; facilitate informed choice; identify conditions and circumstances that contribute to illness, injury, and disease; foster healthy life styles; and participate in institutional and legislative efforts to protect and promote health. Nurses collaborate to address barriers to health—poverty[,] homelessness, unsafe living conditions, abuse and violence, and lack of access—by engaging in open discussion, education, public debate, and legislative action. Nurses must recognize that health care is provided to culturally diverse populations in this country and across the globe. Nurses should collaborate to create a moral milieu that is sensitive to diverse cultural values and practices.

ANA, American Nurses Association.

Source: From American Nurses Association. (2015). *Code of ethics for nurses with interpretive statements.* Silver Spring, MD: Author.

children, elders living in community resource centers, individuals wanting to stay healthy, the homeless, or communities and populations (They argue that the word "patient" denotes illness and a dependency model when actually today's relationship with recipients of care needs to be more respectful and based on a partnership model, recognizing individual differences, strengths, and values.)

Cathy Crowe (2006), a street nurse who has strongly advocated for the homeless in Canada, pointedly highlights this nursing legacy: "Throughout our history, it has been nurses who, after witnessing injustices spoke out. They responded with words, with research, with action, with the development of programs, with legal action and with new policy proposals."

This has been the case within nursing for hundreds of years. Florence Nightingale, the founder of modern Western nursing, addressed this issue when she discussed nursing's responsibility to not only take care of the patient but also tend to the environment: "that the symptoms or the sufferings generally considered to be inevitable and incident to the disease are very often not symptoms of the disease at all, but of something quite different – of the want of fresh air, or of light, or of warmth, or of quiet, or of cleanliness, or of punctuality and care in the administration of diet, of each or of all of these" (1992, p. 93).

Dozens of other nursing advocates have followed this lead, such as Lillian Wald in 1893 when she worked with a colleague to generate financial support to establish a community-based care center in the Lower East Side of New York; or Anne Ross who was inspired by people she met in her community in the 1950s—"those who lacked food or a steady income, people who lacked parenting skills, those living in situations of domestic abuse or neglect" (Crowe, 2006)—and who pushed for legislation to legalize contraception, including a woman's right to choose. A documentary, *Anne Ross: Rebel With a Cause* (Pryor, 1998), profiles her work. Or Patty Gerrity and her colleagues in 1996 when they entered into an agreement with the Philadelphia Housing Authority to address health issues in Philadelphia's 11th Street Corridor, establishing a Health Center for these historically underserved residents (American Academy of Nursing [AAN], n.d.).

For decades, nursing leaders in the United States and across the globe have written about the particular affinity that nurses share for tackling inequities and disparities. Pauly, MacKinnon, and Varcoe issued a call to include health equity as an explicit arena for nursing focus, including "both the conditions that shape access to health services and the structural conditions that influence health and produce health inequities" (2009, p. 118). Reutter and Kushner stated that "nursing has a clear mandate to ensure access to health and health-care by providing sensitive empowering care to those experiencing inequities and working to change underlying social conditions that result in and perpetuate health inequities" (2010, p. 269). Mary Wakefield noted: "Influencing policy means taking clear positions. Like cars in neutral, nurses who are neutral when it comes to health-related policy miss critically important opportunities to advance the health of patients and communities and to advance the profession" (Patton, Zalon, & Ludwick, 2019, p. 465).

■ The Nursing Lens

One way to think about the perspective that nurses bring to health equity is through the nursing lens. As was noted in an editorial, the nursing lens is "a viewpoint from which [the nurse] sees things holistically, considering the person, population or community in the larger context" (Disch, 2012, p. 170). Nurses are systems thinkers, particularly effective at establishing meaningful relationships, with expertise at seeing the big picture and crafting pragmatic solutions that fit within an individual's lifestyle. Things are not always as they seem—and the skillful nurse uses a broader lens when developing interventions with people. Read in Box 2.2 about an extraordinary nurse practitioner (NP) within the Department of Veterans Affairs (VA) system who used her nursing lens to cocreate an effective intervention for a patient.

We know that providing expert, individualized care to a patient and family is the foundation of nursing care—but we also know that we must assess the impact of the illness or procedure more broadly, including the impact on the family, the mitigating factors that might improve or impede recovery, and on upstream factors that warrant attention to prevent further occurrences to this person or others. As Barnsteiner has noted, "nurses today must accept responsibility for delivering high-quality patient care *and* for identifying and addressing system issues" wherever they occur (Disch, 2019, p. 350).

■ Nursing Actions to Improve Health Equity

Nurses have the requisite skills and an inherent commitment to address health equity, inequity, and disparities. We understand the human condition. We have the ability

Box 2.2: An NP's Effective Use of the Nursing Lens

The cardiology NP and attending physician were jointly seeing a patient with conges-tive heart failure in their clinic. They decided that a change in diuretics was warranted. The physician provided comprehensive education about the drug, its side effects, and asked the patient to give the nurses a call if he gained more than 3 pounds within the week. The patient nodded in understanding and said that he would do this. When the physician left, the NP recalled a key fact about the patient's background—he was homeless and, thus, unlikely to have a scale to weigh himself. After confirming that he was homeless, she asked if they could come up with another approach to assess whether the drug was working: "Could you watch whether your shoes become tight over the next few days—and if they do, can you give us a call?" She also made a note to talk with the social worker about housing.

NP, nurse practitioner.

to forge meaningful relationships with individuals and their families during stressful times. We are pragmatic when designing solutions that will work for individuals, orga-nizations, or communities, and we can be fierce advocates for social justice and raising people's voices. As Claire Fagin and Donna Diers noted: "we think of ourselves as Flor-ence Nightingale—tough, canny, powerful, autonomous, and heroic" (1983, p. 116).

Nursing is also well suited, if not best suited, because of nursing's focus on individ-uals within the context of their families, homes, and communities. The skillful nurse cannot treat the patient without consideration of these interconnected components. What is required is a two-pronged approach. Reutter and Kushner (2010) describe the mandate to (a) provide sensitive empowering care at the individual/community level to those experiencing inequities; and (b) work to change the environmental and social conditions that are the root cause of those inequities. Accomplishing these two goals requires understanding the context, origins, and parameters of inequities as well as how the inequities are experienced.

Other chapters in this text cover the nature and extent of health disparities. Emphasized here are two overarching goals for nurses:

- *Provide sensitive empowering care*: Dexheimer-Pharris (2014) writes powerfully of this challenge when describing the approach that a Black nurse successfully employed when taking care of a critically ill White supremacist. Drawing on the *Code of Ethics for Nurses*, she knew that she had to bring her best and healthiest self to their interactions, and that "she also needed to do the mental and spiritual work that involved an analysis of the social structures that set up and maintain racism in her country, which is necessary core content in schools of nursing so that nurses understand the historical roots of racial conflict" (p. 186). She also knew that she had to practice cultural humility, and not impose her beliefs on the situation but rather seek to better understand what this patient wanted, and to work with him to achieve his goals.
- *Work to change the environmental and social conditions that are the root cause of inequities*: Nurses have several options open to them for addressing this larger

problem. Within one's own organization, nurses can work to raise understanding of the existence of inequities or the unintended consequences of certain barriers. Perhaps the electronic health record (EHR) unintentionally perpetuates stereotyping or fails to allow for adequate personalization of the healthcare plan (e.g., noting that someone is homeless). In another situation, a nurse may have important observations to share about someone's response to treatment and yet no place to chart this. For example, the nurse may assess that the patient is especially responsive to a particular pain medication and so needs a far smaller dose than usual. In yet another situation, organizational practices may allow for physicians and others to overlook these sections of the EHR. Within communities, nurses can band together with colleagues to identify persistent problems that foster inequities, such as when multiple hospitals in a community routinely discharge patients with inadequate pain management or without attention to proper placement. Working collectively to effect change at the state level enabled Mary Chesney, PhD, RN, APRN, CNP, FAAN, and colleagues to achieve success, after 16 years of strategic work, in removing statutory barriers to Minnesota's APRN practice, thus expanding access to Minnesotans of quality healthcare (Sabo, Chesney, Tracy, & Sendelbach, 2017). Disch (2019) outlines several strategies for applying the nursing lens to policy work to improve health equity, along with numerous examples of nurses successfully doing this.

To accomplish these goals, Williams and Phillips (2019) propose five steps to address health disparities with several pragmatic suggestions for each. Box 2.3 highlights these with a few examples.

Additional recommendations are presented here:

1. Practice self-reflection and deepen your political consciousness (Pauly et al., 2009). Health is a relative concept and requires understanding one's own values as well as the multiple factors that shape another's experience of it. Expose yourself to new ways of thinking and understanding others' experiences.
2. Spend time learning about the many ways in which social determinants influence health and those by which your patients are particularly affected. Beyond the traditional factors such as food security, housing, income, and social exclusion, factors such as organizational mandates, community constraints, and financial pressures can also promote inequities.
3. Engage other nurses and colleagues who share your concerns in discussing the issue(s) and developing possible approaches.
4. Join and engage in professional organizations to amplify the impact of action.
5. Participate in community health needs assessment processes and outreach opportunities for innovative care delivery within the communities.
6. Become active in the political process, from writing a letter to the editor to joining a campaign or running for office. Nurses are given credence and respect by virtue of their experiences, perspectives, and trustworthiness.
7. Choose your words wisely. As Rumay Alexander, president of the National League for Nursing, has noted: "Words put you on a path" (personal communication, August 20, 2018). Insensitive language and stereotypical attributions perpetuate inequities.

Box 2.3: Five Steps to Address Health Disparities

Increase awareness about health disparities
- Contact the media with stories about health disparities in your community
- Speak at health fairs, parent–teacher association (PTA) and school board meetings, civic meetings, faith-based events, and other community gatherings

Become a leader for addressing health disparities
- Educate others about disparities and share stories about model programs
- Form coalitions with local organizations representing diverse sectors to ensure relevant agendas are on local and state health agendas

Support healthy and safe behaviors in your community
- Involve your employees or neighbors in a group physical activity or challenge
- Host seminars in your local library, school, workplace or other venues to discuss health disparities in your community

Improve access to healthcare
- Partner with a local healthcare provider or employer to offer free health screenings in your workplace or place of worship
- Ask local healthcare providers to translate health and healthcare information into relevant languages

Create healthy neighborhoods
- Advocate for more sidewalks, bike lanes, and recreation facilities
- Ask your neighborhood supermarkets to provide fresh fruit and vegetables to the local food bank

Source: From National Partnership for Action to End Health Disparities. (2011). *Toolkit for community action.* Washington, DC: U.S. Department of Health and Human Services, Office of Minority Health. Retrieved from http://minorityhealth.hhs.gov/npa/files/plans/toolkit/NPA_toolkit.pdf

8. Gather input from patients, their families, and community residents as to what *they* identify as barriers to accessing healthcare—and then join with others to address them.

9. Strive to fix underlying system issues rather than individual situations. Many years ago, nurses at Children's Hospital of Philadelphia would bring in clothes to give to family members who had need. While laudable, this resulted in unequal distribution—and usually family members to whom the nurses felt particularly connected received the donations, inadvertently perpetuating imbalances. Nursing leaders worked with the social work department to establish a coordinated system by which nurses could bring in clothing and family members could equitably receive the items (J. Barnsteiner, personal communication, 1990).

10. Nurse educators should ensure that nursing curricula help nursing students understand contemporary realities and develop sensitive and effective approaches for using their nursing lens to improve health equity.

11. Nurse researchers should engage in community-based research, where appropriate, or at least actively include the people most affected in designing interventions and evaluating improvements.

■ Conclusion

Integral to professional nursing practice is the responsibility to promote health equity and the dignity and worth of each individual. In a seminal document, Margretta Styles (1982) issued a *Declaration of Belief About the Nature and Purpose of Nursing*. In this document, she outlined several beliefs about nursing's role, responsibility, and special position within society. "I believe in nursing as an occupational force for social good, a force that, in the totality of its concern for all human health states and for mankind's responses to health and environment, provides a distinct, unique, and vital perspective, value orientation and service."

While the context of nursing practice has changed from that time, the call to service and the obligation to provide both excellent individualized nursing care and system change remain. Nurses must embrace the stance that "I will make a difference." Paradoxically, making this difference may have become more difficult, given the unrealized promises of technology and the pursuit of standardization of care and efficiency. Consistent application of standards, regardless of individual differences, can actually set back personalized care and certainly undermine health equity. What is needed is an individualized approach in the context of best practice standards.

■ Critical Thinking Exercise

"It just happened again! This time it was Mr. Dombrowski who told the clinic supervisor that he didn't want me taking care of him. I know it's because I'm gay. I don't think that's right—but I don't know what to do about it."

- What information would you want to gather to better understand the situation?
- With whom would you talk?
- What would you say?
- What resources (e.g., organizational, regional, national) could help inform you about the broader issue(s)?
- What could be the first step to develop/amend the organization's practices or policies?

■ Discussion Questions

1. What particular skills or perspectives do nurses bring to policy formation and policy implementation?
2. Why is it not sufficient to provide good patient care in today's healthcare environment?
3. What are the greatest barriers to nurses becoming politically active?
4. What content and skill sets need to be added to nursing curricula to better equip nurses to be politically active?

■ Resources

American Hospital Association. (2017). 2018 *equity of care toolkit* http://www.equityof care.org/resources/resources/2018%20EOC%20Toolkit.pdf

Andermann, A. (2016). Taking action on the social determinants of health in clinical practice: A framework for health professionals. *CMAJ, 188*(17–18), E474–E483. doi:10.1503/cmaj.160177

Lowe, J. (2015). Health equity research. *Nursing Research, 64*(1), 1–2. doi:10.1097/NNR.0000000000000075

■ References

American Academy of Nursing. (n.d.). Behavioral health. Retrieved from http://www.aannet.org/initiatives/edge-runners/behavioralhealth

American Nurses Association. (2015). *Code of ethics for nurses with interpretive statements*. Silver Spring, MD: Author.

Barnsteiner, J., Disch, J., & Walton, M. (Eds.). (2014). *Person and family centered care*. Indianapolis, IN: Sigma Theta Tau International.

Commission on Social Determinants of Health. (2008). *Closing the gap in a generation: Health equity through action on the social determinants of health*. Geneva, Swizterland: World Health Organization. Retrieved from http://apps.who.int/iris/bitstream/handle/10665/43943/9789241563703_eng.pdf

Cronenwett, L., Sherwood, G., Barnsteiner, J., Disch, J., Johnson, J., Mitchell, P., . . . Warren, J. (2007). Quality and safety education for nurses. *Nursing Outlook, 55*(3), 122–131. doi:10.1016/j.outlook.2007.02.006

Crowe, C. (2006). The poor will always be with us? Not if nurses have a role! Retrieved from http://tdrc.net/resources/public/Crowe_Speech_june_16_06.htm

Dexheimer-Pharris, M. (2014). Patient-centered care in the face of cultural conflict. In J. Barnsteiner, J. Disch, & M. K. Walton (Eds.), *Person and family centered care* (pp. 185–202). Indianapolis IN: Sigma Theta Tau International.

Disch, J. (2012). The nursing lens. *Nursing Outlook, 60*(5), 170–171. doi:10.1016/j.outlook.2012.05.004

Disch, J. (2019). Applying a nursing lens to shape policy. In P. M. Patton, M. L. Zalon, & R. Ludwick (Eds.), *Nurses making policy: From bedside to boardroom* (2nd ed., pp. 329–356). New York, NY: Springer Publishing Company.

Fagin, C., & Diers, D. (1983). Nursing as metaphor. *New England Journal of Medicine, 309*, 116–117. doi:10.1056/nejm198307143090220

Health Resources and Services Administration. (2018). *Health equity report 2017*. Retrieved from https://www.hrsa.gov/sites/default/files/hrsa/health-equity/2017-HRSA-health-equity-report.pdf

Institute of Medicine. (2001). *Crossing the quality chasm: A new health system for the 21st century*. Washington, DC: National Academies Press.

National Advisory Council on Nurse Education and Practice. (2013). *Achieving health equity through nursing workforce diversity*. Retrieved from https://www.hrsa.gov/advisorycommittees/bhpradvisory/nacnep/Reports/eleventhreport.pdf

National Medical Association. (2018). New study provides critical insights on unique health needs of African Americans. Retrieved from https://www.nmanet.org/news/413336/NEW-STUDY-PROVIDES-CRITICAL-INSIGHTS-ON-UNIQUE-HEALTH-NEEDS-OF-AFRICAN-AMERICANS.htm

National Partnership for Action to End Health Disparities. (2011). *Toolkit for community action*. Washington, DC: U.S. Department of Health and Human Services, Office of Minority Health. Retrieved from http://minorityhealth.hhs.gov/npa/files/plans/toolkit/NPA_toolkit.pdf

Nightingale, F. (1992). *Notes on nursing: What it is, and what it is not* (A commemorative edition). Philadelphia, PA: Lippincott.

Patton, R. M., Zalon, M. L., & Ludwick, R. (2019). Taking action: Shaping the future. In P. M. Patton, M. L. Zalon, & R. Ludwick (Eds.), *Nurses making policy: From bedside to boardroom* (2nd ed., pp. 447–474). New York, NY: Springer Publishing Company.

Pauly, B. M., MacKinnon, K., & Varcoe, C. (2009). Revisiting "Who gets care?" Health equity as an arena for nursing action. *Advances in Nursing Science, 32*(2), 118–127. doi:10.1097/ans.0b013e3181a3afaf

Pryor, H. (Director). (1998). *Anne Ross: Rebel with a cause* [Documentary]. Montreal, QC, Canada: National Film Board of Canada.

Reutter, L., & Kushner, K. E. (2010). 'Health equity through action on the social determinants of health': Taking up the challenge in nursing. *Nursing Inquiry, 17*(3), 269–280. doi:10.1111/j.1440-1800.2010.00500.x

Robert Wood Johnson Foundation. (n.d.). Achieving health equity. Retrieved from https://www.rwjf.org/en/library/features/achieving-health-equity.html

Sabo, J. S., Chesney, M., Tracy, M. F., & Sendelbach, S. (2017). APRN consensus model implementation: The Minnesota experience. *Journal of Professional Nursing, 8*(2), 10–16. doi:10.1016/s2155-8256(17)30093-5

Smith, G. R. (2007). Health disparities: What can nursing do? *Policy, Politics and Nursing Practice, 8*(4), 285–291. doi:10.1177/1527154408314600

Styles, M. (1982). *On Nursing: Toward a new endowment.* St Louis, MO: CV Mosby.

U.S. Department of Health and Human Services. (2011). *HHS action plan to reduce racial and ethnic ealth disparities: A nation free of disparities in health and health care.* Retrieved from https://minorityhealth.hhs.gov/npa/files/Plans/HHS/HHS_Plan_complete.pdf

Weinstein, J. N., Geller, A., Negussie, Y., & Baciu, A. (Eds.). (2017). *Communities in action: Pathways to health equity.* Washington, DC: National Academies Press. Retrieved from https://www.nap.edu/read/24624/chapter/1

Williams, S. D., & Phillips, J. M. (2019). Eliminating health inequities through national and global policy. In P. M. Patton, M. L. Zalon, & R. Ludwick (Eds.), *Nurses making policy: From bedside to boardroom* (2nd ed., pp. 339–422). New York, NY: Springer Publishing Company.

World Health Organization. (1978). *Primary health care: Report of the International Conference on Primary Health Care: Alma-Ata, USSR.* Geneva, Switzerland: Author.

3 Evidence-Based Policy Making

Myra Michelle DeBose, Ejim Sule, and Debbie Ann Jones

CHAPTER OBJECTIVES

- Define evidence-based policy making
- Articulate the role of nurses in informing the health policy–making process
- Identify key sources of evidence used by lawmakers to inform the health policy–making process

KEY CONCEPTS

Evidence-based nursing practice   Legislative influences
Evidence-based policy making

KEY TERMS

The Congressional Legislative Branch   National Academy of Medicine
Congressional Budget Office   Library of Congress
Government Accountability Office

■ Introduction

Just as nurses use evidence to inform nursing practice, policy makers must also rely on evidence to shape the policy discourse and policy-making process. Such evidence is derived from expert testimony, consumer advocacy groups, case studies, think tanks, previous legislative initiatives, professional and voluntary organizations, as well as evidence from a number of federal and nonfederal agencies. This chapter addresses evidence-based health policy making, highlights key sources of evidence on which policy makers depend during the policy-making process, and articulates implications for nurses in shaping the health policy–making process. We reviewed literature across three main concepts: evidence-based nursing practice (EBNP), evidence-based policy making, and legislative influence. We reviewed several blogs, books, position papers, research articles, and articles of interest that met our inclusion criteria for this discussion.

Evidence-based policy making involves using evidence to establish policies that will improve healthcare and client outcomes. Evidence-based policy making is a:

> discourse or set of methods which informs the policy process, rather than aiming to directly affect the eventual goals of the policy. It advocates a more rational, rigorous and systematic approach. The pursuit of EBP is based on the premise that policy decisions

should be better informed by available evidence and should include rational analysis. This is because policy which is based on systematic evidence is seen to produce
better outcomes. The approach has also come to incorporate evidence-based
practices. (Sutcliffe & Court, 2005, p. iii)

Thus, evidence is critical for developing, implementing, and evaluating health policy
(Cookson, 2005).

The decision-making process in creating health policy should be rigorous
enough to address sensitive and complex issues that will influence populations and
ensure equitable access to healthcare. Known barriers to achieving health equity
can include limited to no access to care, escalating healthcare costs, lack of healthcare resources especially in underserved areas, and lack of culturally competent
providers along with a variety of social and economic factors. Therefore, policy
makers must secure credible evidence from a variety of sources regarding these
issues, sources that will enable policy makers to turn complex decisions into equitable policies for all.

Policy making is not for the faint of heart and requires commitment to seeing
policy development through its many stages of development. Though policy makers
may have access to scientific evidence, many factors may influence how policy makers use this information and what finally influences their decisions. These barriers
may include competing priorities, funding issues, and the lack of constituent input.
Constituent input is particularly important when it comes to some of our most underserved and impoverished communities. The following discussion highlights several
sources of evidence used to help inform the policy-making process.

■ The Pew-MacArthur Results First Initiative

According to the Pew-MacArthur Results First Initiative (The Pew Charitable Trusts
[Pew], 2018), evidence-based policy making can be most effective when governmental
agencies adopt key components of their initiative. These components include program
assessment, budget development, implementation oversight, outcome monitoring,
and targeted evaluation. State and local policy makers can use key components as a
framework to align their decision-making process to evaluate their actions.

- *Program assessment* assists policy makers to ensure projects are original and nondu-
  plicated and ensure taxpayer investments are wisely used.
- *Budget development* should rely on researching an inventory of programs already
  funded and determine their effectiveness.
- *Implementation oversight* allows the policy makers and project managers to guarantee execution of initiatives as planned. Many programs may be new and require
  support to build capacity to implement their projects.
- *Outcome monitoring* helps to pinpoint any challenges faced by projects and to
  determine whether the solutions they have in place will make a difference.
- *Targeted evaluation* helps policy makers compare measured outcomes of funded
  programs to new programs in an effort to determine community-level impact.
  Finally, impact evaluations allow policy making to key in on how effective the project was to be able to meet its outcomes (Pew, 2018).

The Pew-MacArthur Results First Initiative guides policy makers in identifying programs that yield a stronger return on investment. Policy makers seeking the best return on taxpayer dollars are increasingly focusing on cost-effective programs that have demonstrated outcomes. Evidence-based policy making is one strategy to gain support among public leaders who want to reduce wasteful spending, expand successful programs, and strengthen accountability. Evidence-based policies centered on research inform policy development. Results suggesting that an intervention will be favorable for the community will have a better chance of passing into law by policy makers (Pew, 2017).

This Pew-McArthur Initiative (Pew, 2017) also provides an online tool that allows government officials to estimate which funded programs are a worthwhile investment. Government officials can analyze programs and compare program benefits and costs of various federally funded programs (Dube, 2019).

The Milbank Memorial Fund is a foundation created to improve population health. The foundation participates in "nonpartisan analysis, collaboration, and communication on significant issues in health policy" (Milbank Memorial Fund, n.d., para. 1). The fund publishes reports and issues briefs and case studies that are available for policy makers to review to assist with decision-making. This resource is available for developing policy leaders focused on improving population health and eliminating health disparities (Hiatt, 2018). One such partner of Milbank Memorial Fund is the Robert Wood Johnson Foundation Health & Society Scholars (HSS).

A group of six case studies that may be helpful can be accessed at Milbank Memorial Fund in order to get a better understanding of decision-making and policy development. Although the HSS Scholar Program is no longer in existence, the Milbank Memorial Fund has made these case studies available for students, lawmakers, and those interested in policy development. The Milbank Memorial Fund published these case studies in the hope that many audiences, including students, would use them to learn about the connections among research, decision-making, and policy (Hiatt, 2018).

■ Resources Available to Support the Policy-Making Process

There are numerous sources of evidence available to policy makers during the policy-making process. These sources include but are not limited to the following:

- Congressional Budget Office (CBO)
- Congressional Legislative Offices
- Government Accountability Office (GAO)
- National Academy of Medicine (NAM)
- Library of Congress (LOC)

The CBO prepares Congressional reports and cost estimates for budgetary and economic considerations. The CBO can predict the cost of supporting proposed legislation and its impact on the federal budget. This office is nonpartisan, which allows it to conduct an impartial and unbiased analysis (CBO, 2019).

The law requires the CBO to determine a formal cost estimate for most bills approved by the House or Senate Committees. Only appropriation bills are exempt from formal written cost estimates. In addition, CBO will generate informal cost estimates for several Congressional committee legislative proposals. Additional information on the CBO and cost estimates can be found in the literature (CBO, 2019).

The Congressional Legislative Branch is composed of the Senate and the House of Representatives (lawmakers). This body is responsible for making decisions including health policy decisions that affect the nation. Every policy begins with an idea that can go to any elected official. If the elected official shares interest or is convinced of the idea's value, a bill can be written and introduced to the legislative body. The bill is discussed by the legislative bodies, and its pros and cons are debated. After much discussion, the bill is voted on and accepted or rejected. When the bill is passed, it reaches the president to be written into law.

Just like nurses depend on evidence-based research to make decisions, lawmakers also depend on various kinds of evidence to make decisions. Such evidence is derived from leading nursing organizations, expert testimony, consumer advocacy, expert witnesses, case studies, think tanks, and professional and voluntary organizations along with a number of federal and nonfederal agencies.

Nurses play a major role in the passage or support of the bills through their professional and specialty organizations. This is one of the reasons why nurses must join and participate in these organizations. When proposed legislation is up for voting or support, the American Nurses Association (ANA), for example, calls/emails and texts nurses to call or email their representatives to support or not to support the bill. Many organizations have pretyped rationales sent to legislative officials to support the organization's position on an issue. The lawmakers review the rationales to help inform their decision-making when drafting legislation. It is not enough to create health policies based on what policy makers like or want. They must have evidence from the constituents in order to bring the legislation forward.

The GAO is an independent and nonpartisan legislative branch support agency that provides various services to Congress. These services include providing oversight investigation and evaluation of executive operations, activities, and programs. In addition, it establishes standards that guide the provision of reports related to federal budgets and education (Kaiser, 2008).

The GAO is a good source for lawmakers because of their oversight responsibility when it comes to health policy. Reports from the GAO are structured, detailed, and reliable and provide valuable insights during the policy decision-making process. Reports also outline ways to prevent waste in the management of government programs. Congressional members may also call on the GAO to do a report on an issue in which Congress needs more information. To illustrate, on June 13, 2019, the GAO released the report GAO-19_433 on the need for proper oversight on nursing home patients. The report posited the need for the Centers for Medicare and Medicaid Services (CMS) to institute oversight on state agencies, while the Congress analyzes CMS data. The findings and recommendations can be seen in Table 3.1.

The NAM is a resource that nurses can use to obtain scientific evidence-based data, which can be used to help policy makers make decisions. The NAM, formerly known as the Institute of Medicine (IOM), was founded in 1970. The reports provided by the National Academy of Medicine can lead to pathways for the making of federal laws, regulations, and policies. The reports provided by the NAM are regarding identified medical care issues as well as education and research (NAM, 2019a).

The National Academy of Medicine (2019b) partnered with several public and private groups and organizations to form a collaborative action plan to fight the opioid

TABLE 3.1 GAO FINDINGS AND RECOMMENDATIONS FOR PROPER OVERSIGHT ON NURSING HOME PATIENTS

GAO FINDINGS	GAO RECOMMENDATIONS TO CMS
Mental and physical abuse increased over sexual abuse	Report all abuse and the perpetrator type into CMS database using the required guideline and forms. CMS to monitor trends of the reports
Abuse deficiency doubled from 2013 to 2017	Conduct oversight of state survey agencies to ensure that abuse cases are timely reported to law enforcement
Gaps in state agency timely reporting process of reporting	Require all state survey agencies to refer suspected cases of abuse against nursing home residents to law enforcement Develop guidance for state survey agencies when seeking clarification that verified allegations should be reported to law enforcement where it is not possible to cite a federal deficiency to the facilities
Lack of guidance on the content of the report submitted by nursing homes	Develop guidance and a standardized form for reporting by all state survey agencies Provide guidance on the content of the referral that should be sent to law enforcement

CMS, Centers for Medicare and Medicaid Services; GAO, Government Accountability Office.
Source: Data from Governmental Accountability Office. (2019). *Nursing homes: Improved oversight needed to better protect residents from abuse.* Retrieved from https://www.gao.gov/assets/700/699721.pdf

crisis. Five expert panelists presented case scenarios and discussed the challenges of pain control from the perspectives of patients and their caregivers. The evidence presented by the expert panelists illustrates gaps in the current literature and informs best practices. Each panelist provided recommendations that can be used for informing new policies regarding the tapering of opioids in pain management (NAM, 2019c). Nurses can use the information gathered in reports from National Academy of Medicine to shape policy.

The LOC is a resource that lawmakers use to obtain health policy information. It is the oldest and largest library in the world and the main research arm of the U.S. Congress (LOC, n.d.). Lawmakers depend on this library to obtain vital information required to help them in decision-making polices. The library can be accessed online, and materials can be requested through interlibrary loan (www.loc.gov/rr/loan). The LOC houses the Law Library, which makes it possible for lawmakers to view historical legislative information and activities. It provides policy consults where Congressional members can meet via technology, such as Skype and Zoom. Lawmakers also view legal reports, transcripts, webcasts, and videos from previous Senate committee hearings (LOC, n.d.).

The LOC houses archives of judiciary committee hearings and meetings. A number of hearings are archived at the LOC. The hearings and meetings can be viewed and used as evidence to illustrate or showcase issues of concern. These hearings can be instrumental in shaping related policies.

Recommendations on the use of evidence to inform policy decisions are provided. Health policy derived from people who will be affected by policy should be the starting place for policy development. It is not enough to create health policies based on what policy makers like or want. Reviewing a single journal article is not as robust as evaluating a systematic review of the literature. The systematic review is designed to provide a complete summary of current evidence and upon review can play a major role in informing health policy decisions. The evidence must be reviewed by policy makers and must be relevant, transparent, and robust (Innvaer, Gunn, Trommald, & Oxman, 2002; Oxman, Lavis, Lewin, & Fretheim, 2009). There are several links to be found at the home page of the LOC that can be useful in gathering information about current legislative activities. One can also find links to bills to be considered and ways to contact local and state representatives.

■ Implications for Nurses

EBNP allows nurses to use clinical expertise along with the most up-to-date research available on a given topic to provide quality care for clients. Quality improvement interventions that are based on appraisal of "high quality studies and statistically significant research finding" can also be beneficial in policy formation. In addition, review of community-based participatory research (CBPR) outcomes can assist in addressing health inequities and developing policies (Cacari-Stone, Wallerstein, Garcia, & Minkler, 2014).

The role of nurses in early health policy and policy making can be traced to public health movements, like modern-day community-based health initiatives. For example, the need for children to be protected from child labor abuse gave rise to the Federal Children's Bureau. Policy initiatives credited from public health placed nurses in schools and in occupational health settings due to evidence learned from previous initiatives (Ridgway, n.d.). Other policy initiatives such as those for preventing violence against women and federal policies to boost health literacy have the potential to impact client outcome and healthcare access (Kilpatrick, 2000; Koh et al., 2012).

Nurses found themselves implementing policy rather than being a primary influence in shaping policy. The latter would allow better control over nursing practice. There has been an acknowledgment in recent times of how valuable nurses can be in influencing health policies. The evidence-based influence in health policies to which nurses contribute can be seen in care coordination, case management, and patient safety to promote quality healthcare and healthy communities (Almaguer, Law, & Young, 2014; Ferguson, 2001; Spann, 2009; Taft & Nanna, 2008; Toofany, 2005).

Healthcare policies help support standards of care (Burke, 2016). Nurses in leadership roles collaborate to influence health policy issues that affect healthcare and client outcomes nationally and globally (Burke, 2016). Nurses who participate in policy development can impact how care is delivered today as well as tomorrow. Nurses should participate in policy making at local, state, and federal levels of government using their academic and professional experiences to inform health policy process and to enhance policies passed into law (IOM, 2011).

Communication is one of the processes utilized to disseminate evidence-based projects to policy makers and stakeholders, including academicians and professional colleagues. Sharing quality improvement and research projects helps to advance clinical practice, provide optimal care, and improve client outcomes (LoBionda-Wood & Haber, 2018, p. 244). Most often, academicians use traditional methods (e.g., journals, posters, and oral publications) to disseminate these projects. Today, nontraditional venues, such as social media, have become alternative methods of dissemination. The most popular venues are Twitter, YouTube, Vimeo, SlideShare, and Web 2.0 (LoBionda-Wood & Haber, 2018, p. 245).

Collaboration between clients and healthcare providers is instrumental to ensuring that client's healthcare outcomes are improved. This alliance allows clinicians and clients to work together on evidence-based treatment plans. Hence, shared decision-making provides an opportunity for positive impact on clinical outcomes (Arora, Moriates, & Shah 2015; de Wit et al., 2017).

The implications of this chapter may assist health professionals and others in shaping their understanding of how evidence is needed to inform all aspects of the policy-making process. Program outcome data from initiatives that address health inequity have the potential to inform policy makers in critical decision-making. These decisions can create policy actions in both healthcare systems and nonhealth sectors that will contribute to the eradication of health inequities (Artiga & Hinton, 2018; Lee et al., 2018).

◼ Conclusion

This is by no means an exhaustive list of information on evidence-based practice, health policy making, or the role of nursing in informing policy. This chapter can serve as groundwork for further inquiry. Policy makers are instrumental in acting in a manner that best benefits the constituents that they serve.

Healthcare organizations and government entities must be vigilant in their policy formation efforts. Policy makers must engage in the process of consultation and reviewing research. This process allows the policy maker to understand prior initiatives, prior events related to the policy, and the voices of those whom the policy may influence. Without considering how a policy will influence a community, policy makers do a disservice to their constituents. To that end, lawmakers must ensure that every policy and law that is put into place will lead to the best outcome for the general population (Braveman, Arkin, Orleans, Proctor, & Plough, 2017; Dodson, Geary, & Brownson, 2015).

◼ Critical Thinking Exercise

The Future of Nursing: Leading Change, Advancing Health is an outgrowth of a partnership between the IOM (2011) and the Robert Wood Johnson Foundation in 2009. The initial report was released in 2010, and it is one of the most frequently downloaded IOM reports. Three regional town hall meetings presented by the Committee on the Future of Nursing were created out of concern to advance professional nursing to improve the health of all citizens. The meetings featured expert nursing scholars and open dialogue from community members and stakeholders. These meetings are captured in the following link with activities to assist you with a greater understanding of the challenges faced by the nursing profession.

Exercise 1: Visit https://nam.edu/publications/the-future-of-nursing-2020-2030 and listen to one of the town hall meetings.

Exercise 2: Identify how you would use your nursing knowledge to inform the policy-making process.

Exercise 3: Deliberate with team members on the use of information provided in the town hall meetings to help inform lawmakers in the policy-making process.

Exercise 4: How might nurses use this information to advocate for funding to support nursing education and research?

Exercise 5: What are some other policy implications that may result from these town hall meetings?

■ Discussion Questions

■ What resources would you use to advocate to increase funding for nursing education and research?

■ What local, state, and federal data are available to shape policy making around health equity?

■ How would you encourage nurses to engage in the health policy–making process?

■ Resources

Arnold, R. W. (2018). How CBO produces its 10-year economic forecast: Working paper 2018-02. Retrieved from https://www.cbo.gov/publication/53537

Bipartisan Policy Center. (2018). *Evidence-based policymaking primer.* Retrieved from https://bipartisanpolicy.org/wp-content/uploads/2019/03/Evidence-Based-Policymaking-Primer.pdf

Congressional Budget Office. (n.d.). Frequently asked questions about CPO cost estimates. Retrieved from https://www.cbo.gov/about/products/ce-faq

Congressional Budget Office. (2018). How CBO prepares baseline budget projections. Retrieved from https://www.cbo.gov/publication/53532

Institute of Medicine Committee on Health and Behavior: Research, Practice, and Policy. (2001). *Health and behavior: The interplay of biological, behavior, and societal influences.* Washington, DC: National Academies Press. doi:10.17226/9838

Institute of Medicine Committee on Assuring the Health of the Public in the 21st Century. (2002). *The future of the public's health in the 21st century.* Washington, DC: National Academies Press. Retrieved from https://www.nap.edu/download/10548

Institute of Medicine. (2012). *An integrated framework for assessing the value of community-based prevention.* Washington, DC: National Academies Press. doi:10.17226/13487

Jessie's Law: https://www.govtrack.us/congress/bills/115/s581/text

Milbank Memorial Fund publications: https://www.milbank.org/resources/?fwp_resource_type=case-studies

Pew-MacArthur Results First Initiative. (2014). *Evidence-based policymaking: A guide for effective governement.* Retrieved from https://www.pewtrusts.org/~/media/assets/2014/11/-evidencebasedpolicymakingaguideforeffectivegovernment.pdf

Rudolph, L., Caplan, J., Ben-Moshe, K., & Dillon, L. (2013). Health in all policies: A guide for state and local goverments. Washington, DC and Oakland, CA: American Public Health Association and Public Health Institute. Retrieved from http://www.phi.org/uploads/application/files/udt4vq0y712qpb1o4p62dexjlgxlnogpq15gr8pti3y7ckzysi.pdf

United States Government. (n.d.). How a bill becomes a law lesson plan. Retrieved from https://www.usa.gov/bill-law-lesson-plan

U.S. Department of Health and Human Services. (n.d.). Help, resources and information: National opioids crisis. Retrieved from http://www.hhs.gov/opioids

U.S. Department of Health and Human Services. (n.d.). HHS FY 2017 budget in brief—General departmental management. Retrieved from https://www.hhs.gov/about/budget/fy2017/budget-in-brief/gdm/index.html

U.S. Department of Health and Human Services, Office of Disease Prevention and Health Promotion. (n.d.). *Healthy People 2020.* Retrieved from http://www.healthypeople.gov

U.S. Department of Health and Human Services, Office of Minority Health. (2018). *State and territorial efforts to reduce health disparities: Findings of a 2016 Survey by the U.S. Department of Health and Human Services Office of Minority Health.* Washington, DC: U.S. Department of Health and Human Services.

■ References

Almaguer, S. B., Law, Y., & Young C. (2014). *Healthier corner stores: Positive impacts and profitable changes.* Philadelphia, PA: The Food Trust.

Arora, V., Moriates, C., & Shah, N. (2015). The challenge of understanding health care costs and charges. *American Medical Association Journal of Ethics, 17*(11), 1046–1052. doi:10.1001/journalofethics.2015.17.11.stas1-1511

Artiga, S., & Hinton, E. (2018). *Beyond health care: The role of social determinants in promoting health and health equity.* Retrieved from https://www.kff.org/disparities-policy/issue-brief/beyond-health-care-the-role-of-social-determinants-in-promoting-health-and-health-equity

Braveman, P., Arkin, E., Orleans, T., Proctor, D., & Plough, A. (2017). *What is health equity? And what difference does a definition make?* Princeton, NJ: Robert Wood Johnson Foundation. Retrieved from https://www.buildhealthyplaces.org/content/uploads/2017/05/health_equity_brief_041217.pdf

Burke, S. A. (2016). *Influence through policy: Nurses have a unique role.* Retrieved from https://www.reflectionsonnursingleadership.org/commentary/more-commentary/Vol42_2_nurses-have-a-unique-role

Cacari-Stone, L., Wallerstein, N., Garcia, A., & Minkler, M. (2014). The promise of community-based participatory research for health equity: A conceptual model for bridging evidence with policy. *American Journal of Public Health, 104*(9), 1615–1623. doi:10.2105/ajph.2014.301961

Congressional Budget Office. (2019). Introduction to CBO. Retrieved from https://www.cbo.gov/about/overview

Cookson, R. (2005).Evidence-based policy making in health care: What it is and what it isn't. *Journal of Health Services Research & Policy, 10*(2), 118–121. doi:10.1258/1355819053559083

de Wit, L., Fenenga, C., Giammarchi, C., di Furia, L., Hutter, I., de Winter, A., & Meijering, L. (2017). Community-based initiatives improving critical health literacy: A systematic review and meta-synthesis of qualitative evidence. *BMC Public Health, 18*, 40. doi:10.1186/s12889-017-4570-7

Dodson, E., Geary, N., & Brownson, R. (2015). State legislators' sources and use of information: Bridging the gap between research and policy. *Health Education Research, 30*(6), 840–848. doi:10.1093/her/cyv044

Dube, S. (2019). Results first cost-benefit model aids policymakers in funding decisions. Retrieved from https://www.pewtrusts.org/en/research-and-analysis/fact-sheets/2019/05/results-first-cost-benefit-model-aids-policymakers-in-funding-decisions

Ferguson, L. (2001). An activist looks at nursing's role in health policy development. *Journal of Obstetrics, Gynecology Neonatal Nursing, 30*, 546–551. doi:10.1111/j.1552-6909.2001.tb01575.x

Governmental Accountability Office. (2019). *Nursing homes: Improved oversight needed to better protect residents from abuse.* Retrieved from https://www.gao.gov/assets/700/699721.pdf

Hiatt, R. (Ed.). (2018). Population health: The translation of research to policy. Retrieved from https://www.milbank.org/publications/population-health-the-translation-of-research-to-policy

Innvaer, S., Gunn, V., Trommald, M., & Oxman, A. (2002). Health policy-makers' perceptions of their use of evidence: A systematic review. *Journal of Health Services Research & Policy, 7*(4), 239–244. doi:10.1258/135581902320432778

Institute of Medicine. (2011). *The future of nursing: Leading change, advancing health.* Washington, DC: National Academies Press.

Kaiser, F. (2008). *CRS Report for Congress: Government Accountability Office & General Accounting Office.* Retrieved from https://fas.org/sgp/crs/misc/RL30349.pdf

Kilpatrick, D. (2000). *Definitions of public policy and the law.* Retrieved from https://mainweb-v.musc.edu/vawprevention/policy/definition.shtml

Koh, H., Berwick, D., Clancy, C., Baur, C., Brach, C., Harris, L., & Zerhusen, E. (2012). New federal policy initiatives to boost health literacy can help the nation move beyond the cycle of costly 'crisis care'. *Health Affairs, 31*(2), 434–443. Retrieved from https://www.healthaffairs.org/doi/pdf/10.1377/hlthaff.2011.1169

Lee, J., Schram, A., Riley, E., Harris, P., Baum, F., Fisher, M., & Friel, S. (2018). Addressing health equity through action on the social determinants of health: A global review of policy outcome evaluation methods. *International Journal of Health Policy and Management, 7*(7), 581–592. doi:10.15171/ijhpm.2018.04

Library of Congress. (n.d.). About the Library. Retrieved from https://www.loc.gov/about

LoBionda-Wood, G., & Haber, J. (2018). *Nursing research: Methods and critical appraisal for evidence-based practice* (9th ed.). St Louis, MO: Elsevier.

Milbank Memorial Fund. (n.d.). *About the Milbank Memorial Fund.* Retrieved from https://www.milbank.org/about

National Academy of Medicine. (2019a). *About the National Academy of Medicine.* Retrieved from https://nam.edu/about-the-nam

National Academy of Medicine. (2019b). Action collaborative on countering the U.S. opioid epidemic. Retrieved from https://nam.edu/programs/action-collaborative-on-countering-the-u-s-opioid-epidemic

National Academy of Medicine. (2019c). Tapering guidance for opioids: Existing best practices and evidence standards [Public Webinar Video]. Retrieved from https://nam.edu/event/webinar-tapering-guidance-for-opioids-existing-best-practices-and-evidence-standards

Oxman, D., Lavis, J., Lewin, S., & Fretheim, A, (2009). Support tools for evidence-informed health policymaking (STP)1: What is evidence- informed policymaking? *Health Research Policy and Systems, 7*(Suppl. 1), S1 doi:10.1186/1478-4505-7-S1-S1

The Pew Charitable Trusts. (2017). Pew-MacArthur Results First Initiative. Retrieved from https://www.pewtrusts.org/en/projects/pew-macarthur-results-first-initiative

The Pew Charitable Trusts. (2018). Evidence-based policymaking resource center. Retrieved from https://www.pewtrusts.org/en/projects/pew-macarthur-results-first-initiative

Ridgway, S. (n.d.). *Profiles in nursing: Lillian Wald founded public health nursing.* Retrieved from https://www.workingnurse.com/articles/Lillian-Wald-Founded-Public-Health-Nursing

Spann, J (2009). Addressing the Quality and Safety Gap – Part I. In M. D. Ladden & S. B. Hassmiller (Eds.), *Charting Nursing's Future.* Florida: Spann Communications. Retrieved from https://www.rwjf.org/en/library/research/2009/07/cnf-addressing-the-quality-and-safety-gap-part-one.html

Sutcliffe, S., & Court, J. (2005). *Evidence-based policymaking: What is it? How does it work? What relevance for developing countries?* Retrieved from https://www.odi.org/sites/odi.org.uk/files/odi-assets/publications-opinion-files/3683.pdf

Taft, S., & Nanna, K. (2008). What are the sources of health policy that influence nursing practice? *Policy Politics Nursing Practice, 9*, 274–287. doi:10.1177/1527154408319287

Toofany, S. (2005). Nurses and health policy. *Journal of Nurse Management, 12*, 1226–1230. Retrieved from https://go.gale.com/ps/anonymous?p=AONE&sw=w&issn=13545760&v=2.1&it=r&id=GALE%7CA133081700&sid=googleScholar&linkaccess=fulltext

4 Health Equity and Nursing Education: Past, Present, and Future

Wrenetha A. Julion and Monique Reed

CHAPTER OBJECTIVES

- ⊙ Differentiate among the principles of health equity, health disparities, social justice, and social determinants of health
- ⊙ Describe nursing's social mandate as a guiding principle in providing ethical care of diverse populations
- ⊙ Synthesize principles important to understanding health equity, health disparities, and social justice in nursing education across classroom and clinical settings
- ⊙ Analyze how nurse's social mandate for social justice is informed by historical injustices
- ⊙ Summarize the interface between social justice and health equity in nursing education
- ⊙ Synthesize the tenets of health equity for nursing research, education, and practice
- ⊙ Describe a range of creative learning activities designed to address the social determinants of health

KEY CONCEPTS

Health equity

Nursing education

Social justice

Health disparities

Social determinants of health and
   cultural competence

KEY TERMS

Health equity

Ethics

Diversity

Social justice

Social determinants/environmental
   determinants of health

Health advocacy

Health policy

Health disparities

Minority healthcare providers

Competencies/essentials for BSN, PhD,
   Doctor of Nursing Practice

National Institute for Minority Health
   Disparities Health Disparities
   Research Framework

Cultural competence

■ Introduction

Nurses are called to address the health needs of society with the goal of helping individuals, families, groups, and communities achieve their optimum state of wellness (Perry, Willis, Peterson, & Grace, 2017). As such, nurses have a social mandate to address health equity, which is defined by *Healthy People 2020* as "the attainment of the highest level of health for all people" (Office of Disease Prevention and Health Promotion [ODPHP], n.d.-a, para. 5). Inherent in the concept of health equity is that everyone is valued equally and societal efforts must be focused on addressing inequalities, historical and contemporary injustices, and transforming healthcare to eliminate disparities. This chapter begins by defining principles important to addressing health equity and highlight the historical importance of past nursing efforts aimed at addressing health and healthcare inequities. Next, this chapter delineates the current state of nursing education and the myriad of contextual factors that influence nursing education focused on health equity. Exemplars from current nursing curricula focused on promoting health equity and resources for faculty are highlighted; future considerations for nursing students, clinicians, practitioners, and researchers are described.

■ The Past

HEALTH EQUITY

The concept of health equity means that every individual must have a fair chance to attain his or her full health potential, and that no one should be disadvantaged in the pursuit of health. Further, "Achieving health equity requires valuing everyone equally with focused and ongoing societal efforts to address avoidable inequalities, historical and contemporary injustices, and the elimination of health and healthcare disparities" (U.S. Department of Health & Human Services Office of Minority Health, 2011, p. 9). In order to truly understand the importance of health equity, nursing educators must insure that students leave academia prepared to consider how social justice, social determinants of health (SDOH), health disparities, and cultural competence influence health equity. An exemplar of a curricular activity focused on historical inequity in healthcare is provided in Exemplar 4.1.

SOCIAL JUSTICE

Social justice implies that each individual and group is entitled to fair and equal rights that contribute to their fair share of societal benefits (Marmot et al., 2008). The American Association of Colleges of Nursing (AACN) includes social justice as one of its core values and defines it as "acting in accordance with fair treatment regardless of economic status, race, ethnicity, age, citizenship, disability, or sexual orientation" (AACN, 2008b, p. 28). Similarly, the American Nurses Association (ANA) 2015 *Code of Ethics* defines social justice as "a form of justice that engages in social criticism and social change because social structures, policies, laws, and customs can contribute to disadvantage and harm to vulnerable groups" (the ANA *Code of Ethics for Nurses*, 2015a, p. 46). Nursing faculty must be prepared to teach students about social justice

---

Exemplar 4.1. Example of Learning Activity Focused on Historical Healthcare Inequity

Focus: Faculty in the Women and Children's Nursing course for pre-licensure students developed a learning activity based upon *"The Immortal Life of Henrietta Lacks"* (Skloot, 2010)

Activity: Students are required to read the 2010 bestseller by Rebecca Skloot that recounts the experience of salvaging HeLa cells without her knowledge or consent in 1951. These cells became one of the most important tools in medicine, vital for developing the polio vaccine, cloning, gene mapping, and in vitro fertilization, among others. This was done during the era where the medical field was known for experimenting on African Americans. As a result of participating in this classroom activity, students learn about health disparities, medical ethics, and social injustice. This assignment aligns with course objective: 4. Analyze the impact of healthcare policy, culture, technology, and ethics on women's health.

Source: From T. Davis, R. Hunter, & J. Rousseau, personal communication, May 2, 2019.

---

because it instills in students the importance of active engagement to address the underlying causes of SDOH and health-related inequities.

Historically, social justice has been rooted in the very fabric of the nursing profession. Social justice can be traced decades back in nursing to the work of the founders of the National Association of Colored Graduate Nurses (NACGN). The founding members included Mary Eliza Mahoney, the first African American registered nurse, Estelle Massey Riddle and Mabel K. Staupers, who, in addition to promoting social justice in the care of vulnerable patients and communities, also worked to promote greater justice in the nursing profession by advancing the fair and equitable treatment of African American nurses (Hine, 2003). Similarly, historically African American nurses such as Sojourner Truth (Isabella Baumfree) and Harriet Tubman were abolitionists and women's rights activists who worked to promote social justice and equitable treatment of nurses, women, and slaves (Carnegie, 1995).

HEALTH DISPARITIES

According to Truman et al. (2011), health disparities are defined as "differences in health outcomes and their determinants between segments of the population, as defined by social, demographic, environmental, and geographic attributes." There is indisputable evidence that health disparities exist, and that they have grown over time (ODPHP, n.d.-b). Health disparities are often narrowly interpreted as racial or ethnic differences in health outcomes that are seen to a lesser or greater extent among populations (ODPHP, n.d.-a). In the United States, there are many dimensions of disparity, such as race/ethnicity, sex, sexual identity, age, disability, socioeconomic status, and geographic location (ODPHP, n.d.-b). While significant efforts have been taken to reduce health disparities in the United States, gaps are still evident. Populations most negatively impacted are ethnic minorities, low-income families, and those without a high school education (Weinstein, Geller, Negussie, & Baciu, 2017). Even so, disparities in health outcomes have been noted in various diverse groups which include, for example, people who are elderly; have limited literacy, disabilities, or mental health conditions; who live in poverty; and who have varying sexual orientations.

As far back as the 1900s, health disparities have been recognized as a contributor to broad gaps in health and life expectancy between African Americans and Whites. Noted educator Booker T. Washington and sociologist William Edward Burghardt (W.E.B.) DuBois expressed discontent with the lack of access to healthcare experienced by Black people (Srinivasan & Williams, 2014). These racial/ethnic differences contributed to decreased access to healthcare, worse health outcomes, increased morbidity and mortality, and shorter life expectancy (Ansell, 2017; Srinivasan & Williams, 2014). Nursing educators' awareness of historical injustices can inform current and future learning in clinical and classroom settings.

SOCIAL DETERMINANTS OF HEALTH

Health outcomes are significantly impacted by the SDOH, which are the conditions in which people are born, grow, live, work, and age that influence health (SDOH, n.d.). Socioeconomic status, education, neighborhood and physical environment, employment, social support networks, and access to healthcare are examples of SDOH. Furthermore, SDOH can include the availability of, and access to high-quality education, nutritious food, decent and safe housing, affordable and reliable public transportation, culturally sensitive healthcare providers, health insurance, and clean water and air (ODPHP, n.d.-a). Inequalities in health outcomes that are linked to nonmodifiable factors such as race and ethnicity have also been linked to SDOH (Walker, Williams, & Egede, 2016). The concept of SDOH should be introduced early and often across all levels of the curricula.

Lillian Wald is commonly referred to as the founder of Public Health Nursing because of her efforts to move healthcare beyond the walls of healthcare institutions and consider how social factors influence health (Buhler-Wilkerson, 1993). Over 100 years ago, in 1893, Ms. Wald joined forces with her classmate Mary Brewster to take healthcare to the community. She and Ms. Brewster moved into a house in the neighborhood and provided healthcare within the community. This is particularly relevant to the SDOH because the neighbors who visited their home sought help with health, education, jobs, and housing—all of which are known to influence health and health outcomes. This early work was the genesis of both public health and community health nursing.

CULTURAL COMPETENCE

Healthcare provider cultural competence can be associated with health equity, health disparities, and social justice. Cultural competence is defined as integrated knowledge, behaviors, attitudes, skills, and policies that can enable professionals to enact "cross-cultural communication and appropriate effective interactions with others" (Harkess & Kaddoura, 2016). When nurses exhibit cultural competence, they are more likely to provide care that overcomes barriers to optimal health (Garneau,

2017). Didactic and clinical course work as well as experiential learning experiences can effectively help students to increase awareness of the importance of cultural competency in their future encounters with patients, families, and communities (Thornton & Persaud, 2018).

Cultural competence was initially conceptualized in the United States as the healthcare system sought to improve access to quality care for the increasing diversity of the population and to address inequities in the delivery of social services in American Indian/Alaska Native populations (Anderson, Scrimshaw, Fullilove, Fielding, & Normand, 2003; Brach & Fraser, 2002). The concept of cultural competency first became apparent in Leininger's transcultural nursing theory (Leininger, 1988). Nurses have played a key role in developing conceptual models and theoretical frameworks that have been implemented in nursing and nursing education. Other terminology such as "cultural humility" (Thackrah & Thompson, 2013) has been used to frame nursing school curricula. For example, Lonneman (2015) describes the concept of reflective journaling as a curricular strategy to raise cultural awareness. Reflective journaling involved students completing weekly journal entries about the thoughts, feelings, and actions related to the content and activities of the week.

By 2004, several other models such as Leininger's Cultural Care and Diversity and Universality theory, Purnell's Model for Cultural Competence/Transcultural Health Care, Spector's HEALTH Traditions Model, and Giger and Davidhizar's Model of Transcultural Nursing gained attention (AACN, 2008c). Subsequently, Lipson and DeSantis (2007) called attention to the need to consider important issues such as the selection of content, standard, and tools for evaluating the effectiveness of coursework on culture, the nurse–patient encounter, and faculty support.

The National Culturally and Linguistically Appropriate Services (CLAS) Standards in Health and Health Care began to serve as a guideline for cultural competency in nursing schools and healthcare settings (National CLAS Standards, n.d.). The National CLAS Standards, endorsed by the AACN, are a series of action steps to improve health equity and quality, while seeking to end health disparities (AACN, 2008c).

Health equity can be optimized when nurse educators can successfully prepare students to understand and act upon the inextricable linkages among health disparities, SDOH, and cultural competence. Social justice is at the heart of the pursuit of equitable care and serves as the cornerstone for improving the health of society. For the past 17 years and counting, the profession of nursing has been named the most trusted health profession (Demarinis, 2019). In order to maintain this trust and ensure the health of all populations, nurse educators must prepare future nurses to tackle the wicked problems (Rittel & Webber, 1973) that influence the health and well-being of all groups. Wicked problems have multiple causes, are difficult to describe, typically do not have a single right answer, and extend beyond conventional answers because they may lead to negative consequences. Such is the case of policy that serves as a barrier to employment for the poor (Bakst & Tyrrell, 2017). One example is African-style hair braiding, which requires no scissors, heat, or chemicals, and yet, braiders in 16 states have been required to obtain cosmetology licenses in order to braid hair. Cosmetology licensing, which requires training, costs thousands of dollars and hours. Hair braiding has a few startup costs and is a feasible occupation for individuals with limited capital, and yet, without the necessary resources, they are precluded from earning an income.

■ The Present

In light of existing and new challenges related to promoting health equity, nursing education must evolve to keep pace. The vision for the nursing profession must simultaneously advocate for quality and optimal outcomes, while considering efficient models for joining the healthcare workforce. Such models include entry into the profession; disparities in the nursing workforce; persistent disparities in health outcomes; listening to the voices of patients, communities, and providers; and promoting cultural competence. Thus, nursing educators must provide curricula that are dynamic and responsive to the current healthcare climate, while also anticipating tomorrow's healthcare needs (Jeffries, 2015).

ENTRY TO THE NURSING PROFESSION

The preferred vision for nursing education includes generalist, advanced generalist, and advanced specialty nursing education. Generalist nurse education occurs at a minimum in baccalaureate degree nursing programs. Advanced generalist education occurs in master's degree nursing programs, including the Clinical Nurse Leader (CNL®), which is an advanced generalist nursing role. Advanced specialty education occurs at the doctoral level in Doctor of Nursing Practice (DNP) or research-focused degree programs (PhD, DNS, or DNSc). End-of-program outcomes for the baccalaureate, master's, and doctoral nursing programs build on each other. The Doctor of Nursing Tool Kit provides information on faculty and student expectations (AACN, n.d.-b). DNP-prepared nurses are prepared to enhance population health across a variety of settings including acute and long-term care settings, as well as care across a continuum that includes chronic care, rehabilitation, home care, palliative care, hospice, and complex care (Zaccagnini, & White, 2017)

In light of the varying entry points to the profession for registered nurses (associates, baccalaureate, master's, and DNP), nurse educators must be aware of the varying health equity–related competencies across the spectrum of nursing education. According to the AACN, the bachelor's degree should be considered the optimal entry point into the profession (AACN, 2001). Even so, Associate's Degree Nursing (ADN) graduates help to fill the breach in the number of nurses who are needed to keep pace with the healthcare demands. The essentials of nursing education outline the necessary curricular content, competencies, and clinical support of graduates across these levels that must be reflected in academic nursing.

Nursing action is needed to address health equity and can also be considered through explicit actions in which nursing can engage, such as health advocacy, community organization, and innovation through roles such as the CNL (Bender, 2014). The hallmark of the CNL's role is to provide and manage care at the level of the microsystem, the point of care to individuals, clinical populations, and communities. Additional roles include coordinating and overseeing team activities, while also being responsible for improving individual care in an effective and cost-effective way.

DISPARITIES IN HEALTH OUTCOMES

The acceptance by healthcare providers around the existence and causes of healthcare disparities is mixed. Providing nursing students with current evidence of the prevalence and contributing factors of health inequity during their academic careers would likely contribute to their acceptance of the existence of racial health disparities. Acknowledging the existence of health disparities can open the door for open dialog and stimulate discussion and action among nursing educators, clinicians, and researchers to address the disparities that extend beyond nurses educating patients on what they think patients need to know or what patients need to do.

Health conditions that include high blood pressure, diabetes, kidney disease, and cancer are highly prevalent in racial minority populations (Raghupathi & Raghupathi, 2018). More than 40% of African American men and women have high blood pressure, which develops earlier in life and is usually more severe than in Whites (Roger et al., 2012). African American adults are 80% more likely than White adults to have diabetes and twice as likely to die from diabetes (Cunningham et al., 2017). The American Cancer Society reports that African American males are twice as likely to die from prostate cancer–related deaths than White men. The most typical types of cancer are prostate, lung, and colorectal (Alcaraz et al., 2016). African Americans are also more likely to experience health disparities across a number of health conditions as compared to non-Hispanic Whites (Families USA, n.d.; see the infographic in Figure 4.1). In addition to morbidity disparities, differences are also evident in life expectancy. In Chicago, the highest life expectancy was observed among Hispanics at 84.6 years and the lowest life expectancy was observed among African Americans at 71.7 years—a difference of about 13 years (Hunt, Tran, & Whitman, 2015)

In addition to racial/ethnic health disparities, health inequities are also gender and neighborhood related. For example, despite the fact that Whites have higher incidence of breast cancer, mortality rates for African Americans are higher (Srinivasan & Williams, 2014). Similarly, maternal mortality represents a significant health disparity among ethnic and racial minorities (Howell & Zeitlin, 2017), with the rates being more than twice the rate of White women. The United Nations Millennium Development Goal called for a 75% reduction in maternal mortality by 2015 (Creanga & Callaghan, 2017), and yet, the estimated maternal mortality rate for 48 states and Washington, DC increased from 2000 to 2014; the international trend was in the opposite direction (MacDorman, Declercq, Cabral, & Morton, 2016). Maternal mortality and morbidity rates for ethnic/minority groups, in particular African Americans, have increased to staggering rates regardless of the socioeconomic status (MacDorman, Declercq, & Thoma, 2017).

Currently, there exists a 16-year life expectancy gap in Chicago between the city's central business district and a nearby minority community that is just 7 miles away (Ansell, 2017). Life expectancy varies substantially across the 77 community areas of Chicago, from a low of 68.2 to a high of 83.3—a difference of 15 years (Hunt et al., 2015). Efforts have been intensified to understand the factors associated with disparities in health outcomes, and without a proper understanding of the multiple, diverse, and long-standing nature of the disparities, progress will remain slow. Zimmerman and Anderson (2019) provide evidence to support the notion that despite multiple initiatives to promote health equity, progress has remained stagnant over the past 25 years.

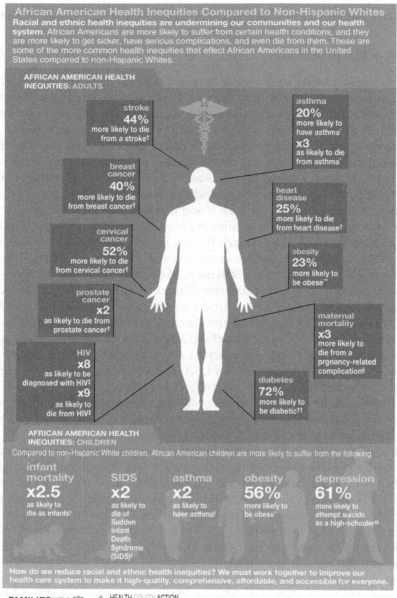

FIGURE 4.1   HEALTH DISPARITIES IN AFRICAN AMERICANS VERSUS WHITES INFOGRAPHIC.

*CDC. Most Recent Asthma Data. 2016

†CDC. National Vital Statistics Reports. Deaths: Final Data for 2016

‡CDC. HIV Surveillance Report Vol. 29. Diagnosis of HIV Infection in the United States and Dependent Areas 2017

§CDC. Pregnancy Mortality Surveillance System. Pregnancy-Related Mortality Ratios. 2011–2014

**CDC. National Center for Health Statistics Data Brief No. 288 (October 2017). Prevalence of Obesity Among Adults and Youth: United States. 2015–2016

††CDC. National Diabetes Statistics Report. 2017

‡‡CDC. Youth Risk Behavior Surveillance – United States. 2017

Source: Reprinted with permission from Families USA: The Voice for Health Care Consumers. (2019). *African American health inequities compared to non-Hispanic Whites*. Retrieved from https://familiesusa.org/wp-content/uploads/2019/08/HSI-Health-disparities_african-americans-infographic.pdf

DISPARITIES IN THE NURSING WORKFORCE

The lack of minority nurses in the nursing workforce coincides with persistent gaps in health outcomes and health equity among minority populations (National Center for Health Statistics [NCHS], 2017). Increasing the number of minority nurses is important to address disparities in minority populations (Pfefferle & Gibson, 2013) because minority nurses experienced with the cultural and contextual circumstances of diverse populations are more likely to be prepared to address the root causes of health disparities. These root causes include environmental factors, SDOH, health behaviors, health literacy, racism, and discrimination (Pfefferle & Gibson, 2013). Efforts have been made to increase the number of minority nurses who practice, as well as the number of research studies focused on issues affecting disparate populations (Phillips & Malone, 2014). According to the Pathways to Doctoral Education, 2009, increasing the racial, ethnic, and gender diversity of faculty and students in research-focused doctoral programs is a priority because of the White women forming a majority in the nursing profession. This is not to say that diversity in the form of culture, gender, religion, ability, age, and sexual orientation is unimportant. According to the AACN Task Force on the Research-Focused Doctorate in Nursing (2009), it is essential to increase diversity in nurse researchers.

The nursing profession is projected to need an additional 1 million nurses by 2030. Most notably, the number of non-Hispanic African American and Hispanic nurses does not currently mirror the demand of the working-age patient population (Health Resources and Services Administration [HRSA], 2017). The percentage of non–Hispanic African American and Hispanic nurses in the workforce increased to 17% in 2014, which is less than the 28% patient demand for non–Hispanic African American and Hispanic nurses projected for 2030. Even so, the number of minority nurses remains low as compared to 31.5% of the U.S. population who are non–Hispanic African Americans and Hispanics (Colby & Ortman, 2015).

An increase in the number of minority nurses in the workforce must begin by increasing the number of minority nursing students. Minority nursing students' recruitment efforts can begin with early exposure through K–12 pipeline programs that promote science, technology, engineering, and math (National Advisory Council on Nurse Education and Practice, 2013), and continuous inclusive efforts at recruitment such as holistic admissions. Holistic review is an admission strategy that seeks to recruit a diverse group by acknowledging an applicant's unique experiences or road traveled, along with his or her traditional academic achievements such as grade point average and performance of standardized tests. The road traveled may be different for each student, but can include challenges that students have overcome, such as managing full-time employment while being a full-time student, learners with English as the second language, caregiver responsibilities, or unique experiences such as professional careers, military experiences, and service opportunities. In order to assess the road traveled, institutions should host candidates in on-campus or virtual one-on-one or small group interviews. Oral communication with the applicants can help to establish a sense of awareness about a candidate's unique contributions to the nursing profession. Faculty should create a holistic interview guide to standardize the point value system that applicants receive for their unique experiences and road traveled.

Once attracted to entry-level programs, minority nursing students have a better chance for retention, satisfaction, and matriculation in environments that promote diversity and have diverse faculty representation. Institutions can promote their commitment to diversity and inclusion by embedding health equity, health disparities, social justice, and cultural competency content within and across the curricula. Furthermore, the institution should establish a diversity mission that aligns with the broader institutional mission, vision, and strategic plan/initiatives. This diversity mission should be considered the responsibility of the institution, rather than relegated to a diversity committee. Finally, there should be an allocation of funds and resources to support the diversity mission and initiatives (US. Department of Education, Office of Planning, Evaluation and Policy Devleopment, 2016). The institutional commitment can then translate into program objectives, course objectives, learning outcomes, and assignments. Universities can further their ability to recruit and retain students by establishing an Office of Diversity and Inclusion. This office should be instrumental in overseeing that faculty and student development programs meet the needs of minority students as well as prepare them to address the needs of minority populations for which they serve. Minority student recruitment and retention can also be influenced by factors such as microaggressions from both fellow students and nursing faculty. Microaggressions, defined as perceived slights based on an unalterable characteristic such as race, age, or gender identity (Hall & Fields, 2012), can hinder academic performance, marginalize students, and interfere with students' willingness to engage with nursing faculty (Hall & Fields, 2013).

Given the relationship of barriers to achieving equity and the lack of minority representation, the need for implementation of retention and recruitment efforts and the need for creating inclusive environments, nurse educators, researchers, and practitioners must advocate for additional funding to support entry-level nursing students, similar to the degree of funding for advanced practice nursing education. Accrediting bodies should also assume responsibility for evaluating recruitment and retention efforts for any initiatives designed to help diverse students to be successful. Thus, the HRSA programs that fund initiatives to diversify the nursing workforce are essential (Phillips & Malone, 2014).

DIVERSE WORKFORCE LIKELY TO WORK WITH DIVERSE POPULATIONS

Diversity in the nursing workforce matters because ethnic and minority groups are projected to compose 57% of the population in 2060 (Poghosyan & Carthon, 2017). The total minority population would more than double, from 116.2 million to 241.3 million, over the period, with those who are foreign born making up one in five of the population (U.S. Census Bureau, 2018). It is essential to have a nursing workforce that will reflect the population of the United States, so as to deliver cost-effective, quality care and improve patients' satisfaction and health outcomes, especially among ethnic and racial minorities.

Diversity in the nursing workforce provides opportunities to deliver quality care which promotes patient satisfaction and emotional well-being. For example, a significant barrier to health among Latinos is the lack of access to healthcare and lack of access to culturally appropriate care. Critical efforts are needed to engage more people from the Latino community into healthcare careers ("Overcoming Barriers," 2012). This has the dual benefits of bringing more healthcare options to underserved communities as well as increasing the cultural competency of care delivered.

EVIDENCE THAT DIVERSE WORKFORCE IMPROVES OUTCOMES

In a recent systematic review of the literature of the effect of race and ethnic concordance on patient and physician communication, authors described that African American patients with non–African American physicians consistently experienced poor communication, information-giving, patient participation, and participatory decision-making than when paired with concordant physicians (Shen et al., 2018). Evidence on the effects of a diverse nursing workforce on health disparities are limited (Phillips & Malone, 2014). Consequently, further investigation is warranted that can (a) determine whether diverse nurses indeed care for minority populations, (b) determine whether racial/ethnic concordance between nurses and patients influences healthcare outcomes, and (c) examine how diversity influences whether nurses are willing to serve as patient advocates.

VOICES OF PATIENTS, COMMUNITIES, AND PROVIDERS

Provision 8.3 of the ANA *Code of Ethics* (2017) charges nurses to acknowledge an obligation to advance health and human rights and reduce disparities. Nurses must fulfill this obligation by reducing barriers to health equity which can include SDOH. These determinants can include education, access to healthcare, safe housing, transportation, and neighborhood crime (SDOH, n.d.). Nursing education should provide students an opportunity for an experiential, hands-on approach to allow them to hear barriers to health outcomes, such as SDOH, from patients themselves (Thornton & Persaud, 2018). The voices of patients and communities have been minimal in conversations around health disparities. It is essential to consider patient-identified barriers and priorities. Nurses can support patients in making informed decisions around selecting providers and dealing with poor healthcare delivery. For example, nurses can counsel patients to voice their dissatisfaction with inefficient medical visits, provider miscommunication, and stressful treatment settings (Gaston-Johansson, Hill-Briggs, Oguntomilade, Bradley, & Mason, 2007). For example, Jack, Liburd, Tucker, and Cockrell (2014) provide an exemplar of methods that healthcare providers can use to obtain insight into the perceptions and experiences of their patients living with diabetes. The cultural perspectives of patients can help explain health behaviors and contribute to collaborative partnerships among patients, providers, health systems, and community resources.

Little is known about nursing's response to patients' narratives about health disparities despite the nursing profession composing a significant sector of the healthcare workforce. A barrier to entertaining patient perspectives is the debate by some providers about the existence of healthcare disparities. Burgess et al. (2017) conducted qualitative interviews with medical healthcare providers about the issues of racial healthcare disparities and health providers' roles in healthcare inequality. The providers who did not believe that providers contributed to healthcare inequality were resistant to the idea that the problems of patients of color were associated with racism. The study provides guidance on developing effective narrative communication strategies that engage providers in conversations focused on efforts to reduce healthcare disparities. An exemplar course that prioritizes the voice of patients and the community is illustrated in Exemplar 4.2.

Exemplar 4.2. Example of Course to Promote Interprofessionalism and Address Disparities

Focus: An interprofessional course has been developed for every student across four colleges (Nursing, Medicine, Health Sciences, Graduate) when he or she enters university in fall. This is a group of over 700 students. Community health mentors are recruited from the neighboring communities to essentially help train health professionals to understand the SDOH.

Activity: Students work in interprofessional teams to interact with health mentors in community settings, examine the barriers to health services for an underserved patient population with a chronic care condition, and identify strategies to overcome these barriers.

SDOH, social determinants of health.

Source: From J. Odiaga, personal communication, May 2, 2019.

PROMOTING CULTURAL COMPETENCE

In addition to training nursing students on assessing the SDOH, cultural competency training must be included in nursing education curricula. The AACN (2008c, 2011b) developed cultural competency tool kits for baccalaureate and graduate nursing education. The competencies were developed to support nursing's social mandate to address health disparities (AACN, 2008c, 2011b). Similarly, theoretical perspectives such as Rachel Spector's HEALTH Traditions Model provide an example of a cultural competency framework for nursing education. Spector's model includes three components: heritage consistency, HEALTH traditions, and cultural phenomena affecting health (AACN, 2008). However, a consideration related to cultural competency is measurement of the concept itself. The current literature identifies that the instruments to assess cultural competence in nurses and nursing students are self-administered and based on individuals' perceptions (Loftin, Hartin, Branson, & Reyes, 2013). The instruments are commonly utilized to test the effectiveness of educational programs designed to increase cultural competence. Even so, there are no objective measures of cultural competence from the patient's perspective. Since the instruments are based on a variety of conceptual frameworks, multiple factors will need to be considered when deciding which instrument to use with students, nurses, and patients in the future.

According to the AACN (2008c), culturally competent baccalaureates exhibit three characteristics: personal awareness of one's own culture, values, beliefs, attitudes, and behaviors; the skills to communicate effectively with individuals from other cultures; and the ability to assess cross-cultural variation. These characteristics are awareness of personal culture, values, beliefs, attitudes, and behaviors; skill in assessing and communicating with individuals from other cultures; and assessment of cross-cultural variations. Graduate-level competencies build upon the bachelor's-level competencies to also include increased leadership capacity in education, research, practice, and policy (AACN, 2011b). The AACN guidelines have been used to design nursing curricula focused on culturally competent nursing education that facilitates the care of diverse patient populations (AACN, n.d.-a). Curricula in the form of both classroom and clinical training that enable nurses to see the patient experience through the eyes of the patient can be integrated into educational strategies and learning experiences that advance caregiving skills (Powell Sears, 2012).

Educators must also remain cognizant that health equity and cultural competency extend beyond racial/ethnic groups. Meade, Mahmoudi, and Lee (2015) have proposed a framework to address health disparities and promote health equity in individuals with disabilities. Again, patient perspectives can inform healthcare professionals about the personal and environmental factors that contribute to reduced access to healthcare and quality and decreased functioning and participation among individuals with disabilities. This model informs researchers, health providers, policy makers, and community advocate groups focused on addressing disparities in individuals with disabilities. The AACN (2008b) recommends integrating cultural competency education across the curricula. Similarly, researchers contend that cultural competency education has the greatest impact when all faculty embrace this curricula content and students encounter the material through a wide variety of experiences (Lonneman, 2015). An example of cultural competency content in CNL and DNP students is included in Exemplar 4.3.

The intersecting linkages among nursing education, health disparities, and diversity of the healthcare workforce represent a current challenge for nursing academia. In order to address this challenge, intentional efforts that include mentoring of diverse students

---

Exemplar 4.3. Example of Course to Promote Cultural Competence in Student Learners – Interprofessional Community-Based Service Learning

Focus: This interprofessional course is designed to provide post-licensure CNL and DNP students with the knowledge and skills to provide care within diverse populations and communities

Activity: Students will be asked to examine personal attitudes and beliefs as they relate to cultural competency and charged with developing a cultural competency framework that can be used to guide their professional practices. The communities neighboring Rush University Medical Center will engage with students in facilitating a service-learning experience that is mutually beneficial. Students will develop and implement a service-learning project in conjunction with and in accordance with the needs of the community settings where they will be placed. Finally, students will reflect upon their experiences as they examine their personal beliefs, values, and views and also reflect upon their experiences interacting with each other and their community-based service-learning site. Examples of projects that have been mutually selected by the student and the service-learning site include: parenting classes, community health assessment, intergenerational reading/mentoring program, development of a patient safety checklist and discharge educational brochure and video for a pain clinic, and evaluation of a high school–college readiness program for minority students.

CNL, Clinical Nurse Leader; DNP, Doctor of Nursing Practice.

Source: From W. Julion, personal communication, May 2, 2019.

and faculty, university-level support by deans and administrators, and transparency in diversity-related hiring and promotion practices are needed (Julion et al., 2019). Additionally, nursing curricula and classroom and clinical activities that promote cultural competency, while considering the voices of patients, communities, and interprofessional healthcare providers, must be developed, implemented, and evaluated.

◼ The Future

EQUIPPING NURSES TO ADDRESS HEALTH EQUITY, SOCIAL JUSTICE, AND SDOH IN NURSING EDUCATION

The future of attaining health equity must include an adequate and purposeful implementation of nursing curricula and experiences. These activities must build on lessons of the past and incorporate the best practices of the present to effectively train the next generation of the nursing workforce. In this chapter, we differentiated and described the basic definitions of the principles affecting health equity and the current state of healthcare and the healthcare workforce. Successful implementation in nursing education must consider a curriculum that describes how nursing students and faculty can address health equity, social justice, and SDOH. For example, in order for nurses to practice effectively, the scope of practice must be expanded to include political competence and policy advocacy to address the social conditions that contribute to disparities. Thus, political advocacy is a legitimate and important nursing role and, therefore, needs to be a focus for nursing education.

The nursing discipline of Public Health Nursing has taken the lead in advancing the principles of health equity and social justice. For example, the Quad Council of Public Health Nursing, founded in 1988, is composed of the Alliance of Nurses for Healthy Environments (AHNE), the Association of Community Health Nursing Educators (ACHNE), the Association of Public Health Nurses (APHN), and the American Public Health Association – Public Health Nursing Section (Swider, Krothe, Reyes, & Cravetz, 2013). The Quad Council serves as the national voice of public health nursing to address priorities for public health nursing education from the generalist to executive level in the areas of practice, leadership, and research. Finally, the National League for Nursing (NLN) has proposed specific recommendations for integrating content on the SDOH into nursing curricula. These recommendations are for faculty, leadership in nursing programs, and for the NLN (NLN, 2019).

TRAINING THE CURRENT AND FUTURE NURSING WORKFORCE TO ENGAGE IN POLITICAL ADVOCACY

Nursing Students
Nursing curricula must equip students at undergraduate and graduate levels to embrace healthcare policy to reduce health inequities. This focus must be expanded to also consider public policy that addresses the SDOH outside of the healthcare system. In order to achieve this, social justice, health equity, and policy must be integrated throughout the nursing curricula at all educational levels (Reutter & Kushner, 2010). While community health nursing courses following the tenets of Quad Council competencies will address the effects of poverty, economic inequities, stress, social exclusion, and job insecurity, this is not, and should not be, the only time it is addressed in nursing curricula

(Mahony & Jones, 2013). Students must be challenged to identify policy implications related to individual client health throughout the health continuum across multiple settings and situations. Entry-level nurses should have the knowledge and skills required to practice nursing in diverse communities; so, nurses must be aware of the influence that social structures and institutionalized power have on health. DNP and PhD students can work to increase and change through scholarly practice and research the understanding of the pathways that link social inequities to health.

Content should begin the first semester; students should be trained to assess clients' SDOH and incorporate them into comprehensive care plans. Social justice must be integrated throughout their educational and professional careers, and into clinical experiences in nursing education (Boutain, 2008). Such an approach would help to socialize students to the idea that it is nursing's responsibility to engage and inform health and social policy in an effort to alleviate social injustices. Structural racism includes societal and institutional influences such as segregation and immigration (Gee & Ford, 2011). Students must be made aware that addressing the impact of structural racism and its effect on illness and injury is as much a part of nursing care as alleviating pain (Thurman & Pfitzinger-Lippe, 2017; Wyman & Henly, 2015).

Efforts to address structural racism can be furthered through active participation in professional affinity organizations. Students should be encouraged to join organizations whose missions and values include the principles of health equity and social justice and expressed commitment to disparities and health equity (e.g., Chi Eta Phi Nursing Sorority, Gay and Lesbian Medical Association [GLMA]). See the select list below:

- American Association for Men in Nursing
- Asian American/Pacific Islander Nurses Association, Inc. (AAPINA)
- Chi Eta Phi Black Nursing Sorority
- National Alaska Native American Indian Nurses Association, Inc. (NANAINA)
- National Association of Hispanic Nurses, Inc. (NAHN)
- National Black Nurses Association, Inc. (NBNA)
- National Coalition of Ethnic Minority Nurse Associations (NCEMNA)
- Philippine Nurses Association of America, Inc. (PNAA)
- GLMA

As active members and student leaders in these organizations, students can participate in research and engage in policy advocacy, service learning, and community engagement to promote health equity. A list of potential organizations explicitly focused on advancing nursing is as follows:

- National Student Nurses Associations
- APHN
- American Psychiatric Nurses Association
- Sigma Theta Tau International Nursing Association
- Association of Women's Health, Obstetric and Neonatal Nurses
- Society of Pediatric Nurses

Students can also seek professional fellowships through a competitive merit-based process that is typically designed to serve a specified goal for the organization. These goals can include providing access to a new career, funding international service or work experiences, developing emerging leaders, or supporting social initiatives. Examples of professional fellowships in nursing are:

- American Academy of Nursing Jones Policy Scholars Program
- National Hartford Center of Gerontological Nursing Excellence: Patricia G. Archbold Scholars and Claire M. Fagin Fellows

Finally, individual colleges of nursing can also develop and implement health equity or policy scholars programs focused on social justice, health equity, and health disparities to allow students to jump-start their advocacy efforts while they are still in nursing school or pursuing advanced degrees (Wyman & Henly, 2015). For example, the Rush University College of Nursing implemented the Public Health Nursing Scholars mentorship program to create a cadre of scholars with a passion for public health nursing based on the mission of Public Health Nursing Section of the American Public Health Association. The Faculty Scholars program has now spread to the departments of Women, Children & Family Nursing, and Adult & Gerontological Health Nursing.

The United States far exceeds other developed countries in healthcare spending, yet has some of the worst health outcomes (Squires & Anderson, 2015). For example, the United States spends 17% of the gross domestic product on healthcare, compared to 10.7% spent by its closest neighbor Canada. Both countries experience racial and ethnic disparities in health, and both have developed guiding principles to address health equity that should be included in nursing education.

The AACN, the ANA, Quad Council Coalition (Quad Council), and Canadian Nurses Association (CNA) each provide guiding principles that should be included in entry-level education. The CNA developed Framework for the Practice of Registered Nurses of Canada (CNA, n.d.). Canada is composed of provinces and territories, or jurisdictions; each jurisdiction establishes its own regulatory body. The executive directors of the jurisdictions work collaboratively to develop entry-level registered nurse competencies. There are five competency categories, three of which include specific competencies related to the SDOH and social justice. In addition to the framework, in 1954, the CNA introduced a *Code of Ethics* which had several subsequent revisions, of which the most recent was in 2017 (CNA, n.d.). The CNA *Code of Ethics*, a standard of ethical values for nurses to adhere to, dedicates an entire section to "Promoting Justice," which describes the guiding principles of justice that nurses should uphold. Relevant AACN, ANA, Quad Council, and CNA principles are described in Table 4.1.

These guiding principles suggest the outcomes expected of graduates of bachelor's- and master's-level nursing programs. The ANA's guiding principles are informed by the *Code of Ethics* and the *Scope and Standards of Practice* (ANA Center for Ethics and Human Rights, 2016). The *Code of Ethics* was created to guide nurses' actions in a manner consistent with quality nursing care and ethical obligations. The ANA *Code of Ethics* has nine provisions. The ANA *Scope and Standards of Practice* has 17 standards (ANA, 2015b).

A number of nursing schools have published on their approaches to meet the AACN's (2008a, 2008c) five cultural competencies for nursing education (see Table 4.2). The AACN (2008a, 2008c) suggests cultural knowledge, cultural care of patients, promotion of culturally congruent skills, cultural awareness and advocacy, and professional development to be included in nursing education to achieve cultural

TABLE 4.1. AMERICAN- AND CANADIAN-RELATED HEALTH EQUITY GUIDING STANDARDS

ORGANIZATION	HEALTH EQUITY GUIDING STANDARDS
AACN (2009, 2017) essentials	Bachelors Essential VIII Professionalism and Professional Values, suggests that professionalism and values such as altruism, autonomy, human dignity, integrity, and social justice are fundamental to the discipline of nursing. Masters Essential VI Health Policy and Advocacy, suggests that the master's-prepared nurse should intervene at the system level by developing policy and being advocates to influence health and health care.
AACN (2008a) Cultural competencies	Competency 1: Apply knowledge of social and cultural factors that affect nursing and health care across multiple contexts. Competency 2: Use relevant data sources and best evidence in providing culturally competent care. Competency 3: Promote achievement of safe and quality outcomes of care for diverse populations. Competency 4: Advocate for social justice, including commitment to the health of vulnerable populations and the elimination of health disparities. Competency 5: Participate in continuous cultural competence development.
ANA (2015a) provisions	Provision 9 The profession of nursing, collectively through its professional organizations, must articulate nursing values, maintain the integrity of the profession and integrate principles of social justice into nursing and health policy.
ANA (2015b) competencies	Standard 8. Culturally Congruent Practice and Associated Competencies For Registered nurse: 1. Demonstrates respect, equity, and empathy in actions and interactions with all healthcare consumers. 2. Participates in lifelong learning to understand cultural preferences, worldview, choices, and decision-making processes of diverse consumers. 3. Creates an inventory of one's own values, beliefs, and cultural heritage. 4. Applies knowledge of variations in health beliefs, practices, and communication patterns in all nursing practice activities. 5. Identifies the stage of the consumer's acculturation and accompanying patterns of needs and engagement. 6. Considers the effects and impact of discrimination and oppression on practice within and among vulnerable cultural groups. 7. Uses skills and tools that are appropriately vetted for the culture, literacy, and language of the population served. 8. Communicates with appropriate language and behaviors, including the use of medical interpreters and translators in accordance with consumer preferences. 9. Identifies the cultural-specific meaning of interactions, terms, and content. 10. Respects consumer decisions based on age, tradition, belief and family influence, and stage of acculturation. 11. Advocates for policies that promote health and prevent harm among culturally diverse, under-served, or under-represented consumers. 12. Promotes equal access to services, tests, interventions, health promotion programs, enrollment in research, education, and other opportunities. 13. Educates nurse colleagues and other professionals about cultural similarities and differences of healthcare consumers, families, groups, communities, and populations.

(continued)

TABLE 4.1. AMERICAN- AND CANADIAN-RELATED HEALTH EQUITY GUIDING STANDARDS (*CONTINUED*)

ORGANIZATION	HEALTH EQUITY GUIDING STANDARDS
	Additional competencies for the graduate-level prepared registered nurse: 14. Evaluates tools, instruments, and services provided to culturally diverse populations. 15. Advances organizational policies, programs, services, and practices that reflect respect, equity, and values for diversity and inclusion. 16. Engages consumers, key stakeholders, and others in designing and establishing internal and external cross-cultural partnerships. 17. Conducts research to improve healthcare and healthcare outcomes for culturally diverse consumers. 18. Develops recruitment and retention strategies to achieve a multicultural workforce. Additional competencies for the advanced practice registered nurse: 19. Promotes shared decision-making solutions in planning, prescribing, and evaluating processes when the health care consumer's cultural preferences and norms may create incompatibility with evidence-based practice. 20. Leads interprofessional teams to identify the cultural and language needs of the consumer.
Quad Council Coalition (2018) Domains	Domain 1: Assessment and Analytic Skills Domain 4: Cultural Competency Skills Domain 6: Public Health Sciences Skills

College of Nurses Ontario CA (2014) competencies	Category: Specialized Body of Knowledge
	  Competency 30—Demonstrates knowledge about human growth and development, role transitions and population health, including the social determinants of health.
	
	Category: Competent application of Knowledge
	  Competency 41—Incorporates knowledge of the health disparities and inequities of vulnerable populations (e.g., sexual orientation, persons with disabilities, ethnic minorities, poor, homeless, racial minorities, language minorities) and the contributions of nursing practice to achieve positive health outcomes.
	
	Category: Service to the public
	  Competency 93—Advocates and promotes healthy public policy and social justice.

CNA (2017) Code of Ethics	Promoting Justice. Nurses uphold principles of justice by safeguarding human rights, equity and fairness and by promoting the public good. Ethical responsibilities: 1. Nurses do not discriminate on the basis of a person's race, ethnicity, culture, political and spiritual beliefs, social or marital status, gender, gender identity, gender expression, sexual orientation, age, health status, place of origin, lifestyle, mental or physical ability, socio-economic status, or any other attribute. 2. Nurses respect the special history and interests of Indigenous Peoples as articulated in the Truth and Reconciliation Commission of Canada's (TRC) Calls to Action (2012). 3. Nurses refrain from judging, labelling, stigmatizing and humiliating behaviours toward persons receiving care or toward other health-care providers, students and each other.

(continued)

TABLE 4.1. AMERICAN- AND CANADIAN-RELATED HEALTH EQUITY GUIDING STANDARDS (*CONTINUED*)

ORGANIZATION	HEALTH EQUITY GUIDING STANDARDS
	4. Nurses do not engage in any form of lying, punishment or torture or any form of unusual treatment or action that is inhumane or degrading. They refuse to be complicit in such behaviours. They intervene, and they report such behaviours if observed or if reasonable grounds exist to suspect their occurrence. 5. Nurses provide care for all persons including those seen as victims and/or abusers and refrain from any form of workplace bullying (CNA, 2016a). 6. Nurses make fair decisions about the allocation of resources under their control based on the needs of persons receiving care. They advocate for fair treatment and fair distribution of resources. Nurses advocate for evidence-informed decision-making in their practice including, for example, evidence for best practices in staffing and assignment, best care for particular health conditions and best approaches to health promotion. 7. Nurses work collaboratively to develop a moral community. As part of this community, all nurses acknowledge their responsibility to contribute to positive and healthy practice environments. Nurses support a climate of trust that sponsors openness, encourages the act of questioning the status quo and supports those who speak out in good faith to address concerns (e.g., whistle-blowing). Nurses protect whistle-blowers who have provided reasonable grounds for their concerns.

competence. The current scope of curricular approaches includes elective courses, professional development hours and simulation activities, experiential learning, interprofessional education and collaboration, and motivational interviewing (Thornton & Persaud, 2018; see Table 4.2).

Nursing Clinicians and Practitioners

Part of the social mandate for nursing and nursing education should address the need to activate the current nursing workforce. Of the approximately 3 million registered nurses in the United States, 62.2% work in a hospital, 10.5% work in ambulatory care, and around 8% work in public health settings including schools and public health departments (Akparawa, 2018). Past deficits in integrating health equity, health disparities, and social justice content in nursing education may leave practicing nurses unprepared to engage in sociopolitical activities aimed at alleviating health inequities, particularly for patients who receive care beyond the walls of the hospital. Thus, continuing education and professional development are needed for practicing nurses that offer information on what nurses can do before patients enter the hospital. This should be mandatory information for all practicing nurses (Thurman & Pfitzinger-Lippe, 2017).

Nursing Researchers

Nurse researchers from ethnic and racial minority groups tend to have lived experiences and understanding of the experiences of others in their ethnic and racial groups, which position them to make relevant contributions to designing and conducting studies among minorities. It is especially important to include such nurses

TABLE 4.2 EXEMPLARS FOR MEETING THE AACN'S CULTURAL COMPETENCIES IN NURSING EDUCATION

AUTHOR, YEAR	STUDENT	PLACEMENT IN CURRICULUM	LEARNING STRATEGY	TOPIC
Amerson (2010)	Undergraduate BSN	Community health nursing course	Service-learning projects with local and international communities	Cultural competence
Ballestas and Roller (2013)	Undergraduate BSN	Elective course	Study abroad program	Cultural competence
Boutain (2008)	Undergraduate BSN	Entire program of study	Curriculum revision and clinical evaluation tool	Social justice
Einhellig, Hummel, and Gryskiewicz (2015)	Undergraduate BSN	Elective research study; simulation activity	Missouri Association for Community Action Poverty Simulation	Social justice
Hatchett, Elster, Wasson, Anderson, and Parsi (2015)	Undergraduate BSN/graduate	Leadership/ bioethics course (online)	Course discussion and assignments	Social justice
Kaminski (2008)	Fourth year BSN students	Nurses influencing change course	Web-based teaching *tools*	Social justice
Kaplan (2010)	Masters	One of three required core courses	Small group assignment, web-based modules, reflective assignment	Cultural competence
M. Reed (personal communication, May 15, 2019)	Graduate entry, Masters	Terms 1 and 2 professional development hours	Six-session diversity and inclusion certificate program	Cultural competence
Rutledge, Garzon, Scott, and Karlowicz (2004)	Nurse practitioner students	Health assessment course	Standardized patients with culturally enhanced patient cases	Cultural competence

AACN, American Association of Colleges of Nursing.

in designing studies and interventions that are culturally relevant and acceptable. For example, the National Institute of Nursing Research (NINR) has done work in this regard through the Minority Supplement Program for Research and Research Training, Mentored Research Scientist Development Award for Minority Investigators, and the NINR AREA award for Health Disparities Research at Minority Serving Institutions (Phillips & Grady, 2002). The National Institutes of Health (NIH) has also implemented initiatives designed to promote and support the careers of women in biomedical science (Plank-Bazinet et al., 2016). Nursing postdoctoral training is another example of an important initiative that can propel the research career of minority researchers forward. The findings from this initiative reveal that nurses who complete an NINR-supported postdoctoral program have greater success obtaining future research dollars than their peers without postdoctorals, and that receipt of a postdoctoral training award results in a 20% increase in scholarly productivity in the form of published manuscripts (Ponte, Hayman, Berry, & Cooley, 2015).

Analysis of policies focused on processes, contexts, and content can inform advocacy efforts and solidify the links between evidence and policy. Such analyses that connect policies to health inequities across populations and locations can validate that unequal distribution of resources contributes to inequity. Research can also be conducted to determine why current policy advocacy related to SDOH has been ineffective. Studies that evaluate policies and programs or their impact on health and healthcare could enhance advocacy efforts. Furthermore, research that examines the attitudes, beliefs, and actions of how those with privilege view those who are vulnerable may also be helpful to raise awareness and inform policy advocacy work (Artiga & Hinton, 2018; Reutter & Kushner, 2010). The research agenda on SDOH must also examine competencies and scope of practice. For example, "Do states with broad nurse-practice acts have better or poorer outcomes among patients with particular chronic illnesses or among underserved and Medicaid populations than states with more restrictive practice acts?" (Mahony & Jones, 2013, p. 283). Other potential research examples related to scope of practice are: "How have physician relative value units (RVUs) impacted the scope of practice for APRNs?" "What is the impact of the implementation of the Affordable Care Act, and its potential repeal on nursing scope of practice?" "[How have] reductions in the work hours of resident physicians [impacted the scope of practice of APRNs]?" and "[What is] the impact of APRN's role expansion on care cost and physician/nursing workload?" (Institute of Medicine Committee on the Robert Wood Johnson Foundation Initiative on the Future of Nursing, 2011, p. 107).

The National Institute for Minority Health Disparities (NIMHD) Minority Health and Health Disparities Research Framework (Maillart & Mayorga, 2018) can serve as an overarching guide for research that examines the multipronged nature of minority health and health disparities (see Figure 4.2). This framework, which considers the domains of influence (biological, behavioral, physical/built environment, sociocultural environment, healthcare system, and health outcomes) and the levels of influence (individual, interpersonal, community, and societal), allows for the classification of data and data analyses to measure progress, gaps, and opportunities to address health disparities.

In recognition of the importance of addressing health equity, national legislation has been proposed. In May 2018, the House of Representatives introduced a bill to improve the health of minority individuals, among other purposes (Health Equity and Accountability Act of 2018 [HEAA], 2018). Among the components of the legislation are Titles that focus on culturally and linguistically appropriate health and healthcare; health workforce diversity; improving healthcare access and quality; improving health outcomes for women, children, and families; mental health; and addressing high-impact minority diseases (see Table 4.3). At the first look, the wide-scoping focus of the HEAA can be perceived as unrealistic in the depth and breadth of the focus of this legislation. However, the sponsors of the bill have taken steps to present a highly comprehensive piece of legislation that, if fully implemented, could truly address the root and extenuating factors that influence health inequity, health disparities, as well as SDOH. This legislation was introduced in the U. S. House of Representatives but died in Congress (GovTrack.us, 2019a). Even when approved, the bill will require intensive resources to implement. A previous version of the bill, HR 2954, was also unsuccessful in procuring the necessary approval (GovTrack.us, 2019b).

The HEAA (2018) and other healthcare legislation can be integrated into nursing curricula. For example, in a doctoral-level health policy nursing course, students are taught how to conduct a policy analysis through small weekly assignments. The

Levels of influence*

Domains of influence (Over the lifecourse)	Individual	Interpersonal	Community	Societal
Biological	Biological vulnerability and mechanisms	Caregiver–child interaction Family microbiome	Community illness Exposure Herd immunity	Sanitation Immunization Pathogen exposure
Behavior	Health behaviors Coping strategies	Family functioning School/work functioning	Community functioning	Policies and laws
Physical/built environment	Personal environment	Household environment School/work environment	Community environment Community resources	Societal structure
Sociocultural environment	Sociodemographics Limited English Cultural identity Response to discrimination	Social networks Family/peer norms Interpersonal discrimination	Community norms Local structural discrimination	Social norms Societal structural discrimination
Healthcare system	Insurance coverage Health literacy Treatment preferences	Patient–clinician relationship Medical decision-making	Availability of services Safety net services	Quality of care Healthcare policies
Health outcomes	Individual health	Family/ organizational health	Community health	Population health

FIGURE 4.2 NIMHD HEALTH DISPARITIES RESEARCH FRAMEWORK.

*Health Disparity Populations: race/ethnicity, low SES, rural, sexual/gender minority. Other fundamental characteristics: sex/gender, disability, geographic region. NIMHD, National Institute for Minority Health Disparities; SES, socioeconomic status.

Source: From National Institute on Minority Health and Health Disparities. (2018). *National Institute on Minority Health and Health Disparities research framework.* Retrieved from https://www.nimhd.nih.gov/about/overview/research-framework/nimhd-framework.htm

TABLE 4.3 H.R. 5942 – HEALTH EQUITY AND ACCOUNTABILITY ACT OF 2018

TITLES	DESCRIPTION AND SUBTITLE
Title I Data collection and reporting	
Title II Culturally and linguistically appropriate health and health-care	
Title III Health workforce diversity	
Title IV Improving health care access and quality	**Subtitle A:** expansion of coverage **Subtitle B:** expansion of access **Subtitle C:** advancing health equity through payment and delivery reform **Subtitle D:** health empowerment zones **Subtitle E:** at-risk community coverage
Title V Improving health outcomes for women, children, and families	**Subtitle A:** in general **Subtitle B:** pregnancy screening
Title VI Mental health	
Title VII Addressing high-impact minority diseases	**Subtitle A:** cancer **Subtitle B:** viral hepatitis and liver cancer control and prevention **Subtitle C:** acquired bone marrow failure disease **Subtitle D:** cardiovascular disease, chronic disease, and other disease issues **Subtitle E:** HIV/AIDS **Subtitle G:** lung disease **Subtitle H:** tuberculosis **Subtitle I:** osteoarthritis and musculoskeletal diseases **Subtitle J:** sleep and circadian rhythm disorders **Subtitle K:** sickle cell disease research, surveillance, prevention, and treatment
Title VIII Health information technology	**Subtitle A:** reducing health disparities through health IT **Subtitle B:** modifications to achieve parity in existing programs **Subtitle C:** additional research and studies **Subtitle D:** closing gaps in funding to adopt certified EHRs
Title IX Accountability and evaluation	
Title X Addressing social determinants and improving environmental justice	**Subtitle A:** in general **Subtitle B:** gun violence

EHRs, electronic health records; IT, information technology.
Source: Data from Health Equity and Accountability Act of 2018, H.R. 5942, 115th Cong. (2018). Retrieved from https://www.congress.gov/bill/115th-congress/house-bill/5942/text

analysis culminates in a final memo that is written to a key stakeholder policy maker or organizational leader (see Exemplar 4.4).

In January 2015, in recognition of the importance of Equity in Health Care, the American Hospital Association (AHA), in conjunction with the Institute for Diversity in Health Management, released the Equity of Care Toolkit for eliminating healthcare

---

Exemplar 4.4. Example of Social Justice and Policy Learning Activity for DNP students

Focus: Exemplars are used to promote social justice for students to become involved in the legislative process and public policy formation by developing a policy memo. The policy memo will be used to address a relevant policy maker or interest group/individual to discuss an issue.

Activity: Students create a memo that addresses the issue relevant to the target audiences' organizational policy environment and provides strategic recommendations regarding the selected policy. Students are referred to written guidelines for writing a policy memo. "Writing an Effective Policy Memo" includes a sample memo that should be used as a template for formatting and includes Introduction, Background, and Conclusion. Students are evaluated based upon a grading rubric which accesses whether their document reflects proficient, competent, or novice for the following domains: introduction, policy analysis, strategic recommendations, relevance, and formatting, for a total of 20 points.

DNP, Doctor of Nursing Practice.

Source: From K. Osborne, personal communication, May 2, 2019.

---

disparities (AHA, 2015a). Alongside this important tool kit, the AHA implemented a strategic initiative called "123forEquity," designed to promote health equity and promote diversity (AHA, 2015b). To date, over 1,816 local/regional and 51 state organizations have signed the pledge (AHA, 2015b). This focuses on "increasing the collection and use of race, ethnicity, language preference, and other socioeconomic data, increasing cultural competency training, increasing diversity in leadership and governance, and improving and strengthening community partnerships" (AHA, 2015c, p. 3). This organizational commitment to addressing health equity and promoting diversity is promising.

Dr. David Ansell, the senior vice president for Community Health Equity of Rush University Medical Center and lifelong advocate for health equity and social justice, describes the importance of "employing a health equity frame to pedagogy and practice" (D. Ansell, personal communication, November 19, 2018). Dr. Ansell asserts that "all trainees in every discipline must have the competency to perform a structural analysis in addition to a biological and psychosocial analysis of illness and health." In clinical practice, it will require looking not only at data across various clinical measures by race, ethnicity, and language (REAL), but also neighborhood-level data. According to Dr. Ansell, "this would make visible potential health disparities and identify opportunities for improvement....Such an approach would amplify the ways in which well-meaning systems and structures actually perpetuate historical injustices like structural racism and sexism." The use of a racial equity framework would provide students, faculty, and researchers with the tools to disrupt or dismantle these malfunctioning systems and structures (D. Ansell, personal communication, November 19, 2018).

■ Conclusion

Nursing's rich legacy of caring positions nurses squarely at the center of the entire healthcare system. Therefore, all nurses and nursing faculty must be equipped to lead the charge that will help drive change in the areas of health equity, social justice, SDOH, health disparities, and cultural competence. Adequate preparation for these key roles must take place in nursing academia with nursing students, faculty, and practicing nurses across all disciplines and levels of practice. In order to prepare nursing faculty to meet the challenge, professional development must be implemented with all faculty, including clinical instructors, mentors, and preceptors, through entities such as the ANA, the AACN, and the Association of American Medical Colleges (AAMC; Thornton & Persaud, 2018). Consultation outside of the home institution with experts in the field and ongoing evaluation may also be needed in order to improve the campus and classroom climate in nursing academia (Julion et al., 2019). Faculty can then be appropriately prepared to educate nursing students on the complex tenets of health equity at all levels of nursing academia (associate, bachelor, and doctoral).

■ Critical Thinking Exercises

- Identify at least three groups of people within your local community at risk of poor health outcomes. Describe how the SDOH or structural racism contributes to their adverse risks.
- Read *The Immortal Life of Henrietta Lacks* (Skloot, 2010); describe and discuss the impact of health disparities, medical ethics, and social injustice in women's health.
- Use role play to understand how members of an interprofessional team may address team members when confronted with racism and stereotyping (AACN, 2008).
- Describe the prevalence of racial, gender, or neighborhood health inequities in your community.
- Identify institutional commitments to health equity in your institution. Examples can include holistic admissions, mission, vision and strategic plans/initiative, program objectives, course objectives, learning outcomes and assignments, Office of Diversity and Inclusion, mentorship, and others.
- Review Provision 8.3 of the ANA Code of Ethics (2015a). Write down your personal statement of obligation to advance health and human rights and reduce disparities.
- Identify a community-based organization in your neighborhood. Establish a rapport with the organization, and develop and implement a service-learning project in conjunction with and in accordance with the needs of the community organization. Reflect upon your experience and examine personal beliefs, values, and views, and also reflect upon your experiences interacting with each other and your community-based service-learning site.
- Review the list of professional affinity organizations and nursing organizations provided in this chapter. Identify and attend a local chapter meeting in your community. Describe a research, social justice, or health disparities initiative related to the organization.

■ Discussion Questions

1. What are the historical events that affected health disparities in the communities you serve?

2. What individual and community strengths exist in health disparity populations that could be used to increase health equity?

3. Why is it important to build a diverse and inclusive culturally competent workforce in the fight against health disparities?

4. How does the concept of structural racism factor into health inequity and health-care disparities?

5. What do you need to learn in order to be effective in influencing policy change related to health and healthcare inequity?

6. How has your institution integrated the SDOH into the nursing curricula, class-room, and clinical experiences?

7. What core competencies do students need to effectively assess and address the SDOH in clinical practice? How does your nursing program prepare students for this important work?

8. The *Healthy People* Initiative has been in existence since 1979. How has it influenced health equity and health disparities over the past 40 years?

■ Resources

American Nurses Association. (n.d.). ANA advocacy toolkit. Retrieved from https://ana .aristotle.com/SitePages/toolkit.asp

American Psychiatric Nurses Association. (n.d.). Undergraduate education faculty tool-kit. Retrieved from https://www.apna.org/i4a/pages/index.cfm?pageid=6018

Asian & Pacific Islander American Health Forum. (2018). *The Health Equity and Accountability Act: A strategic and comprehensive approach to eliminating racial and ethnic health disparities.* Retrieved from https://www.apiahf.org/wp-content/ uploads/2018/04/October2018_HEAA_Factsheet.pdf

Association of Black Nursing Faculty. (n.d.). *The ABNF Journal.* Retrieved from https:// abnf.net/publications

Barton Smith, D. (2016). *The power to heal: Civil rights, Medicare, and the struggle to trans-form America's health care system.* Nashville, TN: Vanderbilt University Press.

Carpenter, L., Kovatchitch, M., Lewallen, L., & Giddens, J. (2011). Curriculum design: Fac-ulty toolkit for innovation in curriculum design. Retrieved from http://www.nln.org/ professional-development-programs/teaching-resources/toolkits/curriculum-design

National Collaborative for Education to Address the Social Determinants of Health. (n.d.). About NCEAS. Retrieved from https://sdoheducation.org/about

National League for Nursing. (n.d.). Advocacy teaching: Nursing is social justice advo-cacy. Retrieved from http://www.nln.org/professional-development-programs/ teaching-resources/toolkits/advocacy-teaching

National League for Nursing. (2017). *NLN diversity & inclusion toolkit.* Retrieved from http://www.nln.org/docs/default-source/default-document-library/diversity-tool-kit.pdf?sfvrsn=2

■ References

Akparawa, N. (2018, December 0). A vision for the future of nursing: Ten key points in his-tory worth reminiscing. Retrieved from https://transformnursing.com/2018/12/01/ a-vision-for-the-future-of-nursing-ten-key-points-in-history-worth-reminiscing

Alcaraz, K., Bertaut, T., Fedewa, S., Gansler, T., Sauer, A. G., McMahon, C., & Wagner, D. (2016). *Cancer facts & figures for African Americans 2016–2018*. Atlanta, GA: American Cancer Society.

American Association of Colleges of Nursing. (n.d.-a). Curriculum guidelines. Retrieved from https://www.aacnnursing.org/Faculty/Teaching-Resources/Curriculum -Guidelines

American Association of Colleges or Nursing (n.d.-b). Doctor of nursing practice (DNP) tool kit. Retrieved from https://www.aacnnursing.org/DNP/Tool-Kit

American Association of Colleges of Nursing. (2001). The baccalaureate degree in nursing as minimal preparation for professional practice. *Journal of Professional Nursing, 17*(5), 267–269.

American Association of Colleges of Nursing. (2008a). *Cultural competency in baccalaureate nursing education*. Retrieved from https://www.aacnnursing.org/Portals/42/ AcademicNursing/CurriculumGuidelines/Cultural-Competency-Bacc-Edu.pdf

American Association of Colleges of Nursing. (2008b). *Essentials of baccalaureate education for professional nursing practice*. Washington, DC: Author. Retrieved from http://www.aacnnursing.org/portals/42/publications/baccessentials08.pdf

American Association of Colleges of Nursing. (2008c). *Tool kit of resources for cultural competent education for baccalaureate nurses*. Retrieved from https://www .aacnnursing.org/Portals/42/AcademicNursing/CurriculumGuidelines/Cultural -Competency-Bacc-Tool-Kit.pdf

American Association of Colleges of Nursing. (2009). *The essentials of baccalaureate education for professional nursing practice: Faculty tool kit*. Washington, DC: Author. Retrieved from https://www.aacnnursing.org/Education-Resources/Tool-Kits/ Baccalaureate-Essentials-Tool-Kit

American Association of Colleges of Nursing. (2011a). *The essentials of master's education in nursing*. Washington, DC: Author. Retrieved from https://www.aacnnursing. org/Portals/42/Publications/MastersEssentials11.pdf

American Association of Colleges of Nursing. (2011b). *Tool kit for cultural competence in master's and doctoral nursing education*. Retrieved from https://www.aacnnursing. org/Portals/42/AcademicNursing/CurriculumGuidelines/Cultural-Competency -Grad-Tool-Kit.pdf

American Association of Colleges of Nursing. (2017). *The essentials of master's education in nursing: Tool kit*. Washington, DC: Author. Retrieved from https://www .aacnnursing.org/Portals/42/AcademicNursing/Tool%20Kits/Masters-Tool-Kit.pdf

American Association of Colleges of Nursing Task Force on the Research-Focused Doctorate in Nursing. (2009). *The research--focused doctoral program in nursing: Pathways to excellence*. Retrieved from https://www.aacnnursing.org/Portals/42/Publications/ PhDPosition.pdf

American Hospital Association. (2015a). *Equity of care: A toolkit for eliminating health care disparities*. Retrieved from http://www.diversityconnection.org/diversityconnection/ membership/Resource%20Center%20Docs/equity-of-care-toolkit.pdf

American Hospital Association. (2015b). #123forEquity Pledge to Act. Retrieved from http://www.equityofcare.org/pledge/pledge-map.dhtml

American Hospital Association. (2015c). Advancing health in America: Health equity. Retrieved from http://www.equityofcare.org/resources/resources/2018%20EOC%20 Toolkit.pdf

American Nurses Association. (2015a). *Code of ethics for nurses with interpretive statements*. Silver Spring, MD: Author. Retrieved from https://www.nursingworld.org/ coe-view-only

American Nurses Association. (2015b). *Nursing: Scope and standards of practice* (3rd ed.). Silver Springs, MD: Author. Retrieved from https://www.iupuc.edu/health-sciences/ files/Nursing-ScopeStandards-3E.pdf

American Nurses Association Center for Ethics and Human Rights. (2016). *The nurse's role in ethics and human rights: Protecting and promoting individual worth, dignity, and human rights in practice settings* [Position Paper]. Retrieved from https://www.nursingworld.org/~4af078/globalassets/docs/ana/ethics/ethics-and-human-rights-protecting-and-promoting-final-formatted-20161130.pdf

Amerson, R. (2010). The impact of service-learning on cultural competence. *Nursing Education Perspectives, 31*(1), 18–22.

Anderson, L. M., Scrimshaw, S. C., Fullilove, M. T., Fielding, J. E., & Normand, J. (2003). Culturally competent healthcare systems: A systematic review. *American Journal of Preventive Medicine, 24*(3 Suppl.), 68–79. doi:10.1016/s0749-3797(02)00657-8

Ansell, D. A. (2017). *The death gap: How inequality kills.* Chicago, IL: University of Chicago Press.

Artiga, S., & Hinton, E. (2018). Beyond health care: The role of social determinants in promoting health and health equity. *Health, 20,* 10. Retrieved from http://files.kff.org/attachment/issue-brief-beyond-health-care

Bakst, D., & Tyrrell, P. (2017). Big government policies that hurt the poor and how to address them. Retrieved from https://www.heritage.org/poverty-and-inequality/report/big-government-policies-hurt-the-poor-and-how-address-them

Ballestas, H. C., & Roller, M. C. (2013). The effectiveness of a study abroad program for increasing students' cultural competence. *Journal of Nursing Education and Practice, 3*(6), 125–133. doi:10.5430/jnep.v3n6p125

Bauer, K., & Bai, Y. (2015). Innovative educational activities using a model to improve cultural competency among graduate students. *Procedia-Social and Behavioral Sciences, 174,* 705–710. doi:10.1016/j.sbspro.2015.01.605

Bender, M. (2014). The current evidence base for the clinical nurse leader: A narrative review of the literature. *Journal of Professional Nursing, 30*(2), 110–123. doi:10.1016/j.profnurs.2013.08.006

Boutain, D. M. (2008). Social justice as a framework for undergraduate community health clinical experiences in the United States. *International Journal of Nursing Education Scholarship, 5*(1), 1–12. doi:10.2202/1548-923X.1419

Brach, C., & Fraser, I. (2002). Reducing disparities through culturally competent health care: An analysis of the business case. *Quality Management in Health Care, 10*(4), 15–28. doi:10.1097/00019514-200210040-00005

Buhler-Wilkerson, K. (1993). Bringing care to the people: Lillian Wald's legacy to public health nursing. *American Journal of Public Health, 83*(12), 1778–1786. doi:10.2105/AJPH.83.12.1778

Burgess, D. J., Bokhour, B. G., Cunningham, B. A., Do, T., Gordon, H. S., Jones, D. M., . . . Gollust, S. E. (2017). Healthcare providers' responses to narrative communication about racial healthcare disparities. *Health Communication, 34*(2), 149–161. doi:10.1080/10410236.2017.1389049

Canadian Nurses Association. (2017). *Code of ethics for registered nurses* (2017 ed.). Ottawa, ON, Canada. Retrieved from https://www.cna-aiic.ca/html/en/Code-of-Ethics-2017-Edition/index.html#2

Carnegie, M. E. (1995). *The path we tread: Blacks in nursing worldwide, 1854–1994.* New York, NY: National League of Nursing Press.

Colby, S. L., & Ortman, J. M. (2015). Projections of the size and composition of the U.S. population: 2014 to 2060. Retrieved from https://www.census.gov/library/publications/2015/demo/p25-1143.html

College of Nurses of Ontario. (2014). *Entry-to-practice competencies for registered nurses.* Retrieved from http://www.cno.org/globalassets/docs/reg/41037_entrytopracitic_final.pdf

Creanga, A. A., & Callaghan, W. M. (2017). Recent increases in the US maternal mortality rate: Disentangling trends from measurement issues. *Obstetrics & Gynecology, 129*(1), 206–207. doi:10.1097/AOG.0000000000001831

Cunningham, T. J., Croft, J. B., Liu, Y., Lu, H., Eke, P. I., & Giles, W. H. (2017). Vital signs: Racial disparities in age-specific mortality among Blacks or African Americans – United States, 1999-2015. *Morbidity and Mortality Weekly Report, 66*(17), 444–456. doi:10.15585/mmwr.mm6617e1

Demarinis, S. (2019). Nurses outpace other professions for honesty and ethics again. *Explore, 15*(3), 175–177. doi:10.1016/j.explore.2019.02.004

Einhellig, K., Hummel, F., & Gryskiewicz, C. (2015). The power of affective learning strategies on socialjustice development in nursing education. *Journal of Nursing Education and Practice, 5*(1), 121–128. doi:10.5430/jnep.v5n1p121

Families USA: The Voice for Health Care Consumers. (2019). African American Health Disparities Compared to Non-Hispanic Whites. Retrieved from https://familiesusa .org/wp-content/uploads/2019/08/HSI-Health-disparities_african-americans -infographic.pdf

Garneau, A. B. (2016). Critical reflection in cultural competence development: A framework for undergraduate nursing education. *Journal of Nursing Education, 55*(3), 125–132. doi:10.3928/01484834-20160216-02

Gaston-Johansson, F., Hill-Briggs, F., Oguntomilade, L., Bradley, V., & Mason, P. (2007). Patient perspectives on disparities in healthcare from African-American, Asian, Hispanic, and Native American samples including a secondary analysis of the institute of medicine focus group data. *Journal of National Black Nurses' Association: 18*(2), 43–52. Retrieved from https://www.researchgate.net/profile/Felicia_Hill-Briggs/publication/5534570_Patient_perspectives_on_disparities_in_healthcare_from_African-American_Asian_Hispanic_and_Native_American_samples_including_a_secondary_analysis_of_the_Institute_of_Medicine_focus_group_data/links/0c9605281330a5cb93000000.pdf

Gee, G. C., & Ford, C. L. (2011). Structural racism and health inequities: Old issues, new directions. *Du Bois Review: Social Science Research on Race, 8*(1), 115–132. doi:10.1017/S1742058X11000130

GovTrack.us. (2019a). H.R. 5942—115th Congress: Health Equity and Accountability Act of 2018. Retrieved from https://www.govtrack.us/congress/bills/115

GovTrack.us. (2019b). H.R. 2954—112th Congress: Health Equity and Accountability Act of 2011. Retrieved from https://www.govtrack.us/congress/bills/112/hr2954

Hall, J. M., & Fields, B. (2012). Race and microaggression in nursing knowledge development. *Advances in Nursing Science, 35*(1), 25–38. doi:10.1097/ANS.0b013e3182433b70

Hall, J. M., & Fields, B. (2013). Continuing the conversation in nursing on race and racism. *Nursing Outlook, 61*(3), 164–173. doi:10.1016/j.outlook.2012.11.006

Harkess, L., & Kaddoura, M. (2016). Culture and cultural competence in nursing education and practice: The state of the art. *Nursing Forum, 51*(3), 211–222. doi:10.1111/nuf.12140

Harris, M. S., Purnell, K., & Lindgren, K. (2013). Moving toward cultural competency: Dreamwork online summer program. *Journal of Cultural Diversity, 20*(3), 134. Retrieved from https://www.ncbi.nlm.nih.gov/pubmed/24279129

Hatchett, L., Elster, N., Wasson, K., Anderson, L., & Parsi, K. (2015). Integrating social justice for health professional education: Self-reflection, advocacy, and collaborative learning. *Online Journal of Health Ethics, 11*(1). doi:10.18785/ojhe.1101.04

Health Equity and Accountability Act of 2018, H.R. 5942, 115th Cong. (2018). Retrieved from https://www.congress.gov/bill/115th-congress/house-bill/5942/text

Health Resources and Services Administration. (December, 2017). *Nursing workforce projections by ethnicity and race 2014–2030.* Retrieved from https://bhw.hrsa .gov/sites/default/files/bhw/health-workforce-analysis/research/projections/hrsa -bhw-rn-lpn-factsheet-12-17.pdf

Hine, D. C. (2003). Black professionals and race consciousness: Origins of the civil rights movement, 1890–1950. *The Journal of American History, 89*(4), 1279–1294. doi:10.2307/3092543

Howell, E. A., & Zeitlin, J. (2017). Improving hospital quality to reduce disparities in severe maternal morbidity and mortality. *Seminars in Perinatology, 41*(5), 266–272. doi:10.1053/j.semperi.2017.04.002

Hunt, B. R., Tran, G., & Whitman, S. (2015). Life expectancy varies in local communities in Chicago: Racial and spatial disparities and correlates. *Journal of Racial and Ethnic Health Disparities, 2*(4), 425–433. doi:10.1007/s40615-015-0089-8

Institute of Medicine Committee on the Robert Wood Johnson Foundation Initiative on the Future of Nursing. (2011). *The future of nursing: Leading change, advancing health.* Washington, DC: National Academies Press.

Jack Jr, L., Liburd, L. C., Tucker, P., & Cockrell, T. (2014). Having their say: Patients' perspectives and the clinical management of diabetes. *Clinical Therapeutics, 36*(4), 469–476. doi:10.1016/j.clinthera.2014.02.003

Jeffries, P. R. (2015). The evolving health care system: The need for nursing education reform. *Journal of Professional Nursing, 31*(6), 441–443. doi:10.1016/j.profnurs .2015.10.012

Julion, W., Reed, M., Bounds, D. T., Cothran, F., Gamboa, C., Sumo, J. (2019). A group think-tank as a discourse coalition to promote minority nursing faculty retention. *Nursing Outlook, 67*(5):586–595. doi:10.1016/j.outlook.2019.03.003

Kaminski, J. (2008). *Using communicative and creative technologies to weave social justice and change theory into the tapestry of nursing curriculum.* Paper presented at Xi Eta Chapter, Sigma Theta Tau International 13th Annual, Vancouver, British Columbia, Canada.

Kaplan, L. (2010). Promoting cultural competence through a health policy course. *Nurse Educator, 35*(2), 87–89.

Leininger, M. M. (1988). Leininger's theory of nursing: Cultural care diversity and universality. *Nursing Science Quarterly, 1*(4), 152–160. doi:10.1177/089431848800100408

Lipson, J. G., & Desantis, L. A. (2007). Current approaches to integrating elements of cultural competence in nursing education. *Journal of Transcultural Nursing, 18*(1, Suppl.), 10S–20S. doi:10.1177/1043659606295498

Loftin, C., Hartin, V., Branson, M., & Reyes, H. (2013). Measures of cultural competence in nurses: An integrative review. *The Scientific World Journal, 2013,* 289101. doi:10.1155/2013/289101

Lonneman, W. (2015). Teaching strategies to increase cultural awareness in nursing students. *Nurse Educator, 40*(6), 285–288. doi:10.1097/NNE.0000000000000175

MacDorman, M. F., Declercq, E., Cabral, H., & Morton, C. (2016). Recent increases in the U.S. maternal mortality rate: Disentangling trends from measurement issues. *Obstetrics and Gynecology, 128*(3), 447–455. doi:10.1097/AOG.0000000000001556

MacDorman, M. F., Declercq, E., & Thoma, M. E. (2017). Trends in maternal mortality by sociodemographic characteristics and cause of death in 27 states and the District of Columbia. *Obstetrics and Gynecology, 129*(5), 811–818. doi:10.1097/ AOG.0000000000001968

Mahony, D., & Jones, E. J. (2013). Social determinants of health in nursing education, research, and health policy. *Nursing Science Quarterly, 26*(3), 280–284. doi:10.1177/0894318413489186

Maillart, L. M., & Mayorga, M. E. (2018). *Introduction to the Special Issue on Advancing Health Services, "Master's Essentials Tool Kit." American Association of Colleges of Nursing: The Voice of Academic Nursing.* Retrieved from http://www.aacnnursing .org/Teaching-Resources/Tool-Kits/Masters

Marmot, M., Friel, S., Bell, R., Houweling, T. A., Taylor, S., & Commission on Social Determinants of Health. (2008). Closing the gap in a generation: Health equity through action on the social determinants of health. *The Lancet, 372*(9650), 1661–1669. doi:10.1016/S0140-6736(08)61690-6

Meade, M. A., Mahmoudi, E., & Lee, S. (2015). The intersection of disability and healthcare disparities: A conceptual framework. *Disability and Rehabilitation, 37*(7), 632–641. doi:10.3109/09638288.2014.938176

National Advisory Council on Nurse Education and Practice. (2013). *Achieving health equity through nursing workforce diversity.* Retrieved from https://www.hrsa.gov/ advisorycommittees/bhpradvisory/nacnep/Reports/eleventhreport.pdf

National Center for Health Statistics. (2017). *Health, United States, 2016: With chartbook on long-term trends in health.* Hyattsville, MD: Author.

National CLAS Standards—Think Cultural Health. (n.d.). Retrieved from https://think culturalhealth.hhs.gov/assets/pdfs/EnhancedNationalCLASStandards.pdf

National Institute on Minority Health and Health Disparities. (2018). *National Institute on Minority Health and Health Disparities research framework.* Retrieved from https://www.nimhd.nih.gov/images/research-framework-slide.pdf

National League for Nursing. (2019). *A VISION FOR integration of the social determinants of health into nursing education curricula.* Retrieved from http://www.nln.org/docs/ default-source/default-document-library/social-determinants-of-health.pdf?sfvrsn=2

Office of Disease Prevention and Health Promotion. (n.d.-a). Disparities. Retrieved from https://www.healthypeople.gov/2020/about/foundation-health-measures/Disparities

Office of Disease Prevention and Health Promotion. (n.d.-b). Social determinants of health. Retrieved from https://www.healthypeople.gov/2020/about/foundation-health-measures/Disparities

Overcoming Barriers to Achieve Health Equity With Latino Communities. (2012, November). *Culture of Health Blog.* Retrieved from https://www.rwjf.org/en/blog .html

Perry, D. J., Willis, D. G., Peterson, K. S., & Grace, P. J. (2017). Exercising nursing essential and effective freedom in behalf of social justice: A humanizing model. *Advances in Nursing Science, 40*(3), 244–262. doi:10.1097/ANS.0000000000000151

Pfefferle, S. G., & Gibson, T. S. (2010). Minority recruitment for the 21st century: An environmental scan. Cambridge, MA: Abt Associates. Retrieved from https://www .naadac.org/assets/2416/minority_recruitment_environmental_scan2.pdf

Phillips, J., & Grady, P. A. (2002). Reducing health disparities in the twenty-first century: Opportunities for nursing research. *Nursing Outlook, 50*(3), 117–120. doi:10.1067/ mno.2002.123529

Phillips, J. M., & Malone, B. (2014). Increasing racial/ethnic diversity in nursing to reduce health disparities and achieve health equity. *Public Health Reports, 129*(1, Suppl. 2), 45–50. doi:10.1177/00333549141291S209

Plank-Bazinet, J. L., Whittington, K. B., Cassidy, S. K., Filart, R., Cornelison, T. L., Begg, L., & Clayton, J. A. (2016). Programmatic efforts at the National Institutes of Health to promote and support the careers of women in biomedical science. *Academic Medicine, 91*(8), 1057. doi:10.1097/ACM.0000000000001239

Poghosyan, L., & Carthon, J. M. B. (2017). The untapped potential of the nurse practitioner workforce in reducing health disparities. *Policy, Politics, & Nursing Practice, 18*(2), 84–94. doi:10.1177/1527154417721189

Ponte, P. R., Hayman, L. L., Berry, D. L., & Cooley, M. E. (2015). A new model for post-doctoral training: The Nursing Postdoctoral Program in Cancer and Health Dispari-ties. *Nursing Outlook, 63*(2), 189–203. doi:10.1016/j.outlook.2014.11.014

Powell Sears, K. (2012). Improving cultural competence education: The utility of an intersectional framework. *Medical Education, 46*(6), 545–551. doi:10.1111/j.1365-2923.2011.04199.x

Quad Council Coalition Competency Review Task Force. (2018). *Community/public health nursing (C/PHN] competencies*. Retrieved from http://www.quadcouncilphn.org/documents-3/2018-qcc-competencies

Raghupathi, W., & Raghupathi, V. (2018). An empirical study of chronic diseases in the united states: A visual analytics approach to public health. *International Journal of Environmental Research and Public Health, 15*(3), 431. doi:10.3390/ijerph15030431

Reutter, L., & Kushner, K. E. (2010). 'Health equity through action on the social determi-nants of health': Taking up the challenge in nursing. *Nursing Inquiry, 17*(3), 269–280. doi:10.1111/j.1440-1800.2010.00500.x

Rittel, H. W. J., & Webber, M. M. (1973). Dilemmas in a general theory of planning. *Policy Sciences, 4*, 155–169. doi:10.1007/BF01405730

Roger, V. L., Go, A. S., Lloyd-Jones, D. M., Benjamin, E. J., Berry, J. D., Borden, W. B., . . . Turner, M. B.. (2012). Heart disease and stroke statistics--2012 update: A report from the American Heart Association. *Circulation, 125*(1), e2–e220. doi:10.1161/CIR.0b013e31823ac046

Rutledge, C. M., Garzon, L., Scott, M., & Karlowicz, K. (2004). Using standardized patients to teach and evaluate nurse practitioner students on cultural competency. *International Journal of Nursing Education Scholarship, 1*(1), 17. doi:10.2202/1548-923X.1048

Shen, M. J., Peterson, E. B., Costas-Muñiz, R., Hernandez, M. H., Jewell, S. T., Matsoukas, K., & Bylund, C. L. (2018). The effects of race and racial concordance on patient-physician communication: A systematic review of the literature. *Journal of Racial and Ethnic Health Disparities, 5*(1), 117–140. doi:10.1007/s40615-017-0350-4

Skloot, R. (2010). *The immortal life of Henrietta Lacks*. New York, NY: Random House Audio.

Spyder. (n.d.). ANA Nursing: Scope and Standards of Practice. Retrieved from https://www.aaacn.org/article/ana-nursing-scope-and-standards-practice

Squires, D., & Anderson, C. (2015). US health care from a global perspective: Spend-ing, use of services, prices, and health in 13 countries. *The Commonwealth Fund, 15*, 1–16. doi:10.15868/socialsector.25051

Srinivasan, S., & Williams, S. D. (2014). Transitioning from health disparities to a health equity research agenda: The time is now. *Public Health Reports, 129*(1, Suppl. 2), 71–76. doi:10.1177/00333549141291S213

Swider, S. M., Krothe, J., Reyes, D., & Cravetz, M. (2013). The quad council practice competencies for public health nursing. *Public Health Nursing, 30*(6), 519–536. doi:10.1111/phn.12090

Thackrah, R., & Thompson, S. (2013). Refining the concept of cultural competence: Build-ing on decades of progress. *Medical Journal of Australia, 199*(1), 35–38. doi:10.5694/mja13.10499

The Legislative Process. (n.d.). Retrieved from https://www.house.gov/the-house-explained/the-legislative-process

Thornton, M., & Persaud, S. (2018). Preparing today's nurse: Social determinants of health and nursing education. *The Online Journal of Issues in Nursing, 23*(3), Manuscript 5.

Thurman, W., & Pfitzinger-Lippe, M. (2017). Returning to the profession's roots. *Advances in Nursing Science, 40*(2), 184–193. doi:10.1097/ANS.0000000000000140

Truman, B. I., Smith, K. C., Roy, K., Chen, Z., Moonesinghe, R., Zhu, J., . . . Centers for Disease Control and Prevention. (2011). Rationale for regular reporting on health disparities and inequalities-United States. *Morbidity and Mortality Weekly Report Surveillance Summaries, 60*(Suppl. 1), 3–10.

U.S. Department of Education, Office of Planning, Evaluation and Policy Development. (2016). Advancing diversity and inclusion in higher education. Retrieved from https://www2.ed.gov/rschstat/research/pubs/advancing-diversity-inclusion.pdf

U.S. Department of Health and Human Services. (2011). *National stakeholder strategy for achieving health equity.* Washington, DC: Author Retrieved from https://www.minorityhealth.hhs.gov/npa/files/Plans/NSS/CompleteNSS.pdf

Walker, R. J., Williams, J. S., & Egede, L. E. (2016). Influence of race, ethnicity and social determinants of health on diabetes outcomes. *The American Journal of the Medical Sciences, 351*(4), 366–373. doi:10.1016/j.amjms.2016.01.008

Weinstein, J. N., Geller, A., Negussie, Y., & Baciu, A. (Eds.). Communities in action: Pathways to health equity. Washington, DC: National Academies Press. Retrieved from https://www.nap.edu/read/24624/chapter/1

Wyman, J. F., & Henly, S. J. (2015). PhD programs in nursing in the United States: Visibility of American Association of Colleges of Nursing core curricular elements and emerging areas of science. *Nursing Outlook, 63*(4), 390–397. doi:10.1016/j.outlook.2014.11.003

Zaccagnini, M. E., & White, K. W. (2017). *The doctor of nursing practice essentials: A new model for advanced practice nursing.* Burlington, MA: Jones & Bartlett Learning.

Zimmerman, F. J., & Anderson, N. W. (2019). Trends in health equity in the United States by race/ethnicity, sex, and income, 1993-2017. *Journal of the American Medical Association Network Open, 2*(6), e196386–e196386. doi:10.1001/jamanetworkopen.2019.6386

5 Health Equity and Health System Transformation Policy

Sinsi Hernández-Cancio and Noelle Thompson

CHAPTER OBJECTIVES

- ⊙ Learn how healthcare policy affects the delivery of healthcare and the functions of nurses
- ⊙ Understand what health system transformation is and the potential risks and opportunities payment and delivery reform efforts can present for communities of color and other underserved or marginalized communities
- ⊙ Know the six domains of health equity and system transformation policy action and roles they may play in promoting and implementing healthcare policies that advance health equity
- ⊙ Learn why decreasing racial, ethnic, and geographic health inequities require directly addressing interpersonal racism (including implicit bias), institutional and structural racism, and social determinants of health (SDOH) through payment and delivery reform
- ⊙ Understand why equitable, high-quality, culturally centered, and patient-centered care requires cohesive, interdisciplinary teams that include nonclinical care providers, and why nurses have a critical role to play on these teams, given their training, location, and the high level of trust the public has for them

KEY CONCEPTS

Interpersonal, implicit, institutional, systemic, and structural racism

Social determinants of health (SDOHs)

Adverse childhood experiences (ACEs)

Trauma-informed care

Health system transformation

The potential risks and opportunities of health system transformation on health equity

The six policy domains of equity-focused system transformation

KEY TERMS

Evidence

Measurement

Safety net

Community health workers (CHWs)

Community partners

Allostatic load

Cultural competency

■ Introduction

Payment and delivery reform, also known as "health system transformation" (HST), is moving rapidly to change the way we pay for healthcare from a system that pays for volume to one that pays for value. However, the needs of communities of color and other underserved communities struggling with persistent health inequities have not been well represented or adequately considered in the HST enterprise. We review the basics of health equity, health system transformation, and the intersection of the two, and describe the six domains for equity-focused HST policy action: payment, measurement, evidence, the safety net, community partnerships, and workforce. We also discuss the important role nurses can play in these efforts.

■ Defining Health Policy and Healthcare Policy

As a nation, we need an efficient, high-quality, affordable healthcare system that works for everybody. Yet the focus of clinical healthcare practitioners, whether nurses, doctors, or others, is usually on delivering healthcare services to individuals, and in some cases, communities. However, their sphere of action and the options they have with regard to how, when, where, and what kind of care they can provide are determined by a number of overlapping public and private policies, many of which the practitioner may not be aware.

In broad strokes, public policies are the collection of decisions made by government entities regarding how resources will be distributed and used to address collective needs, solve specific public problems, and protect the rights of individuals and communities. Private policies are the collective decisions made by private entities, such as corporations and nonprofit organizations, which determine how their businesses are organized and run, including their workplaces and interactions with their customers. Individuals and groups can organize to influence policy decisions, both in the public and private spheres.

The World Health Organization (WHO) defines "health policy" as the "decisions, plans, and actions that are undertaken to achieve specific healthcare goals within a society" (WHO, n.d.). The U.S. National Institutes of Health expands on this definition as follows:

> [health policy refers to the] development by government and other policy makers of present and future objectives pertaining to health care and the health care system, and the articulation of arguments and decisions regarding these objectives in legislation, judicial opinions, regulations, guidelines, standards, etc. that affect health care and public health. (U.S. National Library of Medicine, 2019)

Health policies can include issues outside of the healthcare system, such as nutrition, physical fitness, and primary prevention.

Healthcare policies are a subset of health policies that directly affect the delivery of healthcare, including the administration of hospitals and medical offices, the specific work of particular clinical practitioners (including nurses) across all settings, drug and medical device safety, and a myriad of aspects of patient care, including patient protections. Healthcare policies can influence the availability of resources, clinician working conditions, and specifics of how care is delivered in terms of treatments available, who delivers care, and how accountable providers are for patient outcomes. The Affordable Care Act (ACA) is one of the many examples of healthcare policy legislation that had wide and extensive influence on the practice of medicine, including providing millions of uninsured people with health insurance, establishing a number of consumer protections, and mandating coverage of preventive care with no additional cost.

Nurses are well positioned to strongly influence health policy. Nursing is one of the largest segments of the U.S. workforce, and it is one of the fastest growing professions in the country. Today, there are an estimated nearly 3.9 million nurses nationwide, including 2.9 million RNs and more than 700,000 LPNs, in addition to specialized nurses such as nurse anesthetists and nurse midwives (U.S. Bureau of Labor Statistics, 2019). Nurses have long been considered one of the most trusted professionals among the U.S. public (Brenan, 2018), which gives them the potential for being powerful and compelling educators for the public and policy makers, and effective advocates on behalf of their patients. In addition, their unique perspectives and insights on many aspects of the healthcare system in a variety of care delivery settings are vital in working toward a more agile and equitable healthcare system. Having a solid understanding of healthcare policy will provide nurses with a greater capacity to influence health policy and to gain better access to resources and opportunities that will enable them to provide the best care to their patients (see Box 5.1 for an overview of the levels of policy decision-making).

■ Health System Transformation

Health system transformation (HST), also known as "payment and delivery reform," focuses on changing how healthcare is delivered and paid for with the goal of

Box 5.1: Levels of Healthcare Policy Decision-Making

Healthcare policy can be set at different levels of decision-making, from the federal government, to state government, down to hospital systems and clinics.

- Federal: Congress (laws), the White House (executive orders, special offices or task forces, etc.), and federal agencies like the Department of Health and Human Services, including the Centers for Medicare and Medicaid Services, the Center for Medicare and Medicaid Innovation, and the Centers for Disease Control and Prevention (rules, regulations, guidelines, etc.)
- State: legislature, governors' offices and state agencies, regulatory entities like the insurance commissioner, and licensing and certification boards
- County and municipal: county public health departments and city and municipal agencies
- Nongovernmental actors: providers (as healthcare systems, community health centers, etc.).

improving the efficiency and value of the healthcare system so that it can produce better health outcomes for patients at lower costs. To a great extent, HST developed as a response to escalating healthcare costs and the recognition that in the United States, we pay far more per capita for healthcare than any other industrialized nation (Organisation for Economic Cooperation and Development [OECD], 2018), yet our health outcomes are comparatively poorer (Schneider, Sarnak, Squires, Shah, & Doty, 2017). Moreover, experts have long recognized that there is much waste in the U.S. healthcare system—up to 20% (Berwick & Hackbarth, 2012), and that up to 30% of treatments are preventable or unnecessary (Wolfson & Mende, 2015). An underlying driver of this waste and unnecessary care that drives up healthcare costs is the fact that generally, the more tests, scans, treatments, and procedures providers give patients, the more they are paid—whether or not they are duplicative or really needed to diagnose and treat patients. This is called "fee-for-service" (FFS) payment.

The driving purpose of HST is to change the way we pay for healthcare in this country—from paying for the *amount* of healthcare provided (FFS) to paying for the *value* of the care provided—also known as "value-based payment." The idea is that over time, paying for *quality instead of quantity* should not only improve people's health but also rein in healthcare costs. To achieve this, efforts often focus on achieving the "Triple Aim": (a) improving the individual's experience of care; (b) improving the health of populations; and (c) reducing per capita cost of care (Berwick, Nolan, & Whittington, 2008). The main pathway has been to incentivize and pay for treatments and approaches that work well and are considered "high value" and disincentivize treatments and approaches that are less effective or provide no value in improving the patient's health (see Box 5.2).

While the federal government initiated some early efforts to shift payment from volume to value in the mid-2000s, the ACA accelerated this process with the creation of the Center for Medicare and Medicaid Innovation (CMMI) and the development of

---

Box 5.2: "Never Events": An Example of Not Paying for Quantity

One concrete example of not paying for low-value care is the "Never Event" policy implemented by the Centers for Medicare and Medicaid Services (CMS) in 2008 for Medicare patients (Agency for Healthcare Research and Quality, 2019). Before this, hospitals were paid for anything they did to a patient, including paying for treating complications that should have easily been avoided, and even to fix their own medical errors. Therefore, the payment system provided no incentive to avoid egregious mistakes, such as giving a patient blood of the wrong type or leaving foreign objects inside patients during surgery. If the patient had to stay in the hospital longer, or have a second surgery to remove foreign objects, the hospital would just bill more and increase its revenue. In 2008, CMS implemented a new policy: It would not pay for treatments caused by "never events," mistakes that were so extreme, expensive, and bad for patients that they literally should never happen. Initially this included a list of eight events, including the two already mentioned. Today the list has grown to 14 (Agency for Healthcare Research and Quality, 2019).

a number of new healthcare delivery and payment models—focused primarily on the Medicare program (Abrams et al., 2015). These included initiatives like:

- **Accountable care organizations (ACOs):** A group "of health care providers that agree to be held accountable for improving patient health while lowering health care costs. Providers in ACOs have financial incentives for achieving these goals, which makes ACOs a powerful tool for improving the quality of care more broadly" (Families USA, 2012, para. 1).
- **Transforming primary care through patient-centered medical homes and other similar models:** These models are aimed at revitalizing primary care, which under FFS has been undervalued for decades. They focus on centering primary care and rewarding these providers for adopting more comprehensive, team-based care, improving care coordination with other providers when needed (including home-based care), improving patient engagement, being more accessible to patients, and enhancing their quality and safety initiatives.
- **A variety of payment innovations:** Primarily through the CMMI and Medicare payment policies, a number of different initiatives and pilots have been rolled out that change how providers, like hospitals, are paid across the board, or support state-level or even smaller experiments in changing the delivery of healthcare. These include programs like:
  - Hospital Readmissions Reduction Program (CMS, 2018a), which penalizes hospitals that have too many patients readmitted within 30 days of an initial discharge for a short list of specific conditions, including heart attack, heart failure, and pneumonia
  - Specific waivers under the Medicaid program intended to support efforts to test delivery innovations (CMS, 2019a), such as the Delivery System Reform Incentive Payment program
  - The State Innovation Model programs (CMS, 2019b), which provide states with grants to work on multipayer initiatives to improve quality and reduce costs

In addition to federal policies, states have also been taking the initiative to transform their healthcare systems, and a number of private health systems have been implementing promising innovations as well.

Critical Thinking Questions: If the goal of HST is to incentivize care that is valuable and disincentivize care that is not valuable, who and how do we decide what is valuable healthcare? Does what is valuable vary according to the needs, desires, cultural context, and socioeconomic background of individual patients? Is it possible for the government, or insurance companies, or even individual practitioners, to establish standard determinations of valuable care that work well for everyone?

■ Health Equity Meets Health System Transformation: The Risk and the Opportunity

Given the escalating costs of healthcare, the clear evidence of inefficiency in the healthcare system, the relatively poor health outcomes we experience as a nation, and the deep racial, ethnic, and geographic health inequities that affect a growing proportion of our population, transforming the way we deliver and pay for health services must be a national priority. The current system is financially unsustainable and is shortchanging patients. Unfortunately, HST efforts so far have been largely missing a critical piece: equity. As low as average health outcomes are in the United States, for some communities they are even worse because of the enormous racial, ethnic, and other health and healthcare inequities that exist. These inequities extend beyond insurance coverage, access to care, and even socioeconomic status. People of color have worse health outcomes even when socioeconomic factors are equal to their White counterparts (Meadows-Fernandez, 2018). Yet decision makers have paid very little attention to solving for equity, and as a result, HST initiatives that have been implemented so far have failed to significantly reduce health inequities. Given that we are but one generation away from a workforce that is a majority of people of color (Esri, 2012), ignoring health equity in HST will fail to create a sustainable, high-quality, high-value healthcare system and will undermine our nation's future prosperity.

Racial and ethnic health disparities are a major contributor of excess healthcare costs, in addition to being a significant drag on our economic productivity. The United States spends an estimated $93 billion in excess medical costs per year due to health disparities and loses roughly $42 billion in lost productivity (Turner, 2018). People of color on average have significantly lower life spans, higher rates of a number of chronic and serious conditions, and higher mortality rates from these conditions (see Figure 5.1). For example, Puerto Ricans have the highest prevalence of asthma compared to all other racial and ethnic groups and suffer from this disease at a rate nearly 75% higher than White people (Centers for Disease Control and Prevention [CDC], 2019c). Compared to their White counterparts, American Indians and Pacific Islanders are twice as likely to develop diabetes; non-Hispanic Black women are three to four times more likely to experience a pregnancy-related death and their babies are twice as likely to die before their first birthday (CDC, 2019a, 2019b, 2019d).

CENTERING HEALTH EQUITY IN HST REQUIRES UNDERSTANDING THE DRIVERS OF HEALTH INEQUITIES

The drivers of health inequities are wide-ranging and diverse. Estimates on the relative value of different factors in influencing health vary. Generally, experts estimate that genetics determine up to 30% of a person's health and healthcare about 10% to 20% (Magnan, 2017). What is clear is that these two factors together have less of an influence on one's health than social factors, and the most important drivers of inequities are socially determined. One's zip code affects one's health much more than one's genes and the healthcare one receives (Artiga & Hinton, 2018). Similarly, one's experiences with trauma, toxic stress, and bigotry (including racism, sexism, colorism, xenophobia, Islamophobia, anti-Semitism, homophobia, ableism, and ageism, to name a few) can have a measurable effect on one's health throughout one's life time (Houshyar, Sanchez, Hernández-Cancio, & Thompson, 2019). This means that to achieve health equity, in addition to ensuring that the healthcare system provides high-quality, culturally centered, accessible, and affordable care for everyone, regardless of their background or identities, we must prioritize strategies that adequately address the SDOHs as well as adverse childhood experiences (ACEs).

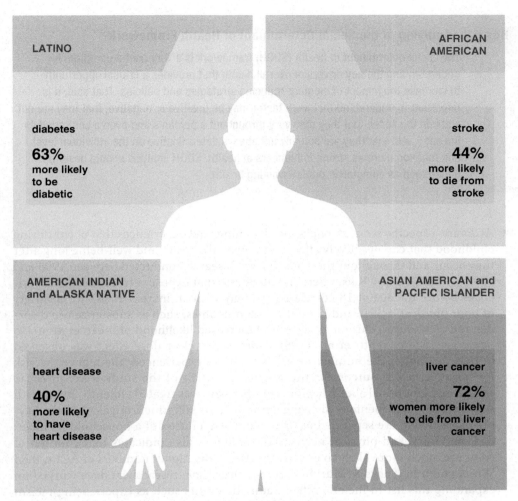

FIGURE 5.1 EXAMPLES OF SOME HEALTH INEQUITIES AS COMPARED TO WHITES.

Source: From Families USA. (2019b). *Racial and ethnic health inequities among communities of color compared to non-Hispanic Whites.*

- *SDOH* are factors apart from medical care and genetics that account for roughly 60% (Schroeder, 2007) to 90% (Magnan, 2017) of overall individual health outcomes. These factors are closely related to where people live, learn, play, pray, work, and age. SDOHs may improve a persons' chances of being healthy or increase their risk of poor health. These include factors such as socioeconomic status, availability of nutritious food, air and water quality, housing, education, transportation, racial segregation, and exposure to racism and violence, among others. One meta-analysis of close to 50 studies found that social factors accounted for over a third of total deaths in the United States yearly (Galea, Tracy, Hoggatt, DiMaggio, & Karpati, 2011). Given the importance of SDOH as drivers of overall health and of health inequities, strategies to address and mitigate the impacts of negative SDOH must be integrated into healthcare policy development, including payment and delivery reform (see Box 5.3).

Box 5.3: Applying of the Social Determinant of Health Framework

The social determinant of health (SDOH) framework is a very useful paradigm for understanding the key drivers of overall health that provides a critical opportunity to increase the impact of inequity-reducing strategies and policies. That said, it is important to understand that each factor may be positive or negative, that they are not static in the sense that they may vary throughout a person's and even a community's life span, and that they are actually not always determinative on the individual level and function more as strong influencers of health. SDOH analysis should never be understood as completely predetermining health.

- *ACEs* are a specific set of strongly socially influenced experiences that occur during childhood that can negatively affect an individual's health and well-being long after they occur and throughout their life course. Research conducted between 1995 and 1997 by the CDC and Kaiser Permanente found that exposure to 10 specific experiences before the age of 18 correlated strongly with an increased risk for a variety of poor physical, social, and mental health outcomes, such as substance use disorder and alcoholism, chronic disease, and increased likelihood of incarceration—to name just a few (Felitti et al., 1998). Moreover, a clear dose effect was observed in that the higher the number of ACEs a person experienced, the higher the risk for negative health outcomes. The original 10 ACEs of the study were: physical, sexual, and emotional abuse; having a mother who was treated violently; living with someone who was mentally ill; living with someone suffering from alcoholism; having parents who are separated or divorced; incarceration of a household member; and emotional and physical neglect. The evidence also indicates that children of color are much more likely to experience ACEs, and higher numbers of ACEs, than White children (Sacks & Murphey, 2018). Over time, researchers have worked on expanding this list to include other traumatic events such as experiencing racism and community violence (The Philadelphia ACE Project, 2019).
- *Toxic stress, trauma, and allostatic load,* while related to ACEs, are distinct. "Toxic stress" and "trauma" are both potential outcomes of exposure to adversity. Toxic stress is defined as the prolonged activation of stress response systems in the absence of protective relationships (Center on the Developing Child at Harvard University, 2019). "Allostasis" refers to the body's ability to adapt to chronic levels of stress (McEwen, Seeman, & Allostatic Load Working Group, 2009). During an acute stress event, the body reacts by flooding the brain with cortisol and adrenalin, heightening the immune response, increasing blood pressure, and producing more glucocorticoids, all of which are useful survival mechanisms in a fight-flight-freeze situation. However, when these physiological conditions become chronic, one ends up with a high allostatic load (McEwen, 2005), which has long-term negative effects on health. A high allostatic load undermines an individual's health in various ways. For example, it is associated with long-term brain wear and tear and reduced cognitive function, chronic hypertension, suppressed immune function, insulin resistance, and overall higher rates of chronic conditions (McEwen et al., 2009).

ACEs, toxic stress, trauma, and high allostatic load have transgenerational health implications. A growing body of research in epigenetics—the modification of gene expressions due to one's interaction with environmental influences—indicates that chronic exposure to toxic stress can produce long-term, harmful changes in brain structure, physiology, and behavior. Moreover, high allostatic load has been shown to affect one's DNA and accelerate aging (Geronimus et al., 2010). There is evidence that these changes can even be passed down to the next generation (Henriques, 2019).

Critical thinking questions: You have a 57-year-old Mexican American patient with diabetes, hypertension, and a body mass index (BMI) of 36 who lives in a ground floor apartment with his daughter and two grandchildren. The apartment is next to a well-maintained park, four blocks from the local community center and six blocks from the church which the whole family attends. He has limited English proficiency, but he has worked consistently in the food service industry most of his life. The neighborhood has no grocery store, and it is bordered by a waste-processing plant. What are the positive and negative SDOH that may contribute to his current and future health status and outcomes? What are the equity implications? What impact could this have on health expenditures?

Racism's Role in Health Inequities

To solve for health equity, it is critical to understand that the experience of racism, in all its forms, is a determinant of health distinct from socioeconomic status—although they do influence each other in either a virtuous or a vicious cycle—depending on the person's race. Experts have described four categories of racism: internalized, interpersonal, institutional, and structural (Hinson, Healey, & Weisenberg, 2019). For purposes of this policy discussion, we want to focus on the following three:

- *Interpersonal racism* (including implicit bias). Interpersonal racism is the kind of discrimination most people usually think about when they hear the word "racism." It is about how people treat each other. Usually we think about overtly, intentional incidences of prejudiced behavior—the use of slurs, purposeful exclusion, and so on. However, there is another type of interpersonal racism—implicit bias. Implicit bias refers to the unconscious stereotypes and beliefs that we associate with particular social groups, which practically everyone has (Kirwan Institute, 2015). As a result, our beliefs and attitudes toward certain individuals, especially those from social groups that we do not personally identify with, can unknowingly negatively affect the way that we treat them. Both these types of racism can be found in healthcare. A recent study conducted by the Robert Wood Johnson Foundation, the Harvard T. H. Chan School of Public Health, and National Public Radio found that people of color, as well as women and people who identify as LGBTQ, reported experiencing discrimination when they sought healthcare services, which in some cases prompted them to forgo seeking care when they needed it. (Robert Wood Johnson Foundation, n.d.).
- *Institutional racism* is the kind of racial discrimination that is built into the policies and practices of social and economic institutions, such as organizations, businesses, schools, universities, police departments, and health systems. This discrimination may be explicit and deliberate, or it may be indirect and unintentional, but in any

case, it limits the rights and opportunities of certain groups. In healthcare, one very damaging expression of institutional racism has been the historic abuse and mistreatment of communities of color by the medical establishment, such as the abuse of enslaved Black women for gynecological experiments (Ojanuga, 1993), the Tuskegee Syphilis Study (Byrd & Clayton, 2001), the case of Henrietta Lacks (Lee et al., 2018), many cases of forced sterilization of women of color (Torpy, 2000), and the testing of oral contraception on Puerto Rican women without their consent (Pendergrass & Raji, 2017), to name just a few.

- *Structural racism* is the cumulative effect of generations of discriminatory laws, policies, and practices that are culturally supported that perpetuate discrimination through mutually reinforcing inequitable, interconnected systems that determine the distribution of resources, risks, and opportunities so that one group is systematically privileged above others. These systems include: housing, education, employment, jobs and earnings, benefits, healthcare, criminal justice, food and water supply, and environmental pollution and degradation, to name a few. Key examples include residential segregation, environmental racism, the school to prison pipeline, and health inequities (Bailey et al., 2017).

■ Achieving Equity-Focused HST: Six Policy Domains for Action

Payment and delivery reform efforts represent a critical crossroads for health equity. On the one hand, if these reforms center on solving for health equity and defining high-value care in a manner that focuses on eliminating inequities proactively, this transformation could support the care delivery models and interventions that would accelerate disparity reduction. However, new payment systems that are designed to address the so-called "average" patient and implemented without consideration of the impact on communities of color, complex patients, and other disadvantaged groups, could further undermine the health of communities that are already struggling. Leveraging HST to advance health equity has been a challenge for providers, researchers, advocates, and decision makers. Unsurprisingly, the voices and interests of communities of color have not been adequately included in this enterprise. In an effort to increase awareness and action in this arena, a number of national- and state-level health equity experts came together as the Health Equity Task Force for Delivery and Payment Transformation to develop a framework of six policy domains for action (Hernández-Cancio, Albritton, Fishman, Tripoli, & Callow, 2018):

- *Payment systems that sustain and reward high-quality, equitable healthcare:* As decision makers develop new ways to pay for value in healthcare, as opposed to volume, these new payment systems must include achieving equity in their definition of value. The financial underpinnings of the healthcare system must align with the goal of eliminating inequities, not just increasing quality overall, and reducing costs. Providing the resources and incentives needed to achieve equity must be explicit.
- *Equity-focused measurement that accelerates reductions in health inequities:* *Measurement* is increasingly important to enable quality improvement, value-based payment, and tracking and improving inequities. Quality measures are used

to evaluate clinical process and outcomes, patient access and experience, and care delivery efficiency. Quality measures are also used as a way to hold healthcare organizations financially accountable if they are not meeting certain standards. Increasingly, payment is being tied to achieving certain standards on particular measures. Payment systems must incorporate equity-sensitive measures to ensure that health systems prioritize equity not just as a goal but also as a requirement of financial sustainability.

- *An evidence base that is representative and transparent:* An important hallmark of value-based care is that it seeks to be evidence based. Quality measures and clinical practice guidelines are developed on the foundation of the existing evidence base. Unfortunately, according to the Institute of Medicine, most of the treatments that we provide in the United States are not well supported by evidence (Institute of Medicine, 2011). Moreover, the evidence that we do have is neither transparent nor representative. Women, children, individuals with disabilities, and communities of color are largely underrepresented in our medical and health systems research evidence base. As a result, treatments have been based largely on what works for White people—primarily adult men. Even when research participants are more diverse, results are rarely stratified by race and ethnicity. When data based on underrepresented groups and communities of color is available, too often it is aggregated and generalized across subgroups—which can mask important variations and limits its value. To achieve health equity we must increase the representation of diverse communities in medical and health systems research, and we need transparency about the limitations of the data that is available and is used to determine treatment guidelines. Only by doing both can we ensure that patients, their doctors, and payers can make more appropriate care decisions that can improve outcomes for everyone.

- *Investments to support safety-net and small community providers in delivery system reform:* Safety-net and small community providers are often the most trusted sources of healthcare in many underserved communities of color. In some cases, they may be the only sources of care. However, due to chronic underfunding, challenging community environments, and lack of scale, among other factors, they often face unique barriers to implementing new value-based payment models. Many of these models require significant up-front investments that these providers may be unable to make. However, they are often essential sources of culturally centered, geographically and language accessible care and should be supported so that they succeed in a value-based healthcare world.

- *Robust and well-resourced community partnerships:* Given our increased understanding of the roles of SDOHs, ACEs, and toxic stress on shaping health, and the limited impact that clinical care has on overall health, health systems that want to move the needle on health outcomes and inequities will need to work beyond the walls of their institutions. They must develop strategies to address social factors that undermine their patients' health. The most effective, and empowering, way for health systems to do this is to partner with trusted community-based organizations that can provide culturally centered, language accessible, nonclinical supports and services to tackle some of the barriers to achieving good health that affect their patients. These partnerships should not be limited to a system of referrals. Rather, health systems should concretely invest in these partnerships, providing direct funding for needed health-related services as well as developing secure platforms to enable appropriate information sharing.

■ *Growing a diverse workforce that drives equity and value:* Ultimately, even the best HST strategies will be meaningless unless we have the workforce to implement them and drive needed transformation. The overall healthcare workforce needs to grow to keep up with the escalating demand, must be more ethnically and racially diverse, better distributed geographically, better trained on issues related to equity, and inclusive of a broader array of jobs—from primary care providers to midlevel providers, to community health workers (CHWs), and to peers. Our current healthcare workforce does not represent the communities that it serves. Only 11% of physicians and 15% of RNs are African American, Hispanic, American Indian, or Alaskan Native (Health Resources & Services Administration, 2013). Moreover, experts predict a shortage of primary care physicians and nurses in the coming years. Health professionals from communities of color are linked to improving both access and quality of care (Marrast, Zallman, Woolhandler, Bor, & McCormick, 2014). Compared to their White counterparts, providers from communities of color are more likely to practice in underserved communities, more likely to go into primary care, and more likely to accept patients covered by Medicaid. Underrepresented communities have also reported increased care satisfaction and an increased utilization of preventive services when treated by someone who shares the same racial or ethnic background (Health Professionals for Diversity Coalition, 2012). In addition, we should think more broadly about who needs to be a part of the healthcare team. The health workforce needs to be expanded beyond clinical care and include other members such as CHWs, systems navigators, interpreters, and peers.

Figure 5.2 provides a summary of these policy domains.

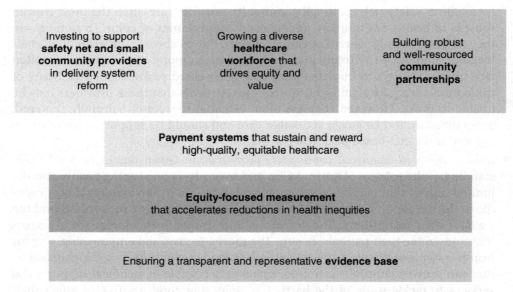

FIGURE 5.2 POLICY DOMAINS FOR ACHIEVING A TRANSFORMED, EQUITABLE, AND HIGH-VALUE HEALTHCARE SYSTEM.

Source: From Families USA. (2019a). *Policy domains for achieving a transformed, equitable, and high value health care system.*

■ Conclusion

Nurses have a powerful role to play in ensuring that payment and delivery reform puts patients first, in all their diversity of backgrounds, experiences, and challenges. Nurses work in many environments: hospitals, clinics, schools, skilled nursing facilities, community health centers, and even in private homes. They are trusted community leaders, key advocates for patients, educators for families, and can help restore trust within communities that have been historically overlooked by or disconnected from the healthcare system. Their unique viewpoint on many aspects of the healthcare system in a variety of settings makes them ideally suited to help lead equity-focused health system transformation efforts. They are able to provide an "on the ground perspective" that can translate what communities need and providers' challenges to decision makers. Their input will contribute to ensuring higher quality care, improving safe practice standards, and advocating for the appropriate allocation of resources.

Nurses have important roles to play in every domain of equity-centered HST. They can be key care team members in the implementation of new payment models and monitor for any unintended consequences that may be affecting particular segments of patients, including communities of color. They can get involved in the development of better, more responsive quality measures, and their application, in their particular clinical practices. Nurses can work directly with clinical and health systems researchers to help design equity-focused studies and even recruit subjects. Many nurses work in safety-net hospitals, community health centers, and with smaller community providers and can support employers' efforts in transformation. Nurses can be the critical link between clinical care teams and community-based service providers to ensure that the totality of patients' health needs are met—not just their clinical care. Nurses are also key leaders in the healthcare workforce and could contribute significantly to recruiting, mentoring, training, and raising awareness about the need for interdisciplinary teams of care that include community-based providers like CHWs. Given nurses' direct knowledge of the healthcare enterprise, their close relationships with patients and their families, and their privileged position of respect and trust in society, they are well positioned to be effective change agents.

■ Critical Thinking Exercise

1. The Hospital Readmissions Reduction Program was implemented under the ACA with the intended goal of decreasing the number of avoidable hospital readmissions by reducing payments to hospitals that have above-average readmission rates for Medicare patients originally admitted for a short list of conditions. What are the factors that influence readmission rates? How could this affect safety-net hospitals and the patients whom they serve? What may the overall health equity implications be?

2. You are working at a hospital labor and delivery department and become concerned about the increasing number of Black babies who are born premature and with low birth weight. Their mothers are also experiencing higher rates of complications during and right after birth. What factors do you think might be contributing to

this trend? What actions do you think could help reverse this trend? Think about what you could try to change within your hospital. How might you work in the larger community to address this? What would you suggest the governor or the Medicaid director do?

■ Discussion Questions

- Give an example of how nurses can get involved with health policy at each level of government—local, state, and federal.
- What are the six domains of equity-focused health system transformation? Choose two of them and give one example in each of how as a nurse you can be an advocate for advancing equity-focused health system transformation within that specific domain.
- Why is the nurse's perspective critical in influencing equity-focused policy?
- Choose a law that was implemented over the past year in your state or local government. Describe how this law hurts or advances health equity or equity-focused health system transformation efforts.

■ Resources

Center for Consumer Engagement in Health Innovation, https://www.community catalyst.org/initiatives-and-issues/initiatives/center-for-consumer-engagement-in -health-innovation/full-description
Center for Medicare & Medicaid Innovation, https://innovation.cms.gov
Center for Youth Wellness, https://centerforyouthwellness.org
Families USA, https://familiesusa.org
Finding Answers, https://www.solvingdisparities.org
Kaiser Family Foundation, https://www.kff.org

■ References

Abrams, M., Nuzum, R., Zezza, M., Ryan, J., Kiszla, J., & Guterman, S. (2015). The Affordable Care Act's payment and delivery system reforms: A progress report at five years. Retrieved from https://www.commonwealthfund.org/sites/default/files/documents/___media_files_publications_issue_brief_2015_may_1816_abrams _aca_reforms_delivery_payment_rb.pdf
Agency for Healthcare Research and Quality. (2019). *Never Events*. Retrieved from https://www.cms.gov/newsroom/fact-sheets/eliminating-serious-preventable-and -costly-medical-errors-never-events
Artiga, S., & Hinton, E. (2018). *Beyond health care: The role of social determinants in promoting health and health equity*. Retrieved from https://www.kff.org/disparities-policy/issue-brief/beyond-health-care-the-role-of-social-determinants -in-promoting-health-and-health-equity
Bailey, Z. D., Krieger, N., Agénor, M., Graves, J., Linos, N., & Bassett, M. T. (2017, April 08). Structural racism and health inequities in the USA: Evidence and interventions. *Lancet, 389*(10077), 1453–1463. doi:10.1016/S0140-6736(17)30569-X

Berwick, D. M., & Hackbarth, A. D. (2012). Eliminating waste in US health care. *Journal of the American Medical Association, 307*(14), 1513–1516. doi:10.1001/jama.2012.362

Berwick, D. M., Nolan, T. W., & Whittington, J. (2008). The Triple Aim: Care, health, and cost. *Health Affairs.* Retrieved from https://www.healthaffairs.org/doi/full/10.1377/hlthaff.27.3.759

Brenan, M. (2018). *Nurses again outpace other professions for honesty, ethics.* Retrieved from https://news.gallup.com/poll/245597/nurses-again-outpace-professions-honesty-ethics.aspx

Byrd, W. M., & Clayton, L. A. (2001). Race, medicine, and health care in the United States: a historical survey. *Journal of the National Medical Association, 93*(3, Suppl.), 11S–34S. Retrieved from https://www.ncbi.nlm.nih.gov/pmc/articles/PMC2593958/pdf/jnma00341-0013.pdf

Centers for Disease Control and Prevention. (2019a). *Diabetes quick facts.* Retrieved from https://www.cdc.gov/diabetes/basics/quick-facts.html

Centers for Disease Control and Prevention. (2019b). *Infant mortality.* Retrieved from https://www.cdc.gov/reproductivehealth/maternalinfanthealth/infantmortality.htm

Centers for Disease Control and Prevention. (2019c). *Most recent asthma data.* Retrieved from https://www.cdc.gov/asthma/most_recent_data.htm

Centers for Disease Control and Prevention. (2019d). *Pregnancy-related deaths.* Retrieved from https://www.cdc.gov/reproductivehealth/maternalinfanthealth/pregnancy-relatedmortality.htm

Centers for Medicare & Medicaid Services. (2018a). Hospital Readmissions Reduction Program (HRRP) archives. Retrieved from https://www.cms.gov/Medicare/Medicare-Fee-for-Service-Payment/AcuteInpatientPPS/HRRP-Archives.html

Centers for Medicare & Medicaid Services. (2018b). ICD-10 HAC list. Retrieved from https://www.cms.gov/Medicare/Medicare-Fee-for-Service-Payment/HospitalAcqCond/icd10_hacs.html

Centers for Medicare & Medicaid Services. (2019a). Section 1332 State Innovation Waivers. Retrieved from https://www.cms.gov/cciio/programs-and-initiatives/state-innovation-waivers/section_1332_state_innovation_waivers-.html

Centers for Medicare & Medicaid Services. (2019b). State Innovation Models Initiative: General information. Retrieved from https://innovation.cms.gov/initiatives/state-innovations

Center on the Developing Child at Harvard University. (2019). *Toxic stress.* Retrieved from https://developingchild.harvard.edu/science/key-concepts/toxic-stress

Esri. (2012). *Minority population growth – The new boom.* Retrieved from https://www.esri.com/library/brochures/pdfs/minority-population-growth.pdf2012

Families USA. (2012). *Implementing accountable care organizations.* Retrieved from https://familiesusa.org/product/implementing-accountable-care-organizations

Families USA. (2019a). *Policy Domains for Achieving a Transformed, Equitable, and High Value Health Care System.*

Families USA. (2019b). *Racial and ethnic health inequities among communities of color compared to non-Hispanic Whites.*

Felitti, V. J., Anda, R. F., Nordenberg, D., Williamson, D. F., Spitz, A. M., Edwards, V., . . . Marks, J. S. (1998). Relationship of childhood abuse and household dysfunction to many of the leading causes of death in adults. The Adverse Childhood Experiences (ACE) Study. *American Journal of Preventive Medicine, 14*(4), 245–258. doi:10.1016/s0749-3797(98)00017-8

Galea, S., Tracy, M., Hoggatt, K. J., DiMaggio, C., & Karpati, A. (2011). Estimated deaths attributable to social factors in the United States. *American Journal of Public Health, 101*(8), 1456–1465. Retrieved from https://ajph.aphapublications.org/doi/10.2105/AJPH.2010.300086

Geronimus, A. T., Hicken, M. T., Pearson, J. A., Seashols, S. J., Brown, K. L., & Cruz, T. D. (2010). Do US black women experience stress-related accelerated biological aging?: A novel theory and first population-based test of Black-White differences in telomere length. *Human Nature, 21*(1), 19–38. doi:10.1007/s12110-010-9078-0

Health Professionals for Diversity Coalition. (2012). *Fact sheet: The need for diversity in the health care workforce.* Retrieved from http://www.aapcho.org/wp/wp-content/uploads/2012/11/NeedForDiversityHealthCareWorkforce.pdf

Health Resources & Services Administration. (2013). *The U.S. health workforce chartbook.* Retrieved from https://bhw.hrsa.gov/sites/default/files/bhw/nchwa/chartbookpart1.pdf

Henriques, M. (2019, March 26). *Future: Can the legacy of trauma be passed down the generations?* Retrieved from http://www.bbc.com/future/story/20190326-what-is-epigenetics

Hernández-Cancio, S., Albritton, E., Fishman, E., Tripoli, S., & Callow, A. (2018). *A framework for advancing health equity and value.* Retrieved from https://familiesusa.org/sites/default/files/product_documents/FamiliesUSA_Policy-Options_Report.pdf

Hinson, S., Healey, R., & Weisenberg, N. (2019). *Race, power and policy: Dismantling structural racism.* Retrieved from https://www.racialequitytools.org/resourcefiles/race_power_policy_workbook.pdf

Houshyar, S., Sanchez, D., Hernández-Cancio, S., & Thompson, N. (2019). *Helping our children grow and thrive: Leveraging the health care system to prevent and mitigate adverse childhood experiences and advance equity in childhood.* Retrieved from https://familiesusa.org/resources/helping-our-children-grow-and-thrive-leveraging-the-health-care-system-to-prevent-and-mitigate-adverse-childhood-experiences-and-advance-equity-in-childhood

Institute of Medicine Roundtable on Value & Science-Driven Health Care. (2011). *Learning what works: Infrastructure required for comparative effectiveness research: Workshop summary.* Washington, DC: National Academies Press. Retrieved from https://www.ncbi.nlm.nih.gov/pubmed/22013609

Kirwan Institute. (2015). *Understanding implicit bias.* Retrieved from http://kirwaninstitute.osu.edu/research/understanding-implicit-bias

Lee, M., Reddy, K., Chowdhury, J., Kumar, N., Clark, P., Ndao, P., . . . Song, S. (2018). Overcoming the legacy of mistrust: African Americans' mistrust of medical profession. *The Journal of Healthcare Ethics & Administration, 4*(1), 16–40. doi:10.22461/jhea.1.71616

Magnan, S. (2017). Social determinants of health 101 for health care: Five plus five. *NAM Perspectives.* Discussion Paper, National Academy of Medicine, Washington, DC. doi:10.31478/201710c

Marrast, L., Zallman, L. Woolhandler, S., Bor, D., & McCormick, D. (2014). Minority physicians' role in the care of underserved patients: Diversifying the physician workforce may be a key in addressing health disparities. *JAMA Internal Medicine, 174*(2), 289–291. doi:10.1001/jamainternmed.2013.12756

McEwen, B., Seeman, T., & Allostatic Load Working Group. (2009). *Allostatic load and allostasis.* Retrieved from https://macses.ucsf.edu/research/allostatic/allostatic.php

McEwen, B. S. (2005). Stressed or stressed out: What is the difference? *Journal of Psychiatry & Neuroscience, 30*(5), 315–318. Retrieved from https://www.ncbi.nlm.nih.gov/pmc/articles/PMC1197275

Meadows-Fernandez, R. (2018). *Even as Black Americans get richer, their health outcomes remain poor.* Retrieved from https://psmag.com/social-justice/even-as-black-americans-get-richer-their-health-outcomes-remain-poor

Ojanuga, D. (1993). The medical ethics of the 'Father of Gynecology', Dr. J Marion Sims. *Journal of Medical Ethics, 19*(1), 28–31. doi:10.1136/jme.19.1.28

Organisation for Economic Cooperation and Development. (2018). Health spending. *Health Resources.* doi:10.1787/8643de7e-en

Pendergrass, D., & Raji, M. (2017). *The bitter pill: Harvard and the dark history of birth control.* Retrieved from https://www.thecrimson.com/article/2017/9/28/the-bitter -pill

Robert Wood Johnson Foundation. (n.d.). *Discrimination in America: Experiences and views on affects of discrimination across major population groups in the United States.* Retrieved from https://www.rwjf.org/en/library/research/2017/10/discrimination -in-america--experiences-and-views.html

Sacks, V., & Murphey, D. (2018). *The prevalence of adverse childhood experiences, nationally, by state, and by race or ethnicity* [Blog post]. Retrieved from https://www.childtrends .org/publications/prevalence-adverse-childhood-experiences-nationally-state-race -ethnicity

Schneider, E., Sarnak, D., Squires, D., Shah, A., & Doty, M. (2017). Mirror, Mirror 2017: International comparison reflects flaws and opportunities for better U.S. health care. Retrieved from https://interactives.commonwealthfund.org/2017/july/mirror -mirror

Schroeder, S. (2007). We can do better: Improving the health of the American People. *The New England Journal of Medicine, 357*, 1221–1228. doi:10.1056/NEJMsa073350

The Philadelphia ACE Project. (2019). Philadelphia ACE survey. Retrieved from http:// www.philadelphiaaces.org/philadelphia-ace-survey

Torpy, S. (2000). Native American women and coerced sterilization: On the trail of tears in the 1970s. *American Indian Culture and Research Journal, 24*(2), 1–22. Retrieved from https://www.law.berkeley.edu/php-programs/centers/crrj/zotero/loadfile.php ?entity_key=QFDB5MW3

Turner, A. (2018). *The business case for racial equity: A strategy for growth.* Retrieved from https://altarum.org/RacialEquity2018

U.S. Bureau of Labor Statistics. (2019). *May 2018 occupation profiles.* Retrieved from https://www.bls.gov/oes/current/oes_stru.htm#29-0000

U.S. National Library of Medicine. (2019). *Collection development guidelines of the National Library of Medicine.* Bethesda, MD: Author. Retrieved from https://www. ncbi.nlm.nih.gov/books/NBK518690

Wolfson, D. B., & Mende, S. (2015). To reduce unnecessary care, choosing wisely moves from awareness to implementation. *Health Affairs.* Retrieved from https://www .healthaffairs.org/do/10.1377/hblog20150701.049032/full

World Health Organization. (n.d.). *Health policy.* Retrieved from https://www.who.int/ topics/health_policy/en

6 Genetics, Social Determinants of Health, and Policy Challenges Across the Life Span

Justina A. Trott and Sharon L. Ruyak

CHAPTER OBJECTIVES

⊙ Understand the genetics of health and the environmental impact on health (epigenetics and the social determinants of health [SDOHs])

⊙ Apply that understanding to delineate the complex interactions of genetics, epigenetics, SDOHs (exposome), and the human microbiome to individual and population health across the life span

⊙ Contribute to health policy by analyzing the practice of medicine, research, policy, programs, education, and services using a diversity/sex/gender/health equity lens

KEY CONCEPTS

Social determinants of health	Ableism
Life span	Social ecology model
Racism	Intersectionality
Sexism	Interprofessional teams/collaboration
Classism	Transformative policy
Ageism	

KEY TERMS

Genetics	Ability/disability
Epigenetics	Social determinants of health
Race	Epigenome/epigenetics
Class	Exposome
Sex	Microbiome
Gender	Genome/genomics

■ Introduction

Effective policy needs to be grounded in accurate information/science. While policy makers do not have to be scientists, their team should include individuals with a sound understanding of science as well as individuals affected by the policy. This chapter provides an overview and

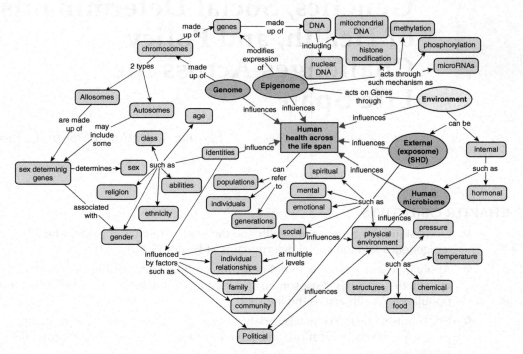

FIGURE 6.1 CONCEPT MAP: HEALTH ACROSS THE LIFE SPAN.

understanding of the biology of health equity and health disparities across the life span. This is not a deep dive into molecular genetics but rather a brief review of the basics of genetics and human growth and development, inheritance, and how individuals and populations coevolve with their environments. Using real-world examples, we examine the effect of SDOHs on the health and wellness of individuals and populations across the life span through biologic changes mediated by genetics. We also use sex and gender as examples of how we can approach diversity in general. Finally, we highlight how understanding the unique biology of individuals and populations presents challenges and opportunities in crafting health policy for both personalized medicine and population health.

The health of individuals is multidimensional involving biology and multiple aspects of their environment over time. Health across the life span is the result of the interaction of genetic and environmental determinants. Genes are passed on from parents to children over generations. In addition, the environment contributes to health. The external environment consists of physical, emotional, spiritual, mental, social, and political aspects of our lives, while the internal environment consists of hormones, chemicals, and the trillions of bacteria, viruses, and other parasites living in and on bodies. A "concept map" is presented here, which is explored throughout this chapter (see Figure 6.1).

■ A Broader Definition of Life Span: Health Across the Generations

How do we understand the life span? Traditionally we think of our life span as starting at birth and ending with death. However, health can be conceptualized in terms of the thousands of generations that have preceded us and those generations that will come after us.

What contributes to our health? In this context, we can look at the genome and the epigenome, or the environment surrounding genes (the internal and external environments), which affects the expression of genes, and the actions (as individuals and as societies) we take to change our internal and external environments.

Human health across the life span is a function of individual genes/chromosomes. Additionally, the exposome, which is a measure of an individual's cumulative exposures across the lifetime, affects health (Wild, 2005). The exposome includes exposures to such things as physical, social, spiritual, mental, emotional, and political environments and identities. This environment can also include all the organisms living within and on the human body known as the "human microbiome." How do the internal and external environments affect our health? The environment can modify the expression of DNA (deoxyribonucleic acid), which makes up chromosomes and genes (Notterman & Mitchell, 2015). The specific ways the environment affects humans also depend on the timing of the environmental exposure; for example, the same exposure will affect the fetus, youth, adult, or elder differently (Graeter & Mortensen, 1996; Shields, 2017).

■ Basic Genetics: Chromosomes, Genes, Epigenome, and Human Growth and Development

Genetics is the study of genes and inherited traits. Heredity is the transmission of traits from parents to their offspring. DNA is found in each cell nucleus forming genes. Genes are packaged into chromosomes forming the blueprint for cells, organs, and tissues in our bodies, making us uniquely who we are. Each human somatic cell has 46 chromosomes; 22 pairs are autosomes and usually two sex chromosomes (although sex determination is much more complicated than sex chromosomes alone). DNA is also found in another form, mitochondrial DNA inherited only from the mother.

The complete set of genes for humans is known. The human genome consists of 20,000 to 25,000 individual genes. Each gene has one or more variants, which are called "alleles."

Each cell in our body consists of the same genetic material. Yet each cell and tissue is not the same. What causes the differentiation of each cell and tissue type is the expression of the genes in our chromosomal blueprint. Only a subset of genes is expressed in each cell. Gene expression is determined by two main mechanisms: DNA sequence and mechanisms that are separate or independent of the DNA, which are chemical tags known as the "epigenome." Epigenetic changes turn genes on and off in a cell or tissue in a specific manner that is critical to controlling the environment of specific cells with specific functions. Epigenetic mechanisms do not affect the DNA sequence but produce heritable changes in how genes function through well-established mechanisms such as methylation, phosphorylation, and histone modification, which tighten DNA coiling preventing DNA expression. Through these mechanisms, the epigenome responds to internal and external signals and adjusts the expression of specific genes accordingly (Genetic Science Learning Center, n.d.-a, n.d.-b, n.d.-d).

■ Fetal Development

Over the past several decades, increasing emphasis has been placed on the Developmental Origins of Health and Disease (DOHaD). This hypothesis originated in the 1980s with Dr. Barker and colleagues (Barker, Osmond, Golding, Kuh, & Wadsworth, 1989). This theory is also known as "fetal programming" where programming refers to the process through which environmental exposure during critical periods of fetal development can lead to adverse health across the life span (Barker, 1998). This concept of *fetal programming* demonstrates key features of cell and tissue differentiation.

The same genetic information is present in each fetal cell; however, DNA sequences and epigenetic factors determine specific patterns of gene expression.

Fetal development begins at fertilization. Each somatic cell (nonsex cell) has two of each chromosome, and therefore, two alleles for each gene, one from the mother and one from the father. The exception to this is the X and Y chromosomes. These chromosomes have genes that are not present on the other chromosomes. The X chromosome is much larger with approximately 1,500 total genes while the Y chromosome has less than 300 genes. The X genes code for nonsexual functions in both males and females. However, most of the Y genes code for male sexual development. Because female cells contain two X chromosomes while male cells contain one X and one Y chromosome, during early development, X inactivation causes silencing of gene expression on one X chromosome, leading to approximately equal gene expression in males and females. This is a random process in human cells with maternal and paternal X chromosomes being randomly inactivated early in fetal development allowing for sex differences in gene expression in different cells (Wizemann & Pardue, 2001; see Figure 6.2).

In addition to these inherent biological processes, maternal and environmental exposures are powerful upstream contributors to fetal development and health across the life span. The placenta serves as the interface between the mother and the fetus and epigenetics is the likely process through which the maternal environment influences fetal development (Nugent & Bale, 2015). The epigenome controls the expression of specific genes exerting a flexible response to changes in the environment allowing for adaptability and ultimately placental function. Throughout fetal development, exposures like maternal nutrition, stress hormones, social interactions, and environmental toxins can produce epigenetic changes in genes in the placenta. Some of these changes are positive adaptive changes while others are maladaptive leading to adverse health outcomes.

■ Inheritance: Species, Individuals, and Populations Coevolve
  With Their Environments

Humans contain much of the same genetic material as other living organisms. The DNA of all humans is 99.9% the same (The 1000 Genomes Project Consortium, 2015). There is no one gene or even one chromosome that can identify a specific racial/ethnic group of individuals. There are patterns of genetic variants (alleles) that are found in higher frequencies within certain ethnic groups. These occur especially if the groups have been isolated from each other over millennia. If several of these genetic variations are found in one individual, it is more likely for that individual to be identified

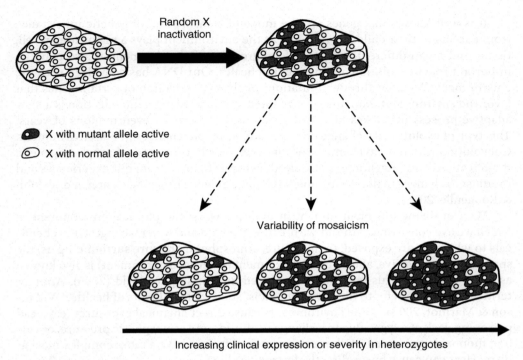

Random X inactivation

● X with mutant allele active
◎ X with normal allele active

Variability of mosaicism

Increasing clinical expression or severity in heterozygotes

FIGURE 6.2 X-CHROMOSOME INACTIVATION COMPENSATES FOR DIFFERENCES IN GENE DOSAGE.

Source: From Wizemann, T. M., & Pardue, M.-L. (Eds.). (2001). *Exploring the biological contributions to human health: Does sex matter?* Washington, DC: National Academies Press. Retrieved from http://www.ncbi.nlm.nih.gov/books/NBK222288

as part of a specific group. There are hundreds of millions of variants in the human genome. There can be as much variation within the group as there is between groups. That means that approximately 85% of human variation occurs within an identified population and approximately 15% variation can be found between populations. This can mean that two individuals from different identified groups may be more genetically like each other than genetically like the group with which they identify (Keita et al., 2004; Hawks, 2013).

Most genetic variation in humans has no biological impact. However, some genetic variation is positive and may increase the chance of survival. An example of this is the single-gene disorder that leads to sickle cell disease. In certain areas where malaria is prevalent, this mutation provides protection, a positive selective adaptation to the environment. Other single-gene disorders, such as cystic fibrosis and Duchenne muscular dystrophy, have adverse health consequences. There are also specific chromosomes associated with specific anatomic and physiologic changes leading to adverse health effects such as trisomy 21 (Down syndrome) and a missing X chromosome in Turner syndrome. However, our susceptibility to most prevalent common chronic conditions is multifactorial and related to the interaction of multiple genes and environment. Even eye color is determined by multiple genes (White & Rabago-Smith, 2011).

It is well-known that genes are the mode of transmission of genetic inheritance from parents to their children. And just as the environment plays a major role in cell, tissue, and organ differentiation, and fetal growth and development, it also plays an important role in evolution and population health. Our DNA has coevolved with the environment. Whether through mutations or through selection of certain genes that favor the environment, humans have adapted and thrived. Genetic selection is a slow adaptive process that takes hundreds of thousands of years, even millions of years. This type of evolutionary change does not address rapid changes in our environment. Coevolution with our environment occurs over shorter time spans through epigenetic modification. The epigenome is flexible allowing us to learn from our experiences and to adjust to changes in the environment (Genetic Science Learning Center, n.d.-c; John & Rougeulle, 2018).

We can define our environment in multiple ways: the physical environment in which we live consisting of the air we breathe, the food and water we ingest, the chemicals to which we are exposed, temperature, atmospheric pressure surrounding us, the spaces in which we live, and so on. Environment (external environment) is also known as the "exposome." This term was introduced by Christopher Wild (2005). Another term often used to refer to the environment is "social determinants of health" (Wilkinson & Marmot, 2003). Some environments cause direct chemical exposures (e.g., lead poisoning, lack of oxygen due to a change in altitude and atmospheric pressure, or carbon monoxide poisoning). Other environmental factors have a more complex mechanism. Heat can cause burns directly destroying skin.

Heat can also alter genetic expression. For example, turtle eggs hatching in sand at 36°C will hatch 50% males and 50% females. If the sand is warmer, more females are hatched and if the sand is colder, more males will hatch. The temperature does not change our DNA. Temperature changes gene expression, thus changing sex. The trillions of organisms living on our skin and in our gut, the microbiome, also contribute to health and disease. There is evidence that autoimmune diseases and allergies are associated with an absence of exposure to important bacteria and viruses and that exposures to local flora and fauna help us adapt to local living conditions (Velasquez-Manoff, 2013).

The environments to which we are exposed are also related to our identities such as race/ethnicity, socioeconomic status (SES), gender, age, abilities, religions, sexual orientation, and so on—either self-defined or assigned by societies and governments. Different identities are associated with inequitable distribution of resources, contribute to differences in population health, and explain many of the health disparities that exist. Our environments also consist of emotional, social, mental, spiritual, and historic dimensions. Our emotional environment includes not only how others feel about and treat us, but it also includes how we feel about ourselves. In *A Gardner's Tale*, Camara Jones, MD, MPH, describes the impact of racism and internalized racism on health (Jones, 2000).

Ancestral historic exposures to physical and emotional environments contribute to health, disease, and resilience in subsequent generations (Brave Heart, Chase, Elkins, & Altschul, 2011; Brave Heart, Elkins, Tafoya, Bird, & Salvador, 2012; Walters et al., 2011). These exposures can lead to epigenetic modifications of genes. For example, the epidemic of diabetes in Native American communities has been associated with historic trauma (Satterfield, DeBruyn, Santos, Alonso, & Frank, 2016).

◼ Policy Challenges

Clinicians, researchers, and policy makers face many challenges in their attempts to improve health and well-being, which are the result of complex interactions between genetics and environment. Premature deaths are attributed to genetics, SDOHs, environment, behaviors, and access to healthcare. Genetic predisposition accounts for approximately 30% of premature deaths, social circumstances 15%, environmental exposures 5%, individual behaviors 40%, and lack of access to adequate healthcare 10% (Schroeder, 2007; see Figure 6.3).

First, underlying inequity is structural, social, and individual and manifests as racism, sexism, ageism, ableism, homophobia, adultism, and so on. The social ecology model creates a context situating individuals within relationships, families, communities, organizations, societies, and governments (Bronfenbrenner, 1977). Contexts create environments in which individuals and groups can make choices. Unfortunately, not all choices are available to every individual or group. Bird and Rieker developed a model of constrained choices that suggests actions and decisions made at the family, work, community, and government policy levels create or limit opportunities. Limited opportunities allow for some choices and not others (Bird & Rieker, 2008).

Clinicians are often faced with the task of treating disease and addressing health at the individual level. And although individual behaviors account for 40% of premature deaths, individual behaviors involve the ability to make choices. Constrained choice presents challenges to individuals and clinicians trying to change behaviors to improve

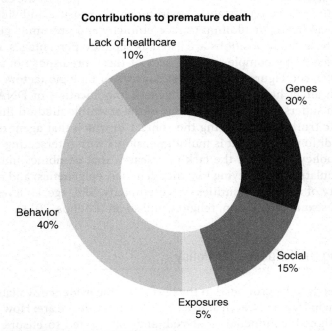

Contributions to premature death

Lack of healthcare 10%

Genes 30%

Social 15%

Exposures 5%

Behavior 40%

FIGURE 6.3 CONTRIBUTIONS TO PREMATURE DEATH.

Source: Adapted from Schroeder, S. A. (2007). We can do better—Improving the health of the American people. *New England Journal of Medicine, 357*(12), 1221–1228. doi:10.1056/NEJMsa073350

health (Bird & Rieker, 2008). Within the limits of constrained choices, patients and practitioners do the best they can to make healthful changes (Vuolo, Kadowaki, & Kelly, 2016).

Furthermore, clinical medicine and research are moving toward personalized medicine focusing on genes and genetic testing. Genetic solutions raise ethical considerations about the full downstream impact on individuals and future generations by introducing genetic alterations into the human genome pool. The scientific community has invested heavily in the idea that personalized medicine can be achieved through identification of every gene and the use of genetic splicing techniques such as CRISPER-Cas9 to replace "disease genes." Although this may work in rare cases, in which the disease is the result of a single-gene disorder, this approach will not work for most common chronic diseases. Additionally, targeting individual genes may result in unintended consequences. Recently, CRISPER-Cas9 was used to replace a gene to protect twins from HIV (*The Lancet*, 2018; Li, Walker, Nie, & Zhang, 2019; Wang et al., 2019). However, it has been noted that removal of this specific gene and replacement increased susceptibility to the West Nile virus (Glass et al., 2005). Most proteins generated by specific genes are used in multiple physiologic systems for different purposes. As in this case, altering specific genes does not alter the body's response to only a single disease vector. Ethical considerations such as equitable access to genetic interventions and misuse of genetic engineering are also concerns (Kolata & Belluck, 2018).

Finally, public health efforts have focused on populations to address the SDOHs (where we live work, play, and pray). Public health efforts have been limited by research that assumed each population was homogeneous with respect to the contributions to premature death: social circumstance, environmental exposure, individual behaviors, and access to healthcare, in addition to race/ethnicity and presumed genetic similarity. Although these predispositions are listed as separate percentages, different populations are affected by complex confluences of these predispositions (Sen, Iyer, & Mukherjee, 2009; see Figure 6.3). This list consists of biologic factors as well as the SDOHs (which affect health through epigenetic modification of DNA). Population health research suffers from the limitations of the scientific method that emphasizes a single empiric truth while ignoring the context in which that agent operates (Phillips, 2011). Additionally, context is multidimensional with intersecting variables. The challenge for policy makers is the lack of research that combines individual health and public/population health tying together genetics, epigenetics, and addressing the intersectionality of multiple identities—race/ethnicity, SES, age, abilities, sex, gender, sexual identity, sexual orientation, religion, and so on (Phillips, 2011).

■ Generating the Evidence for Policy

Good policy needs to be grounded in the best scientific evidence available. Two questions that can help frame research and provide useful evidence are: How does research need to be designed, conducted, analyzed, and interpreted to ensure that similarities and differences in individuals and populations can be understood and applied to policy, programs, services, prevention, screening, diagnosis, and treatment? What is the differential impact of this research, policy, program, and/or service on specific individuals and populations?

It is important to remember that when we ask the second question, we need to establish not only the focus of the research and the individual or population being studied or the target population of the policy but also the context (Sen et al., 2009). Additionally, it is important to remember that the most accurate description and experiences of the individual and/or population come from that individual/population.

Community-based participatory research (CBPR) is invaluable in achieving these aims. CBPR can lead to community-based participatory policy (CBPP; Cacari-Stone, Wallerstein, Garcia, & Minkler, 2014). CBPR ensures that those who establish the research agenda participate in how the research is conducted, and those who analyze and interpret the results include those most impacted by the research and policies that follow.

Approaches to answering the preceding questions include: (a) Improve research methods to produce information that can be analyzed by all the SDOHs. This will include CBPR approaches in designing research, performing data collection, reporting disaggregated data (by sex, gender, race/ethnicity, age, abilities, etc.), and analyzing data using a diversity lens incorporating an intersectional approach. (b) Move upstream through transformative approaches. (c) Increase efficiency by focusing on effective system change implemented through a social justice lens. We cannot improve outcomes in an expensive, unjust, and ineffective system through efficiency. This will only lead to a more efficient, unjust, ineffective system.

SEX AND GENDER AS AN EXAMPLE

There are tools and methods to design research and measure health equity at the individual and group (public health/population) levels. We provide examples using sex and gender to illustrate these tools and methods since most people can understand that women and men are different genetically and that there are certain social roles that are expected of women and men (Phillips, 2011). Sex is an example of true genetic difference and together with gender can serve as a model for understanding the health consequences of genetics, epigenetics (environmental), and bias.

Although there is some disagreement about the exact number, approximately 99.6% of all humans can be divided into one of two groups: XX chromosomes associated with being female or XY chromosomes associated with being male. There are variations in sex beyond XX and XY, which account for approximately 4% of the human population including such variants as XO, XXX, XXY, XYY, XX/XY, and sexually ambiguous genitalia, and so on, resulting in a spectrum of sexual differentiation (Hull & Fausto-Sterling, 2003; Wizemann & Pardue, 2001). Sex, which we think of as binary, is much more complicated. Sexual phenotype results from chromosomal complement, specifically sex chromosomes X and Y, genes not on the X and Y chromosomes, hormones produced from specific genes, hormone receptors, hormone receptor sensitivity, and possibly other factors. Additionally, there is social pressure to conform to roles assigned based on sex determination, which often has been assigned based on external genitalia. Clearly having a different configuration of chromosomes has an impact on growth, development, and health outcomes (Wizemann & Pardue, 2001). Applying a sex/gender lens to research and policy can help sort out the complex interconnections between sex (a genetic determinant of health) and gender (a SDOH mediated by the epigenome and a source of sexism) at both the individual and population levels.

There are many examples of sex and gender differences in prevention, screening, diagnosis, and treatment (Wizemann & Pardue, 2001). Research on breast cancer highlights the importance of both sex and the intersection of multiple SDOHs mediated by epigenetics (Pasculli, Barbano, & Parrella, 2018). Race/ethnicity, SES, age, and rurality have been documented (Hernandez & Blazer, 2006; White, Richardson, Li, Ekwueme, & Kaur, 2014, pp. 1990–2009) as important in the prevention, screening, diagnosis, and treatment of breast cancer demonstrating drastically different health outcomes (Davoudi Monfared et al., 2017; Newman & Kaljee, 2017).

A decade or more of research on women and cardiovascular disease (CVD) illustrates the importance and benefits of addressing health disparities at the right levels of genetics, epigenetics (Cunningham & Eghbali, 2018; Saban, Mathews, DeVon, & Janusek, 2014), and SDOHs using the social ecology model with a transformative approach to mitigate discrimination and bias.

CVD is the leading cause of death in both men and women. The 30-day mortality rate after myocardial infarction (MI) is higher in women than men. Dr. Bernadine Healy speculated possible reasons for the differential rates of death following MIs (Mosca, Barrett-Connor, & Wenger, 2011). Much of this speculation has been borne out by research. Many risk factors for CVD are similar in men and women; however, the prevalence and distribution of risk factors differ. There are many anatomic and physiologic differences such as the following. Women have different presenting symptoms. Microvascular disease and endothelial dysfunction is more common in women. Women have smaller coronary arteries (Bairey Merz et al., 2006). Several gender differences are as follows. Physical activity is higher in men. Women delay seeking treatment and do not recognize the signs and symptoms of heart disease unique to or more common in women. Gender bias also plays a role. Initial research was done only on men and applied to women. Prevention, screening, diagnosis, and treatment protocols were developed based on that research. Delays in treatment occurred because practitioners did not perceive that women were at risk for heart disease (Mosca et al., 2011).

According to the Centers for Disease Control and Prevention, between 1980 and 2000, improvements controlling major risk factors accounted for approximately half of the decrease in rates of death due to heart disease in the United States and the remaining decrease was due to the use of evidence-based secondary prevention and other treatments (Mosca et al., 2011). In the intervening years between 2000 and 2011, additional sex-specific research on women and CVD changed clinical practice prevention recommendations for women. In 2002, results from the Women's Health Initiative clearly demonstrated that hormone therapy did not prevent coronary artery disease in healthy women and, in fact increased the risk of stroke. Similarly, following the Women's Health Study, aspirin was no longer recommended as primary prevention in women (Mosca et al., 2011).

Mosca et al. (2011) recommended a transformative approach to CVD research. Among the recommendations were to include equal numbers of women and men, broaden inclusion criteria, conduct women-only trials for diseases unique to or more common in women, include quality-of-life measures, and disaggregate and report data by sex. Although the recommendations were specific to CVD, they echoed recommendations made a decade earlier by the Institute of Medicine (see Boxes 6.1 and 6.2; Wizemann & Pardue, 2001).

Box 6.1: Summary of Barriers to Progress in Research on Sex Differences

Terminology

- There is inconsistent and often confusing use of the terms "sex" and "gender" in the scientific literature and popular press.

Research Tools and Resources

- The conduct of research on sex differences and longitudinal research may require more complex studies and additional resources.
- Information on sex differences can be difficult to glean from the published literature.
- Useful information on the sex of origin of cell and tissue culture material is often lacking in the literature.
- There is a lack of data from longitudinal studies encompassing different diseases, disorders, and conditions across the life span.
- There is a lack of consideration of hormonal variability.

Interdisciplinary and Collaborative Research

- The application of federal regulations is not uniform.
- Opportunities for interdisciplinary collaboration have been underused.

Non–Health-Related Implications of Research on Sex Differences in Health

- There is a lack of awareness that the consequences of genetics and physiology may be amenable to change.
- The finding of sex differences can lead to discriminatory practices.

Source: From Wizemann, T. M., & Pardue, M.-L. (Eds.). (2001). *Exploring the biological contributions to human health: Does sex matter?* Washington, DC: National Academies Press. Retrieved from http://www.ncbi.nlm.nih.gov/books/NBK222288

RESEARCH METHODS AND TOOLS TO IMPROVE QUALITY OF EVIDENCE FOR POLICY

Some specific research methods and tools to achieve the recommendations of the Institute of Medicine and improve the quality of evidence for policy include complexity modeling, big data, BIAS FREE Framework, and the Gender Integration Continuum Tool (GICT). Complexity modeling (methods used in physics to study complex systems) and big data (data sets so large and complex that usual methods of analysis cannot be used; Gandomi & Haider, 2015) research methods can help address intersectionality moving us closer to personalized medicine. These methods will require an intersectional approach to understanding health; interprofessional teams of healthcare practitioners; inter-/transdisciplinary research teams—including those traditionally thought of as outside of medicine and healthcare; and new voices in policy making in the areas of research, medical programs and services, and models of practice reimbursement. Complexity modeling including research methods such as agent-based modeling, microsimulation models, system dynamics, and hybrid models provide new ways to design, conduct, and analyze data (Kaplan et al., 2017).

Box 6.2: Summary of Major Recommendations to Advance the Understanding of Sex Differences and Their Effects on Health and Illness

- Promote research on sex at the cellular level.
- Study sex differences from womb to tomb.
- Mine cross-species information.
- Investigate natural variations.
- Expand research on sex differences in brain organization and function.
- Monitor sex differences and similarities in all human diseases.
- Clarify use of the terms "sex" and "gender."
- Support and conduct additional research on sex differences.
- Make sex-specific data more readily available.
- Determine and disclose the sex of origin of biological research materials.
- Conduct and construct longitudinal studies so that the results can be analyzed by sex.
- Identify the endocrine status of research subjects (an important variable that should be considered when possible in analyses).
- Encourage and support interdisciplinary research on sex differences.
- Reduce the potential for discrimination based on identified sex differences.

Source: From Wizemann, T. M., & Pardue, M.-L. (Eds.). (2001). *Exploring the biological contributions to human health: Does sex matter?* Washington, DC: National Academies Press. Retrieved from http://www.ncbi.nlm.nih.gov/books/NBK222288

Big data research methods include collecting millions of pieces of personal or population information from multiple sources in real time (Gandomi & Haider, 2015; Kitchin, 2014). For example, Zeevi et al. (2015) collected data on blood tests including continuous blood glucose monitoring, stool tests for microbiome analysis, complete daily food diaries, sleep and physical activity using a smartphone, anthropomorphic data, blood pressure, pulse, medical and lifestyle and nutritional questionnaires. The megadata collected included 46,898 meals and 1.5 million glucose measurements over 5,435 days on 800 individuals. The goal was to create personalized dietary recommendations that would result in optimal postprandial glucose levels (Zeevi et al., 2015). For as big as this database was, more data could have been included in this collection such as psychosocial factors. As with genetic interventions, big data raises ethical issues around confidentiality and unauthorized use of personal data.

The BIAS FREE Framework (Burke & Eichler, 2006) can help to clarify questions of similarities and difference, and power and agency to correct bias and achieve equity. The framework outlines diagnostic questions and solutions for assessing how maintaining an existing hierarchy, failing to examine differences, and using double standards affect research. It also lists types of hierarchies to consider.

Proponents of moving upstream to address population health disparities sometimes argue whether the solutions will be found in changes in laws or changes in social attitudes. To be successful, health policy must focus interventions and allocate resources at all levels simultaneously. The GICT is useful to evaluate any policy for its transformative potential toward equity (see Figure 6.4). Many policies to achieve

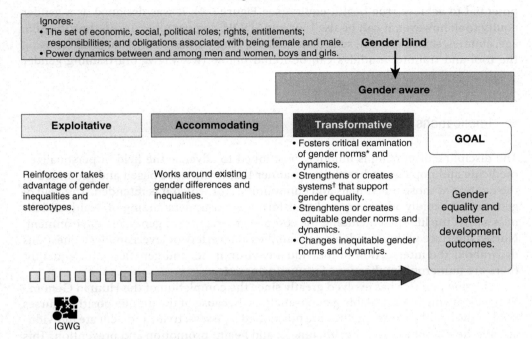

FIGURE 6.4 IGWG'S GENDER INTEGRATION CONTINUUM.

*Norms encompass attitudes and practices.

†A system consists of a set of interacting structures, practices, and relations.

IGWG, Interagency Gender Working Group.

Source: From Interagency Gender Working Group. (2017). *The Gender Integration Continuum user's guide* (Handout #1). Washington, DC: Author. Retrieved from https://www.igwg.org/wp-content/uploads/2017/12/17-418-GenderContTraining-2017-12-12-1633_FINAL.pdf. Reproduced by permission. All rights reserved.

equity at most are harm reduction policies, for example, needle exchange programs, naloxone, and buprenorphine. These programs are useful; however, our goal should be social transformation to eliminate the need for such policies. Policies would be multilevel to achieve individual, family, cultural, community, and societal changes.

The Interagency Gender Working Group's (IGWG) GICT is useful in structuring and evaluating approaches that target multiple levels simultaneously (IGWG, 2017). The tool categorizes interventions and policies as follows:

- Gender exploitative/aggravating approaches:
  Take advantage of rigid gender norms and existing imbalances in power to achieve program objectives.
- Gender accommodating approaches:
  Acknowledge the role of gender norms and inequities while seeking to develop actions that adjust to and often compensate for them.
- Gender transformative approaches:
  Actively strive to examine, question, and change rigid gender norms and imbalance of power as a means of reaching gender equity objectives (Caro, 2009).

The GICT is useful to evaluate research and policies for their transformative potential to achieve true health equity (see Figure 6.4). It was designed as a gender equity tool; however, it can be used for any SDOH demographic: race/ethnicity, SES, age, abilities, sexual identity, sexual orientation, religion, and so on. A manual for using the tool and training modules can be found online (www.igwg.org/training/gender -analysis-and-integration).

■ Implications for Nursing

The discipline of nursing is uniquely positioned to advance the field of personalized medicine and population health in a manner that is evidence based and grounded in the context of those individuals and communities for which it is intended. The field of genomics is rapidly advancing and transforming our understanding of health and illness across the life span including the complex interaction of genes and environment. Nurses interface with individuals and families at a variety of levels and face questions daily about the intersection of individual environments and genetics. Consequently, there are numerous implications for nursing practice.

Nursing practice has evolved greatly since the completion of the Human Genome Project allowing for affordable genetic analysis. Because of the unique position nurses hold in the healthcare arena, they are positioned to assess, treat, and educate individuals and their families about health, illness, and health promotion and prevention. This encompasses a broad range of activities including individual screening, risk assessment, testing, diagnosis, personalized treatment plans, health monitoring across the life span, and public health (Conley et al., 2013).

Additionally, nurse scientists are placing increased emphasis on the incorporation of gene environment interactions into research studies. Important areas identified for exploration by nurse researchers include: (a) strategies to reduce health disparities, (b) lifestyle behavior modification, (c) managing chronic illness, (d) implications for genomic technology to improve health, and (e) end-of-life experiences (Conley & Tinkle, 2007). In addition, nurse researchers are increasingly relying on research approaches such as community-engaged research to eliminate disparities. Furthermore, nurses are using the evidence generated through this research to inform dialogue and address health policy issues.

■ Conclusion

Understanding the contribution of genetics, epigenetics, SDOHs (exposome), the human microbiome, and their complex interactions at the individual and population levels will be necessary to achieve true health equity. This will require inter-/ transdisciplinary teams including those traditionally thought of as "outside" of medicine/healthcare, as well as interprofessional collaboration, and transformative health policy. Additionally, it will require applying the principles of transformative policy making.

■ Critical Thinking Exercise

1. Comment on the intersection of genetics/genomics and the SDOHs and why addressing one concept without addressing the other may be scientifically flawed.

■ Discussion Questions and Exercise

1. What are the social determinants of health?
2. What are health and healthcare disparities?
3. What is the role of epigenetics in health and health equity?
4. Exercise: Related to Sex or Gender?

Please check whether each example is related to sex or gender.

Example	Sex	Gender
1. Women experience different cardiac symptoms of a heart attack than men.		
2. Reasons women do not receive prompt treatment for heart attacks may include women's lack of knowledge of heart attacks in women, providers' lack of awareness of heart attack signs in women, fear of calling an ambulance, responsibility to care for other(s) in the home, and lack of insurance.		
3. Men are less likely than women to use the healthcare system, and this is especially true for the use of preventive services. When men do present for healthcare, they are more likely to be experiencing critical health problems. As a result, the ED is a more common care site for men than for women.		
4. Women's life expectancy is longer than men's.		

Source: From Office on Women's Health. (2010, November 3). Orientation Meeting for the Coalition for a Healthier Community Award. Washington, DC.

■ Resources

Addie, S., Alper, J., & Beachy, S. H. (2018). *Understanding disparities in access to genomic medicine: Proceedings of a workshop.* Washington, DC: National Academies Press. Retrieved from https://www.nap.edu/read/25277/chapter/1

Canadian Institutes of Gender and Health. (2019). Online training modules: Integrating sex & gender in health research. Retrieved from http://www.cihr-irsc.gc.ca/e/49347.html

Government of Canada. (2018). Determinants of health. Retrieved from https://www.canada.ca/en/services/health/determinants-health.html

The Human Exposome Project: https://humanexposomeproject.com/news/taking-on-the-exposome

Institute for Women's Policy Research: https://iwpr.org

National Women's Health Network: https://nwhn.org

National Women's Law Center: https://nwlc.org/issue/health-care-reproductive-rights

Rediscovering Biology: http://www.learner.org/courses/biology/index.html

Sainani, K. (2016). Taking on the exposome: How bioinformatics tools are bringing insight to the environmental side of the health equation. Retrieved from http://biomedicalcomputationreview.org/content/taking-exposome

TED. (2016). *The problem with race-based medicine: Dorothy Roberts* [Video file]. Retrieved from https://www.youtube.com/watch?v=KxLMjn4WPBY

■ References

Bairey Merz, C. N., Shaw, L. J., Reis, S. E., Bittner, V., Kelsey, S. F., Olson, M., . . . Sopko, G. (2006). Insights from the NHLBI-sponsored Women's Ischemia Syndrome Evaluation (WISE) Study. *Journal of the American College of Cardiology, 47*(3, Suppl.), S21–S29. doi:10.1016/j.jacc.2004.12.084

Barker, D. J. (1998). In utero programming of chronic disease. *Clinical Science, 95*(2), 115–128. doi:10.1042/cs0950115

Barker, D. J., Osmond, C., Golding, J., Kuh, D., & Wadsworth, M. E. (1989). Growth in utero, blood pressure in childhood and adult life, and mortality from cardiovascular disease. *BMJ (Clinical Research Ed.), 298*(6673), 564–567. doi:10.1136/bmj.298.6673.564

Bird, C. E., & Rieker, P. P. (2008). *Gender and health: The effects of constrained choices and social policies.* Cambridge; New York: Cambridge University Press.

Brave Heart, M. Y. H., Chase, J., Elkins, J., & Altschul, D. B. (2011). Historical trauma among indigenous peoples of the Americas: Concepts, research, and clinical considerations. *Journal of Psychoactive Drugs, 43*(4), 282–290. doi:10.1080/02791072.2011.628913

Brave Heart, M. Y. H., Elkins, J., Tafoya, G., Bird, D., & Salvador, M. (2012). Wicasa Was'aka: Restoring the traditional strength of American Indian boys and men. *American Journal of Public Health, 102*(Suppl. 2), S177–S183. doi:10.2105/AJPH.2011.300511

Bronfenbrenner, U. (1977). Toward an experimental ecology of human development. *American Psychologist, 32*(7), 513–531. doi:10.1037/0003-066X.32.7.513

Burke, M. A., & Eichler, M. (2006). *The "BIAS FREE" framework: A practical tool for identifying and eliminating social biases in health research.* Geneva, Switzerland: Global Forum for Health Research.

Cacari-Stone, L., Wallerstein, N., Garcia, A. P., & Minkler, M. (2014). The promise of community-based participatory research for health equity: A conceptual model for bridging evidence with policy. *American Journal of Public Health, 104*(9), 1615–1623. doi:10.2105/AJPH.2014.301961

Caro, D. (2009). *A manual for integrating gender into reproductive health and HIV programs: From commitment to action* (2nd ed.). Washington, DC: Population Reference Bureau. Retrieved from https://assets.prb.org/igwg_media/manualintegrgendr09_eng.pdf

Conley, Y. P., Biesecker, L. G., Gonsalves, S., Merkle, C. J., Kirk, M., & Aouizerat, B. E. (2013). Current and emerging technology approaches in genomics. *Journal of Nursing Scholarship, 45*(1), 5–14. doi:10.1111/jnu.12001

Conley, Y. P., & Tinkle, M. B. (2007). The future of genomic nursing research. *Journal of Nursing Scholarship, 39*(1), 17–24. doi:10.1111/j.1547-5069.2007.00138.x

Cunningham, C. M., & Eghbali, M. (2018). An introduction to epigenetics in cardiovascular development, disease, and sexualization. *Advances in Experimental Medicine and Biology, 1065*, 31–47. doi:10.1007/978-3-319-77932-4_2

Davoudi-Monfared, E., Mohseny, M., Amanpour, F., Mosavi-Jarrahi, A., Moradi-Joo, M., & Heidarnia, M. A. (2017). Relationship of social determinants of health with the three-year survival rate of breast cancer. *Asian Pacific Journal of Cancer Prevention: APJCP, 18*(4), 1121–1126. doi:10.22034/APJCP.2017.18.4.1121

Gandomi, A., & Haider, M. (2015). Beyond the hype: Big data concepts, methods, and analytics. *International Journal of Information Management, 35*(2), 137–144. doi:10.1016/j.ijinfomgt.2014.10.007

Genetic Science Learning Center. (n.d.-a). Basic genetics. Retrieved from https://learn.genetics.utah.edu/content/basics

Genetic Science Learning Center. (n.d.-b). Old genes, new tricks. Retrieved from https://learn.genetics.utah.edu/content/basics/newtricks/

Genetic Science Learning Center. (n.d.-c). The epigenome learns from its experiences. Retrieved from https://learn.genetics.utah.edu/content/epigenetics/memory/

Genetic Science Learning Center. (n.d.-d). What is mutation? Retrieved from https://learn.genetics.utah.edu/content/basics/mutation/

Glass, W. G., Lim, J. K., Cholera, R., Pletnev, A. G., Gao, J.-L., & Murphy, P. M. (2005). Chemokine receptor CCR5 promotes leukocyte trafficking to the brain and survival in West Nile virus infection. *The Journal of Experimental Medicine, 202*(8), 1087–1098. doi:10.1084/jem.20042530

Graeter, L. J., & Mortensen, M. E. (1996). Kids are different: Developmental variability in toxicology. *Toxicology, 111*(1–3), 15–20. doi:10.1016/0300-483X(96)03389-6

Hawks, J. (2013). Significance of neandertal and denisovan genomes in human evolution. *Annual Review of Anthropology, 42*(1), 433–449. doi:10.1146/annurev-anthro-092412-155548

Hernandez, L. M., & Blazer, D. G. (Eds.). (2006). *Genes, behavior, and the social environment: Moving beyond the nature/nurture debate.* Washington, DC: National Academies Press. doi:10.17226/11693

Hull, C. L., & Fausto-Sterling, A. (2003). Letter to the Editor. *American Journal of Human Biology, 15*(1), 112–116. doi:10.1002/ajhb.10122

Interagency Gender Working Group. (2017). *The Gender Integration Continuum user's guide* (Handout #1). Washington, DC: Author. Retrieved from https://www.igwg.org/wp-content/uploads/2017/12/17-418-GenderContTraining-2017-12-12-1633_FINAL.pdf

John, R. M., & Rougeulle, C. (2018). Developmental epigenetics: Phenotype and the flexible epigenome. *Frontiers in Cell and Developmental Biology, 6.* doi:10.3389/fcell.2018.00130

Jones, C. (2000). Levels of racism: A theoretic framework and a gardener's tale. *American Journal of Public Health, 90*(8), 1212–1215. doi:10.2105/AJPH.90.8.1212

Kaplan, G. A., Diez Roux, A. V., Simon, C. P., & Galea, S. (Eds.). (2017). *Growing inequality: Bridging complex systems, population health, and health disparities.* Washington, DC: Westphalia Press.

Keita, S. O. Y., Kittles, R. A., Royal, C. D. M., Bonney, G. E., Furbert-Harris, P., Dunston, G. M., & Rotimi, C. N. (2004). Conceptualizing human variation. *Nature Genetics, 36*(11, Suppl.), S17–S20. doi:10.1038/ng1455

Kitchin, R. (2014). Big Data, new epistemologies and paradigm shifts. *Big Data & Society, 1*(1), 205395171452848. doi:10.1177/2053951714528481

Kolata, G., & Belluck, P. (2018, December 5). Why Are Scientists So Upset About the First Crispr Babies? *The New York Times.* Retrieved from https://www.nytimes.com/2018/12/05/health/crispr-gene-editing-embryos.html

The Lancet. (2018). CRISPR-Cas9: A world first? *The Lancet, 392*(10163), 2413. doi:10.1016/S0140-6736(18)33111-8

Li, J., Walker, S., Nie, J., & Zhang, X. (2019). Experiments that led to the first gene-edited babies: The ethical failings and the urgent need for better governance. *Journal of Zhejiang University-SCIENCE B, 20*(1), 32–38. doi:10.1631/jzus.B1800624

Mosca, L., Barrett-Connor, E., & Wenger, N. K. (2011). Sex/gender differences in cardiovascular disease prevention: What a difference a decade makes. *Circulation, 124*(19), 2145–2154. doi:10.1161/CIRCULATIONAHA.110.968792

Newman, L. A., & Kaljee, L. M. (2017). Health disparities and triple-negative breast cancer in African American Women: A review. *JAMA Surgery, 152*(5), 485–493. doi:10.1001/jamasurg.2017.0005

Notterman, D. A., & Mitchell, C. (2015). Epigenetics and understanding the impact of social determinants of health. *Pediatric Clinics of North America, 62*(5), 1227–1240. doi:10.1016/j.pcl.2015.05.012

Nugent, B. M., & Bale, T. L. (2015). The omniscient placenta: Metabolic and epigenetic regulation of fetal programming. *Frontiers in Neuroendocrinology, 39*, 28–37. doi:10.1016/j.yfrne.2015.09.001

Office on Women's Health. (2010, November 3). Orientation Meeting for the Coalition for a Healthier Community Award. Washington, DC.

The 1000 Genomes Project Consortium. (2015). A global reference for human genetic variation. *Nature, 526*(7571), 68–74. doi:10.1038/nature15393

Pasculli, B., Barbano, R., & Parrella, P. (2018). Epigenetics of breast cancer: Biology and clinical implication in the era of precision medicine. *Seminars in Cancer Biology, 51*, 22–35. doi:10.1016/j.semcancer.2018.01.007

Phillips, S. P. (2011). Including gender in public health research. *Public Health Reports, 126*(3, Suppl.), 16–21. doi:10.1177/00333549111260S304

Saban, K. L., Mathews, H. L., DeVon, H. A., & Janusek, L. W. (2014). Epigenetics and social context: implications for disparity in cardiovascular disease. *Aging and Disease, 5*(5), 346–355. doi:10.14336/AD.2014.0500346

Satterfield, D., DeBruyn, L., Santos, M., Alonso, L., & Frank, M. (2016). Health promotion and diabetes prevention in American Indian and Alaska Native communities—Traditional Foods Project, 2008-2014. *Morbidity and Mortality Weekly Report Supplements, 65*(1), 4–10. doi:10.15585/mmwr.su6501a3

Schroeder, S. A. (2007). We can do betterImproving the health of the American People. *New England Journal of Medicine, 357*(12), 1221–1228. doi:10.1056/NEJMsa073350

Sen, G., Iyer, A., & Mukherjee, C. (2009). A methodology to analyse the intersections of social inequalities in health. *Journal of Human Development and Capabilities, 10*(3), 397–415. doi:10.1080/19452820903048894

Shields, A. E. (2017). Epigenetic signals of how social disadvantage "gets under the skin": A challenge to the public health community. *Epigenomics, 9*(3), 223–229. doi:10.2217/epi-2017-0013

Velasquez-Manoff, M. (2013). *An epidemic of absence: A new way of understanding allergies and autoimmune diseases* (1st Scribner paperback ed.). New York, NY: Scribner.

Vuolo, M., Kadowaki, J., & Kelly, B. C. (2016). A multilevel test of constrained choices theory: The case of tobacco clean air restrictions. *Journal of Health and Social Behavior, 57*(3), 351–372. doi:10.1177/0022146516653790

Walters, K. L., Mohammed, S. A., Evans-Campbell, T., Beltrán, R. E., Chae, D. H., & Duran, B. (2011). Bodies don't just tell stories, they tell histories. *Du Bois Review: Social Science Research on Race, 8*(01), 179–189. doi:10.1017/S1742058X1100018X

Wang, C., Zhai, X., Zhang, X., Li, L., Wang, J., & Liu, D. (2019). Gene-edited babies: Chinese Academy of Medical Sciences' response and action. *The Lancet, 393*(10166), 25–26. doi:10.1016/S0140-6736(18)33080-0

White, A., Richardson, L. C., Li, C., Ekwueme, D. U., & Kaur, J. S. (2014). Breast cancer mortality among American Indian and Alaska Native women, 1990-2009. *American Journal of Public Health, 104*(Suppl. 3), S432–S438. doi:10.2105/AJPH.2013.301720

White, D., & Rabago-Smith, M. (2011). Genotype-phenotype associations and human eye color. *Journal of Human Genetics, 56*(1), 5–7. doi:10.1038/jhg.2010.126

Wild, C. P. (2005). Complementing the genome with an "exposome": The outstanding challenge of environmental exposure measurement in molecular epidemiology. *Cancer Epidemiology, Biomarkers & Prevention, 14*(8), 1847–1850. doi:10.1158/1055-9965.EPI-05-0456

Wilkinson, R., & Marmot, M.. (Eds.). (2003). *Social determinants of health: The solid facts* (2nd ed). Copenhagen, Denmark: World Health Organization Regional Office for Europe.

Wizemann, T. M., & Pardue, M.-L. (Eds.). (2001). *Exploring the biological contributions to human health: Does sex matter?* Washington, DC: National Academies Press. Retrieved from http://www.ncbi.nlm.nih.gov/books/NBK222288

Zeevi, D., Korem, T., Zmora, N., Israeli, D., Rothschild, D., Weinberger, A., . . . Segal, E. (2015). Personalized nutrition by prediction of glycemic responses. *Cell, 163*(5), 1079–1094. doi:10.1016/j.cell.2015.11.001

Population Health

7

The Conceptual Model of Nursology for Enhancing Equity and Quality: Population Health and Health Policy

Jacqueline Fawcett

CHAPTER OBJECTIVES

⊙ Present a new conceptual model of nursology for enhancing population health equity and quality through development and implementation of health policies

⊙ Discuss the quadruple foci of the new conceptual model of nursology: equity, quality, population health, and health policy

⊙ Identify the environments, population factors, and stakeholders that influence the attention given to population health concern and development and implementation of health policies

⊙ Identify the influence of health policies and stakeholders on population-centered nursologists' activities

⊙ Identify the link between population-centered nursologists' activities and population quality of life

KEY CONCEPTS

Environments   Population factors
Health policy   Population health concern
Population-centered nursologists'   Population quality of life
   activities   Stakeholders

KEY TERMS

Equity   Population
Health policy   Population health
Nursology   Quality

◼ Introduction

The discipline of nursology is concerned with the discovery, dissemination, and application of discipline-specific knowledge in the form of conceptual models and theories (Fawcett et al., 2015). The purpose of this chapter is to explain the evolution and content of a new conceptual model that is offered as an addition to the literature of the discipline—the Conceptual Model of Nursology for Enhancing Equity and Quality: Population Health and

Health Policy. The quadruple foci of the new conceptual model are equity, quality, population health, and health policy.

■ Background

EQUITY

For the purposes of the new conceptual model, "equity" refers to equitable, or fair, opportunities for a high level of wellness and other aspects of population quality of life. "Health equity" refers to elimination of disparities, inequalities, and inequities in the extent of a population's wellness, illness, and disease (Braverman, 2014). "Health disparities" and "health inequalities" are regarded as a lower prevalence of wellness and a greater prevalence of illness and disease in a population. Health inequities are "systematic differences in the health status [i.e., differences in wellness, illness, and disease] of different population groups" (World Health Organization [WHO], 2017, para. 2). These disparities, inequalities, and inequities are thought to be influenced by societal and institutional structures and systems—including society-based disadvantages and diverse forms of discrimination (Drevdahl, 2018)—and, therefore, result in substantial economic and social costs to the population (WHO, 2017).

QUALITY

The focus on quality draws attention to the need for health policies that mandate the highest possible quality of nursologists' activities. "The highest possible quality of nursologists' activities" refers to excellent, efficient, effective, and safe care of populations that is based on a population-based conceptual model, relevant population-based theories, and the best available empirical evidence (Allen-Duck, Robinson, & Stewart, 2017; Venes, 2013).

POPULATION HEALTH

Population health has been a major research and practice specialty in the discipline of nursology at least since the time of Nightingale (1859/1992). Contemporary emphasis on population health has become a central focus of our discipline, due primarily to growing global awareness of an increase in many chronic diseases, a resurgence of some infectious disease epidemics, and emergence of new epidemics (Fawcett & Ellenbecker, 2015).

The focus on population health starts with an understanding of a population and of health. A population is more than one individual, an aggregate group of people residing in a local, state, national, or international geographic region or an aggregate group of people with common characteristics (Fawcett & Ellenbecker, 2015; Keyes & Galea, 2016). The aggregate is treated as a whole entity, a unity, rather than a collection of individuals (Fawcett & AbuFannouneh, 2017).

"Population health" encompasses the extent of wellness, illness, and disease of the aggregate. This view of health contrasts with the mostly implicit understanding of health as wellness. Wellness is the extent to which a population experiences wellbeing, whereas illness and disease refer to the extent to which the population is sick.

Illness and disease are regarded as separate conditions. Venes (2013) explained, "Disease and illness differ in that disease is usually objective and tangible or measurable whereas illness (and associated pain, suffering, or distress) is subjective and personal" (p. 699).

HEALTH POLICY

Health policy refers to a plan and guidelines for a desirable course of action about a wellness, illness, or disease condition that is regarded as a concern by members of society (Sudduth, 1999). "Health policy," according to Loewit (as cited in Groah & Hader, 2019), "is used to achieve specific health goals within a population on local, state, . . . national [or international] level. Health policy gives clarity and direction to a specific problem with the goal of improving health outcomes" (p. 170).

Health policy has been of explicit interest to the members of the discipline of nursology and has been regarded as a specialty much more recently than the population health nursological specialty (Ellenbecker, Fawcett, & Glazer, 2005). The interest in health policy can be at least in part attributed to the advanced practice movement (Milstead, 1999). In recent years, leaders of professional nursology organizations have called for their members to advocate for health policies that address the discipline's ethical and social mandates (Ellenbecker et al., 2017).

■ THE CONCEPTUAL MODEL OF NURSOLOGY FOR ENHANCING EQUITY AND QUALITY: POPULATION HEALTH AND HEALTH POLICY

The Conceptual Model of Nursology for Enhancing Equity and Quality: Population Health and Health Policy evolved from several sources, including published papers and personal communications. The population health focus owes allegiance to work by Evans and Stoddart (1990), Stiefel and Nolan (2012), Kindig and Stoddart (2003), Stoto (2013), and Fawcett and Ellenbecker (2015). The health policy focus owes its allegiance to work by Fawcett and Russell (2001) and Russell and Fawcett (2005). The evolution of the new conceptual model was greatly facilitated by conversations with colleagues, including doctoral students, in the United States and Holland.

CONCEPTS

The seven concepts of the conceptual model, listed here and displayed in Figure 7.1, are:

1. Environments
2. Population factors
3. Population health concern
4. Health policy
5. Population-centered nursologists' activities
6. Population quality of life
7. Stakeholders

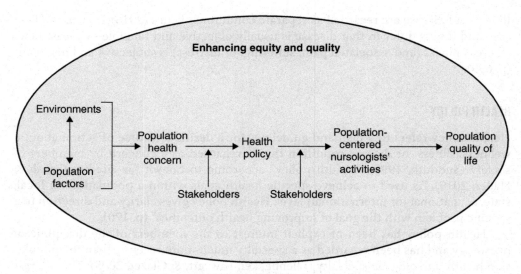

FIGURE 7.1 CONCEPTS AND RELATIONAL PROPOSITIONS.

All seven concepts are multidimensional, and concepts 3 and 5 include subdimensions. The concepts and their dimensions and subdimensions are depicted in Figures 7.2 through 7.8. The definitions of the concepts, dimensions, and subdimensions, which are nonrelational propositions, are given in Tables 7.1 to 7.7.

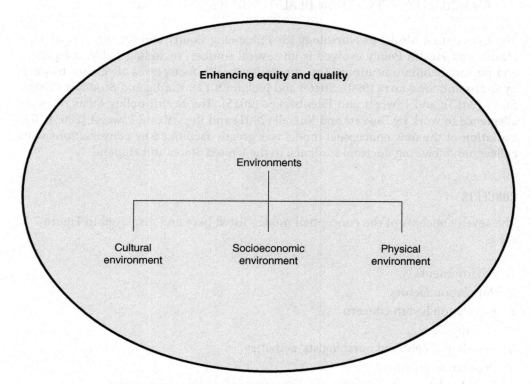

FIGURE 7.2 DIMENSIONS OF ENVIRONMENTAL FACTORS.

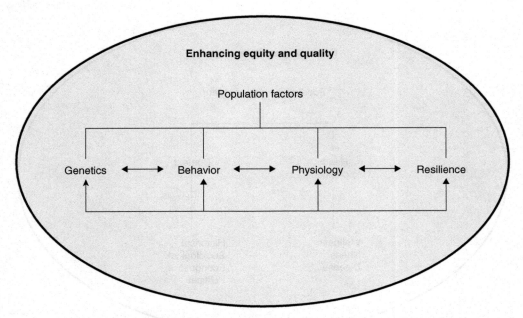

FIGURE 7.3 INTERRELATED DIMENSIONS OF POPULATION FACTORS.

Environments

Environments, sometimes referred to as "upstream factors," are considered structural and system determinants of health, which are "macro-level forces, such as financial, legal, and governmental systems and policies, which exert an effect on human life" (Drevdahl, 2018, p. 152), as well as lifestyles, neighborhoods, geographic segregation, education, limited access to essential services and newer health technology, rates of incarceration, pollution, socioeconomic status, structural stigma, and structural and systematic racism.

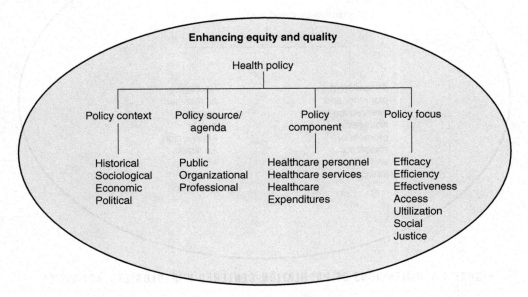

FIGURE 7.4 DIMENSIONS AND SUBDIMENSIONS OF HEALTH POLICY.

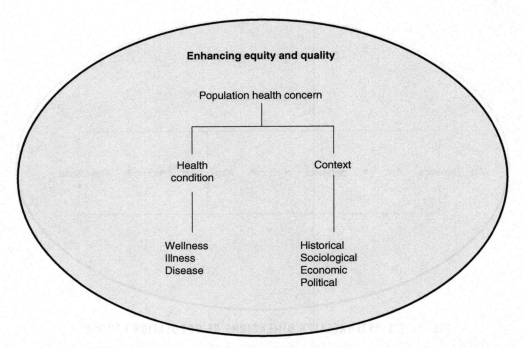

FIGURE 7.5 DIMENSIONS AND SUBDIMENSIONS OF THE POPULATION HEALTH CONCERN.

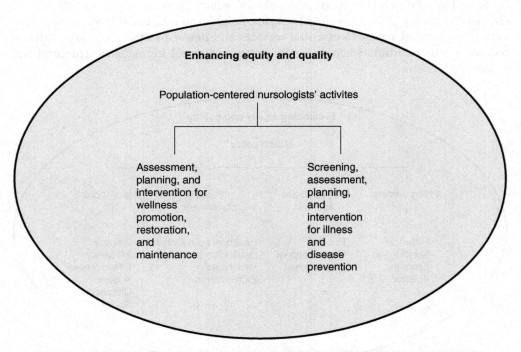

FIGURE 7.6 DIMENSIONS OF POPULATION-CENTERED NURSOLOGISTS' ACTIVITIES.

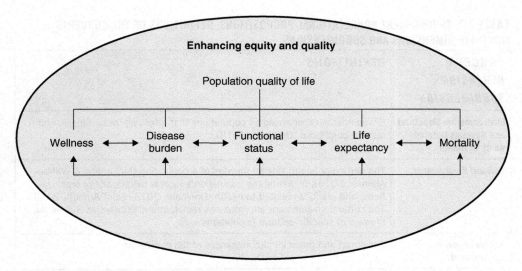

FIGURE 7.7 INTERRELATED DIMENSIONS OF POPULATION QUALITY OF LIFE.

Typical dimensions of environments are socioeconomic environment and physical environment (Fawcett & Ellenbecker, 2015). Although culture could be considered part of the socioeconomic environment, cultural environment was added as a dimension of environments in recognition that nursologists always have at least implicitly taken the culture of a population into account (Drevdahl, 2018).

Population Factors

Population factors—genetics, behavior, physiology, and resilience—are considered social determinants of health, which are conditions in which people are born, grow,

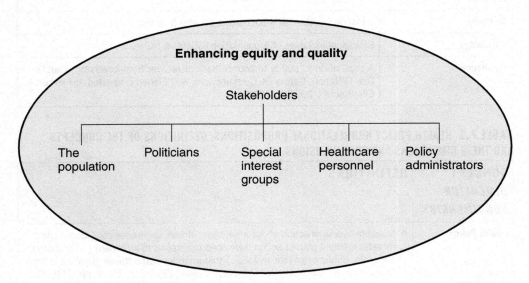

FIGURE 7.8 DIMENSIONS OF STAKEHOLDERS.

TABLE 7.1 ENVIRONMENT NONRELATIONAL PROPOSITIONS: DEFINITIONS OF THE CONCEPTS AND THEIR DIMENSIONS AND SUBDIMENSIONS

CONCEPT *DIMENSION* *SUBDIMENSION*	DEFINITIONS
Environments: Structural and Systems Determinants of Health	Environments experienced by populations that affect wellness, illness, and disease conditions (Drevdahl, 2018)
Cultural Environment	The particular health-related lifeways of a population (McFarland & Wehbe-Alamah, 2015), including the population's values, beliefs, social organizations, and practices related to health (Drevdahl, 2018; Saint Arnault, 2018). The cultural environment encompasses racial, ethnic lifeways as well as the lifeways of specific cultural populations.
Socioeconomic Environment	The social and financial circumstances of the population
Physical Environment	The physical surroundings of the population (Kindig & Stoddart, 2003), including climate and safety

TABLE 7.2 POPULATION FACTORS' NONRELATIONAL PROPOSITIONS: DEFINITIONS OF THE CONCEPTS AND THEIR DIMENSIONS AND SUBDIMENSIONS

CONCEPT *DIMENSION* *SUBDIMENSION*	DEFINITIONS
Population Factors: Social Determinants of Health	Essential elements of populations that affect wellness, illness, and disease conditions (Office of Disease Prevention and Health Promotion, n.d.)
Genetics	Inherited origins of a population
Behavior	Lifestyle variables of a population (Stiefel & Nolan, 2012)
Physiology	Biological variables of a population (Stiefel & Nolan, 2012)
Resilience	A population's "ability to bounce back or recover from adversity" (Garcia-Dia, DiNapoli, Garcia-Ona, Jakubowski, & O'Flaherty, as cited in Fawcett & Ellenbecker, 2015, p. 292)

TABLE 7.3 HEALTH POLICY NONRELATIONAL PROPOSITIONS: DEFINITIONS OF THE CONCEPTS AND THEIR DIMENSIONS AND SUBDIMENSIONS

CONCEPT *DIMENSION* *SUBDIMENSION*	DEFINITIONS
Health Policy	A desirable course of action about a wellness, illness, or disease condition; "The purposeful, general plan of action developed to respond to a concern . . . or matter in either the public or private sector . . . that includes authoritative guidelines. This plan directs human behavior toward specific goals" (Sudduth, 1999, pp. 219, 221)
Policy Context	Disciplinary influences on development and evolution of the health policy

(continued)

TABLE 7.3 HEALTH POLICY NONRELATIONAL PROPOSITIONS: DEFINITIONS OF THE CONCEPTS AND THEIR DIMENSIONS AND SUBDIMENSIONS (*CONTINUED*)

CONCEPT *DIMENSION* *SUBDIMENSION*	DEFINITIONS
Historical	Chronological evolution of the policy
Sociological	Society's influence on development of the policy
Economic	Financial influences on and effects of the policy
Political	Political influences on development of the policy
Policy Source/ Agenda	The origin of the health policy and what is to be done about a wellness, illness, or disease condition; "an agenda is a collection of difficulties or issues and their causes, representations . . . and suggested resolutions that get the attention and consideration of policy makers" (Groah & Hader, 2019, p. 166)
Public	A desirable course of action about a wellness, illness, or disease condition "developed by nations, states, cities, and towns" (Russell & Fawcett, 2005, p. 320); public policy encompasses social policy, which encompasses health policy (Williams & Phillips, 2019)
Organizational	A desirable course of action about a wellness, illness, or disease condition "developed by healthcare institutions, such as hospitals, clinics, and home healthcare agencies, to guide practice at a particular institution" (Russell & Fawcett, 2005, p. 320) in the form of specific practice protocols and "interpretation of state regulations and The Joint Commission standards" (Groah & Hader, 2019, p. 185)
Professional	A desirable course of action about a wellness, illness, or disease condition, in the form of "standards or guidelines developed by discipline-specific and multidisciplinary associations . . . to provide direction for those individuals and groups who work for or with the associations" (Russell & Fawcett, 2005, p. 320)
Policy Component	A part of the health policy
Healthcare Personnel	Provisions about "individuals with the professional and technical education required for the provision of healthcare services" (Russell & Fawcett, 2005, p. 321)
Healthcare Services	Provisions regarding "procedures that nurses and other healthcare personnel provide, which can range from basic screening tests to complex, technology-driven interventions" (Russell & Fawcett, 2005, p. 321)
Expenditures	Financial provisions of the policy, specifically, "the costs of healthcare services incurred by [populations], providers, payers, and society" (Russell & Fawcett, 2005, p. 321)
Policy Focus	The specific aspects addressed by the health policy
Efficacy	Policy-mandated provisions that yield results
Efficiency	Policy-mandated provisions that yield results that require the fewest possible resources and actions in the least amount of time possible
Effectiveness	Policy-mandated provisions that yield substantial desirable results
Access	Policy-mandated provisions that support obtaining healthcare
Utilization	Policy-mandated provisions that encourage use of healthcare services
Social Justice	Policy-mandated processes that emphasize "a state of health equity characterized by both the equitable [and fair] distribution of services affecting health and helping relationships" (Matwick & Woodgate, 2016, p. 182)

TABLE 7.4 POPULATION HEALTH CONCERN NONRELATIONAL PROPOSITIONS: DEFINITIONS OF THE CONCEPTS AND THEIR DIMENSIONS AND SUBDIMENSIONS

CONCEPT *DIMENSION* *SUBDIMENSION*	DEFINITIONS
Population Health Concern	A concern about the extent of wellness, illness, or disease of a population that requires attention
Health Condition	A experience of wellness, illness, or disease
Wellness	"A state of mental [, emotional,] and physical balance and fitness" (Venes, 2013, p. 2501)
Illness	A "subjective and personal [experience] associated [with] pain, suffering, or distress. . . . Sickness . . . An aliment" (Venes, 2013, pp. 699, 1197)
Disease	An "objective and tangible or measurable [condition manifested by] clinical signs and symptoms, and laboratory or radiographic findings" (Venes, 2013, p. 699)
Context	Disciplinary perspectives of the concern
Historical	Chronological evolution of the concern
Sociological	Societal influences on recognition of the concern
Economic	Financial aspects of the concern
Political	Political attention to the concern

TABLE 7.5 POPULATION-CENTERED NURSOLOGISTS' NONRELATIONAL PROPOSITIONS: DEFINITIONS OF THE CONCEPTS AND THEIR DIMENSIONS AND SUBDIMENSIONS

CONCEPT *DIMENSION* *SUBDIMENSION*	DEFINITIONS
Population-Centered Nursologists' Activities	"Actions performed by [nursologists] directed to populations" (Fawcett & Ellenbecker, 2015, p. 292)
Screening, Planning, and Intervention for Wellness Promotion, Restoration, and Maintenance	Provision of nursologists' practice processes directed to enhancing the optimal level of the population's collective "growth, integration of experience, and meaningful connection with others, reflecting [population] valued goals and strengths, and resulting in being well and living values" within the context of the culture of the population (McMahon & Fleury, as cited in Fawcett & Ellenbecker, 2015, p. 293)
Screening, Planning, and Intervention for Illness and Disease Prevention	Provision of nursologists' practice processes directed to avoiding subjective experiences of an illness and objective and tangible clinical signs and symptoms of a disease (Venes, 2013)

TABLE 7.6 POPULATION QUALITY OF LIFE NONRELATIONAL PROPOSITIONS: DEFINITIONS
OF THE CONCEPTS AND THEIR DIMENSIONS AND SUBDIMENSIONS

CONCEPT DIMENSION SUBDIMENSION	DEFINITIONS
Population Quality of Life	The results of population-focused nursologists' activities; a population's "physical, psychological, [mental, emotional,] social, economic, and environmental" well-being (Fulton, Miller, & Otte, as cited in Fawcett & Ellenbecker, 2015, p. 293)
Wellness	A population's condition of overall well-being
Disease Burden	Incidence and/or prevalence of major chronic health conditions in a population (Stiefel & Nolan, 2012); "the total effect of a disease" on a population (Venes, 2013, p. 699), including extent of disability
Functional Status	"A population's optimal level of performing usual activities of daily living" (Fawcett & Ellenbecker, 2015, p. 293)
Life Expectancy	A population's overall "expected years of remaining life at any age" (Stiefel & Nolan, 2012, p. 13)
Mortality	"Years of potential life lost" for a population (Stiefel & Nolan, 2012, p. 4)

TABLE 7.7 STAKEHOLDERS' NONRELATIONAL PROPOSITIONS: DEFINITIONS OF THE CONCEPTS
AND THEIR DIMENSIONS AND SUBDIMENSIONS

CONCEPT DIMENSION SUBDIMENSION	DEFINITIONS
Stakeholders	People and groups "that have a say in what goes on" (Furlong, 1999, p. 43); "Individuals or organizations that are either directly or indirectly affected by [a health policy or a health concern]" (Sudduth, 1999, p. 233)
The Population	More than one individual; an aggregate group of people, including families, residing in a local, state, national, or international geographic region or an aggregate group of people with common characteristics (Fawcett & Ellenbecker, 2015; Keyes & Galea, 2016)
Politicians	People holding an elected political office, who make decisions about population health concerns that need to be addressed by health policies by setting policy priorities and determining specific policy agenda
Special Interest Groups	Collectives of people addressing a specific population health concern or health policy; "Individuals who have organized themselves around some common interest and who seek to influence [health concerns and] policy . . . . They clarify and articulate citizens' preferences, warn policy-makers of problems with their proposals, and suggest ways to make them more palatable" (Weissert & Weissert, as cited in Wakefield, 1999, p. 86)
Healthcare Personnel	People who are engaged in the provision of healthcare; healthcare personnel may organize as a special interest group
Policy Administrators	People charged with overseeing implementation of a health policy, including payers and funders

develop, live, learn, work, play, and age that have an influence on the extent of wellness, illness, and disease of the population. Population factors are influenced by the distribution of money, power, and resources at global, national, and local levels (Office of Disease Prevention and Health Promotion, n.d.).

Environments are structural and system determinants of health. Population factors are social determinants of health.

Health Policy

Health policy encompasses four dimensions, each of which has subdimensions. The separate access and utilization subdimensions of health policy focus underscore that although access is required for utilization of services by a population, access to those services does not necessarily mean that the services will be used by that population. For the purposes of this conceptual model, the emphasis is on what happens at a population level when a health policy is implemented in the form of population-centered nursologists' activities. These activities are targeted to improve population quality of life, rather than on how a policy comes to be.

Although access is necessary for utilization, access does not guarantee utilization.

Population Health Concern and Health Policy

The word "concern" refers to an issue that must be examined and, ideally, resolved. Concerns about health policy encompass issues of wellness, illness, and disease. Inclusion of historical, sociological, economic, and political subdimensions of the concept dimension of both population health concern and health policy highlights the ways in which a population health concern and health policy are understood in multiple disciplines. Ellenbecker et al. (2005) explained:

> Historical context is important because understanding patterns of how and why things happened in the past can shed light on society's plans for the future. . . . A sociological context is required because practices are shaped by beliefs and values of groups. . . . An economic context is required because [population health concerns and] policies are decisions about allocation of society's resources. . . . A political context is required because [population health concerns and] policies [occur] in the political arena. (p. 232)

Context for population health concerns and health policies includes historical, sociological, economic, and political perspectives.

Population-Centered Nursologists' Activities

The idea that nursologists' activities are population-centered extends the shift from patient-centered nursology to person-centered nursology (Clarke & Fawcett, 2013).

Given the importance of the cultural environment (a dimension of environments), nursologists' activities—including screening/assessment, planning, and intervention—must reflect *cultural awareness* ("[Nursologists'] recognition of their own culture and cultural differences among human beings"), *cultural sensitivity* ("Employing one's knowledge, consideration, understanding, respect, and tailoring after realizing awareness of self and others and encountering a diverse [population]"), *cultural humility* ("Actively listening to those from differing backgrounds while at the same time being attuned to what we are thinking and feeling about other cultures"), and *cultural competence* ("[Nursologists] . . . utilize cross-cultural knowledge and culturally sensitive skills in implementing culturally congruent [nursologists'] care"); see Drevdahl (2018, p. 149).

> *Population-centered nursologists' activities must reflect cultural awareness, cultural sensitivity, cultural humility, and cultural competence.*

Inasmuch as health encompasses wellness, illness, and disease, population-centered nursologists' activities are separated into promotion, restoration, and maintenance of wellness and prevention of illness and disease. This separation of activities avoids interpretation of health promotion as promotion (or restoration or maintenance) of illness or disease.

Population-centered nursologists' activities include the typical processes of assessment, planning, and intervention as well as screening. "Assessment" refers to a comprehensive examination of the population's health condition (wellness, illness, and disease), whereas "screening" is more narrowly focused on early diagnosis of illness and disease, often before any signs or symptoms become empirically evident (Venes, 2013).

> *Population-centered nursologists' activities include assessment, screening, planning, and intervention.*

Population Quality of Life

"Population quality of life" refers to the outcome of population-centered nursologists' activities and is used in place of the typical process component of evaluation. Wellness is a dimension of this concept, underscoring the importance of wellness as distinct from the usual elements of quality of life, which tend to emphasize extent of freedom from illness and disease (Venes, 2013).

> *Evaluation of population-centered nursologists' activities is determination of the outcome of population quality of life.*

RELATIONAL PROPOSITIONS

The propositions of the new conceptual model that state relations between the conceptual model concepts are depicted in Figure 7.1. The propositions are as follows:

1. The reciprocal relation between environments and population factors is related to the population health concern.
2. The relation between population factors and the population health concern is moderated by stakeholders.
3. The relation between the health policy and population-centered nursologists' activities is moderated by stakeholders.
4. There is a relation between population-centered nursologists' activities and population quality of life.

Proposition 1 is supported by Drevdahl's (2018) statement that economics, geography, and sociocultural factors (dimensions of environments) are linked with genetics (a dimension of population factors). Propositions 2 and 3 mean that the ideological, ethical, political, and/or pragmatic position taken by stakeholders can change the relation between the other concepts. The relation is nullified if the stakeholders' position is very strongly against the health policy, regardless of the importance or prevalence of the population health concern and the importance of a health policy to address that concern (proposition 2). Similarly, if the stakeholders' position is very strongly against the population-centered nursologists' activities, the desired population-centered nursologists' activities cannot be implemented regardless of the merits of the health policy or the nursologists' activities (proposition 3). Conversely, if the stakeholders' position is very strongly in favor of the health policy, then the importance and prevalence of the population health concern will influence development and implementation of the health policy (proposition 2) and the population-centered nursologists' activities will be developed and implemented in accordance with the mandates of the health policy (proposition 3). Clearly, "it behooves [us] to carefully determine the identity of the stakeholders, their concerns, and the very real pressure they could bring to bear upon [those who are charged with developing and implementing the health policy]" (Sudduth, 1999, p. 235). Proposition 4 links the population-centered nursologists' activities with population quality of life, which is the outcome of the health policy–mandated population-centered nursologists' activities.

In addition to the reciprocal relation between environments and population factors (Figure 7.1), the dimensions of population factors are interrelated (Figure 7.3) as are the dimensions of population quality of life (Figure 7.7).

■ Conclusion

The quadruple foci of the conceptual model emphasize the importance of health policy–mandated equity in population-centered nursologists' activities that lead to a high level of population quality of life. These foci are consistent with the mandates of the codes of ethics of many nursology associations worldwide. The new conceptual model now needs to be used to guide descriptive research to determine the content validity of the concepts and their dimensions and subdimensions. The new conceptual model also needs to be used to guide the derivation of middle range theories and situation-specific theories necessary for correlational and experimental research to test the relational propositions. Theory derivation and research require identification of theory concepts that can be logically linked with the conceptual model concepts and identification of existing or newly developed empirical measures of the theory concepts. Whether the new conceptual model will be a useful guide for evidence-based nursologists' practice depends, of course, on the findings of the research.

■ Critical Thinking Exercise

- Identify a contemporary population health concern.
- Think about how the new conceptual model of nursing for enhancing health equity and quality (The Conceptual Model of Nursology for Enhancing Equity and Quality: Population Health and Health Policy) could be used to guide a study about that population health concern. This will require linkage of specific, relevant theory concepts (variables) to each dimension and subdimension of each concept of the new conceptual model and linkage of the theory concepts to empirical measures.

■ Discussion Questions

1. What revisions would you recommend for the conceptual model, such as fewer or additional concepts, fewer or additional dimensions, and/or fewer or additional subdimensions?
2. Give some examples of the influence of stakeholders' influence on a health policy about an important contemporary population health concern.
3. What is the added value of the new conceptual model for studying population health concerns?
4. Why is health policy an important area of knowledge for all nursologists?

■ Resources

Agency for Healthcare Research and Quality: https://www.ahrq.gov
American Academy of Nursing: http://www.aannet.org/home
American Academy of Nursing Expert Panels: http://www.aannet.org/expert-panels
American Nurses Association Health Policy Page: https://www.nursingworld.org/practice-policy/health-policy
Centers for Disease Control and Prevention—National Center for Health Statistics: https://www.cdc.gov/nchs/nvss/index.htm
Institute for Healthcare Improvement: http://www.ihi.org
National Institutes of Health: https://www.nih.gov
National Institute of Nursing Research: https://www.ninr.nih.gov
Nursology.net: https://nursology.net
Office of Disease Prevention and Health Promotion—*Healthy People 2020*: https://www.healthypeople.gov
World Health Organization: http://www.who.int

■ References

Allen-Duck, A., Robinson, J. C., & Stewart, M. W. (2017). Healthcare quality: A concept analysis. *Nursing Forum, 52,* 377–386. doi:10.1111/nuf.12207

Braverman, P. (2014). What are health disparities and health equity? We need to be clear. *Public Health Reports, 129*(Suppl. 2), 5–8. doi:10.1177/00333549141291S203

Clarke, P. N., & Fawcett, J. (2013). Life as a nurse metatheorist. *Nursing Science Quarterly, 26,* 238–240. doi:10.1177/0894318413489185

Drevdahl, D. J. (2018). Cultural shifts: From cultural to structural theorizing in nursing. *Nursing Research, 67,* 146–160. doi:10.1097/NNR.0000000000000262

Ellenbecker, C. H., Fawcett, J., & Glazer, G. (2005). A nursing PhD specialty in health policy: University of Massachusetts Boston. *Policy, Politics, and Nursing Practice, 6,* 229–235. doi:10.1177/1527154405279146

Ellenbecker, C. H., Fawcett, J., Jones, E. J., Mahoney, D., Rowlands, B., & Waddell, A. (2017). A staged approach to educating nurses in health policy. *Policy, Politics, and Nursing Practice, 18,* 44–56. doi:10.1177/1527154417709254

Evans, R. G., & Stoddart, G. L. (1990). Producing health, consuming health care. *Social Science & Medicine, 31,* 1347–1363. doi:10.1016/0277-9536(90)90074-3

Fawcett, J., & AbuFannouneh, A. (2017). Thoughts about population health nursing research methods: Questions about participants and informed consent. *Nursing Science Quarterly, 30,* 353–355. doi:10.1177/0894318417724461

Fawcett, J., Aronowitz, T., AbuFannouneh, A., Al Usta, M., Fraley, H. E., Howlett, M. S. L., . . . Zhang, Y. (2015). Thoughts about the name of our discipline. *Nursing Science Quarterly, 28,* 330–333. doi:10.1177/0894318415599224

Fawcett, J., & Ellenbecker, C. H. (2015). A proposed conceptual model of nursing and population health. *Nursing Outlook, 63,* 288–298. doi:10.1016/j.outlook.2015.01.009

Fawcett, J., & Russell, G. (2001). A conceptual model of nursing and health policy. *Policy, Politics, and Nursing Practice, 2,* 108–116. doi:10.1177/152715440100200205

Furlong, E. A. (1999). Agenda setting. In J. A. Milstead (Ed.), *Health policy and politics: A nurse's guide* (pp. 43–75). Gaithersburg, MD: Aspen.

Groah, L. K., & Hader, A. L. (2019). Setting the agenda. In R. M. Patton, M. L. Zalon, & R. Ludwick (Eds.), *Nurses making policy: From bedside to boardroom* (2nd ed., pp. 163–191). New York, NY: Springer Publishing Company/American Nurses Association.

Keyes, K. M., & Galea, S. (2016). *Population health science.* New York, NY: Oxford University Press.

Kindig, D., & Stoddart, G. (2003). What is population health? *American Journal of Public Health, 93,* 380–383. doi:10.2105/AJPH.93.3.380

Matwick, A. L., & Woodgate, R. L. (2016). Social justice: A concept analysis. *Public Health Nursing, 34,* 176–184. doi:10.1111/phn.12288

McFarland, M. R., & Wehbe-Alamah, H. B. (2015). The theory of culture care diversity and universality. In. M. R. McFarland & H. B. Wehbe-Alamah (Eds.), *Leininger's culture care diversity and universality: A worldwide nursing theory* (3rd ed., pp. 1–34). Burlington, MA: Jones and Bartlett.

Milstead, J. A. (Ed.). (1999). *Health policy and politics: A nurse's guide.* Gaithersburg, MD: Aspen.

Nightingale, F. (1992). *Notes on nursing: What it is and what it is not* (Commemorative ed.). Philadelphia, PA: Lippincott. [Originally published 1859]

Office of Disease Prevention and Health Promotion. (n.d.). *Healthy people 2020: Social determinants of health.* Retrieved from https://www.healthypeople.gov/2020/topics-objectives/topic/social-determinants-of-health

Russell, G. E., & Fawcett, J. (2005). The conceptual model for nursing and health policy revisited. *Policy, Politics, and Nursing Practice, 6,* 319–326. doi:10.1177/1527154405283304

Saint Arnault, D. (2018). Defining and theorizing about culture: The evolution of the cultural determinants of health-seeking, revised. *Nursing Research, 67,* 161–168. doi:10.1097/NNR.0000000000000264

Stiefel, M., & Nolan, K. (2012). *A guide to measuring the triple aim: Population health, experience of care, and per capita cost. IHI Innovation Series White Paper.* Cambridge, MA: Institute for Healthcare Improvement. Retrieved from http://www.ihi. org/resources/Pages/IHIWhitePapers/AGuidetoMeasuringTripleAim.aspx

Stoto, M. A. (2013, February 21). *Population health in the Affordable Care Act era.* Retrieved from http://www.academyhealth.org/sites/default/files/publications/files/AH2013pophealth.pdf

Sudduth, A. L. (1999). Policy evaluation. In J. A. Milstead (Ed.), *Health policy and politics: A nurse's guide* (pp. 219–256). Gaithersburg, MD: Aspen.

Venes, D. (2013). *Taber's cyclopedic medical dictionary* (22nd ed.). Philadelphia, PA: F. A. Davis.

Wakefield, M. K. (1999). Government response: Legislation. In J. A. Milstead (Ed.), *Health policy and politics: A nurse's guide* (pp. 77–103). Gaithersburg, MD: Aspen.

Williams, S. D., & Phillips, J. M. (2019). Eliminating health inequities through national and global policy. In R. M. Patton, M. L. Zalon, & R. Ludwick (Eds.), *Nurses making policy: From bedside to boardroom* (2nd ed., pp. 391–422). New York, NY: Springer Publishing Company/American Nurses Association.

World Health Organization. (2017). *10 facts on health inequities and their causes.* Retrieved from https://www.who.int/features/factfiles/health_inequities/en

8 Integrating the Social Determinants of Health Into the Clinical Setting

Angela M. Moss and Christopher M. Nolan

CHAPTER OBJECTIVES

- Define the social determinants of health (SDOHs) and their relationship to achieving health equity
- Describe nursing's role in achieving health equity through nursing practice, education, research, and policy advocacy
- Demonstrate how healthcare organizations' prioritization of health equity can improve health outcomes

KEY CONCEPTS

Healthcare systems impacting health equity

Social determinants of health (SDOHs)

KEY TERMS

Academic–practice partnerships

Access

Built environment

Community health

Community partnerships

Health

Health equity

Health disparity

Health inequity

Healthcare systems

Nursing

Population health

Public health

Social determinants of health

Social policies

Politics

Wellness

■ Introduction

At the time of writing (2019), there are major shifts in how U.S. healthcare providers, health systems, insurers, policy makers, and the general public think about health. Consider this: U.S. healthcare costs in 2015 were over $3 trillion, equaling over 17% of the gross domestic product (GDP). In 1960, healthcare costs were only $27 billion, equaling just 5% of the GDP at that time (Amadeo, 2017). Across this same time frame, we have experienced tremendous technological advances in the detection and treatment of the leading causes of death in the

United States, such as cardiovascular disease and cancer. Yet this remarkable spending increase coupled with advances in healthcare technology does not correlate with improved health outcomes, and particularly so for underrepresented groups. Americans still have poorer health outcomes (Kindig, 2015), suggesting that our medical system is insufficient for ensuring better health. In other words, healthcare access and quality alone are not enough to improve health outcomes.

How can this be? Health policy experts suggest the SDOHs—factors such as socioeconomic status, education and employment opportunities, social support networks, and physical environment safety—play a much larger role on health outcomes than does clinical care. This is widely supported in the literature. Pincus, Esther, DeWalt, and Callahan (1998) conducted a 30-year review of studies comparing the United States (without universal healthcare access) and the United Kingdom (with universal healthcare access) and found that persons with lower socioeconomic status and lower education attainment had poorer health outcomes despite adequate access to healthcare. Another study by Zogg, Scott, Jiang, Wolf, and Haider (2016) found racial/ethnic disparities in health outcomes could be largely explained by insurance and income, where those with lower income had poorer outcomes. Lower income greatly increases one's risk for disease and premature death (Woolf et al., 2015), and income is more strongly related to health disparities than other demographic characteristics such as race or ethnicity (Dubay & Lebrun, 2012).

Across countries with widely varying sociopolitical context, economies, and healthcare systems, access to quality healthcare *combined with* improved SDOHs are the two key interrelated factors to improve the health of populations (Flato & Zhang, 2016; Korda, Clements, & Kelman, 2009; Krieger, Barbeau, & Soobader, 2005; Rodney & Hill, 2014). This suggests healthcare organizations must focus attention on social needs in order to achieve healthy outcomes for patients. Naysayers might say it is impossible for healthcare organizations and health professionals alone to impact the social determinants affecting health for *all* of society. This is true. On the macrolevel, societal change must be facilitated by policy makers, researchers, economists, community leaders, and individuals. Collectively these groups can work toward improving social structures to subsequently improve health. However, on the microlevel, healthcare providers have the power to address individual disparities at the point of care, and healthcare organizations can provide the structure and means to do so. The days where healthcare systems and professionals treat individuals only when they are sick are over.

■ CONCEPTS

Over the years, a variety of terms have been used to describe intersecting concepts related to the SDOHs and health equity. To frame our discussion, we present these terms here with their common definitions and brief context.

SOCIAL DETERMINANTS OF HEALTH

The SDOHs are the conditions in which people are born, grow, live, work, and age (World Health Organization [WHO], 2018). SDOH factors are loosely categorized into five main areas. These are: (a) the physical environment and safety or "built

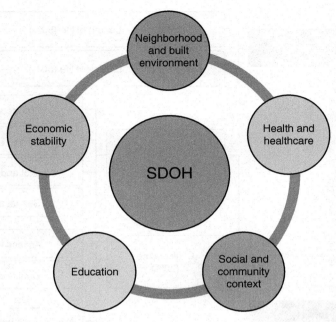

FIGURE 8.1 SOCIAL DETERMINANTS OF HEALTH.

Source: From Office of Disease Prevention and Health Promotion. (n.d.-b). *Social determinants of health.* Retrieved from https://www.healthypeople.gov/2020/topics-objectives/topic/social-determinants-of-health

environment"; (b) economic stability; (c) education access and attainment; (d) family and social support; and (e) access to quality healthcare. See Figure 8.1 for the *Healthy People 2020* diagram depicting common SDOH categories.

The SDOHs are influenced by the distribution of resources and are largely responsible for health inequities. For example, when a community is underresourced regarding food resulting in a food desert, people living in that community are more likely to have poor health outcomes related to poor diet.

SDOHs are greatly influenced by policies, systems, and environments, and it is difficult to quantify their influence on health outcomes. Public health experts generally agree that clinical care accounts for only 10% to 20% of the modifiable contributors to overall health outcomes (Hood, Gennuso, Swain, & Catlin, 2016). According to the University of Wisconsin Population Health Institute (UWPHI, 2018) County Health Rankings Model, 80% of health outcomes are influenced by nonclinical care factors—the physical environment accounts for 10%, social and economic factors for 40%, and health behaviors for 30% (UWPHI, 2018; see Figure 8.2). It is difficult to accurately measure how much any given factor influences health outcomes, but suffice it to say healthcare access and quality have a relatively small influence when considering all influencers of health outcomes.

HEALTH DISPARITY

A "health disparity" is a difference in health outcomes between groups within a population (Dubay & Lebrun, 2012). According to the Centers for Disease Control and Prevention (CDC), health disparities are preventable differences in the burden of disease,

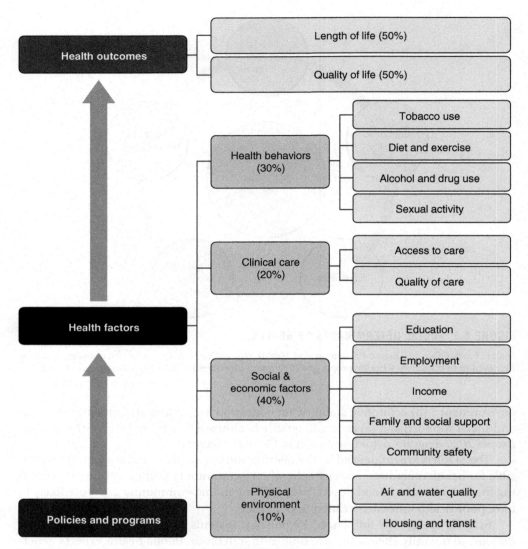

FIGURE 8.2 COUNTY HEALTH RANKINGS AND ROAD MAPS.

Source: From County Health Rankings & Roadmaps. (2016). County Health Rankings model [Image file]. Retrieved from https://www.countyhealthrankings.org/county-health-rankings-model. © 2014 UWPHI. Reprinted with permission from University of Wisconsin Population Health Institute.

injury, violence, or opportunities to achieve optimal health that are experienced by socially disadvantaged populations (CDC, 2008). Health disparities are often caused by SDOHs such as poverty, unemployment, systemic racism, lack of access to healthy food, insecure housing, and low educational attainment (WHO, 2008).

An example of a health disparity is a difference in life expectancy between individuals in one part of a city and those in another. Examples of this phenomenon can be found in many large cities where life expectancy changes dramatically in very small geographic areas such as a few stops on the public transportation system (Ansell, 2017; WHO, 2018). For example in Chicago, the Loop enjoys a life expectancy of 85 years, whereas the community of West Garfield Park, just a few train stops west, is at 69 years (Rush, 2016). Oftentimes microlevel data illuminating health disparities is lost in large aggregated data sets. To help address this problem related to geographic disparities, the Robert Wood Johnson Foundation (RWJF) U.S. Small-area Life Expectancy Estimates Project (USALEEP) created a useful tool to examine health disparities at the hyperlocal or neighborhood levels in the United States (RWJF, n.d.). Similarly, the U.S. Department of Health and Human Services Office of Minority Health has many resources examining health disparities as well as a catalog of what is being done at state and local levels to advance health equity "at every point of contact" (U.S. Department of Health and Human Services Office of Minority Health, 2019).

HEALTH INEQUITY

A "health inequity" is defined as an avoidable and unnecessary systematic difference in health between populations that is unjust (WHO, 2008). You will note the similarity to the definition of a health disparity, and in fact, many experts, including the CDC, use these terms interchangeably (MPH@GW Staff, 2018). A helpful way to think of these terms is health disparities often lead to a lack of health equity, or health inequities. Similar to health disparities, health inequities are considered unfair and unjust and could be reduced by improved policies and resources.

An example of an avoidable health inequity is HIV infection rates among African Americans, whereby almost half of all new infections occur in this group, although African Americans represent only about 13% of the U.S. population and there is no genetic or biological reason for this difference (WHO, 2017). Long-term systemic health disparities, poor public policies, gaps in SDOH needs, and structural racism are factors, among others, that have contributed to this health inequity outcome. In short, health inequities are more than lack of equal resources, but they also refer to the inequalities that infringe on fairness and human rights norms (WHO, 2008).

HEALTH EQUITY

"Health equity" is achieved when everyone has a fair opportunity to attain their full health potential (Wyatt, Laderman, Botwinick, Mate, & Whittington, 2016). No one is disadvantaged because of their socially determined circumstance. This requires removing obstacles to health such as poverty and discrimination while creating access to good jobs with fair pay, quality education and housing, safe environments, and quality healthcare. Health equity is the ultimate goal. It is important to note that some populations or groups need more support in order to achieve health equity. This is due to the socioeconomic structures producing social, economic, or environmental disadvantages, which unfairly and adversely affect groups of people. Therefore achieving equity cannot be accomplished through treating everyone equally, but must be achieved by addressing underlying issues and meeting individual needs of underserved and vulnerable populations (MPH@GW Staff, 2018).

POPULATION HEALTH

"Population health" is defined as the health outcomes of a group of individuals, including the distribution of such outcomes within the group (Kindig & Stoddart, 2003). Groups can be defined based on geography such as nations or communities, but can also be others such as ethnic or age groups, patients, employees, prisoners, gender, and so on. Policy makers and change agents are particularly interested in health outcomes among various populations as these guide and inform health policy and programs.

BUILT ENVIRONMENT

The "built environment" is an umbrella term used to describe where people live, work, and play. Healthcare providers who work in nontraditional healthcare settings, in other words beyond the hospital and clinic walls, are said to work in the built environment or provide localized care. One example is a school nurse partnering with a local high school to teach teens safe-sex principles. Another example is a primary care clinic located in a low-income housing complex for mothers and children.

ECONOMIC STABILITY

Not to be confused with the macroeconomic financial term, in the context of the SDOHs, "economic stability" refers to the financial resources people have available to them. Poor economic stability can limit access to nutritious foods, safe neighborhoods and stable housing, and educational opportunities, which in turn can negatively affect health outcomes. For example, older adults with poor economic stability might live in a neighborhood with frequent criminal activity and so they might not walk outside, which may negatively affect physical and mental health.

EDUCATION ACCESS AND ATTAINMENT

"Education access" refers to the structures and resources available to a group or individual to pursue knowledge and/or formal education. "Educational attainment" refers to the highest degree or level of completed education an individual achieves. In relation to health, an individual with poor education access, and consequently low educational attainment, will more likely have poorer health outcomes (Zimmerman, Woolf, & Haley, 2015).

FAMILY AND SOCIAL SUPPORT

"Social support" means having friends and other people, including family, with whom one communicates and connects regularly in a meaningful way. These regular connections lead to a broader focus on life and more positive self-image. Family and social support networks are also often those to whom individuals might turn in times of need or crisis. It is well established in the literature that individuals with strong family and/or social support networks have improved health outcomes (Reblin & Uchino, 2008).

ACCESS TO QUALITY HEALTHCARE

"Access to healthcare" means "the timely use of personal health services to achieve the best health outcomes" (Millman, 1993, p. 4). Access to care is a key component to promoting and maintaining health, preventing and managing disease, reducing unnecessary disability and premature death, and achieving health equity (Office of Disease Prevention and Health Promotion, 2019).

◼ Individual Practice to Address SDOHs

In 2010, the Institute of Medicine issued a landmark report titled the *Future of Nursing* identifying nurses as integral to America's complex healthcare system (Institute of Medicine, 2011). The report recognized nurses' unique position to promote wellness at individual and population levels, and also highlighted the need for nurses to practice to the full scope of their education and license (Donelan, DesRoches, Dittus, & Buerhaus, 2013; Strout, 2012). The SDOHs easily resonate with nurses given that nursing's educational and practice metaparadigm recognizes that health outcomes are affected by conditions outside the healthcare system. Yet it can be overwhelming and even frightening for clinicians to assume responsibility for issues traditionally outside their expertise or current accountability structure. Let us consider the context of practice, education, research, and policy advocacy for ways individual healthcare providers can address the SDOHs in their patient populations.

PRACTICE

Individuals working in healthcare sectors have an opportunity to assess and address SDOHs with every patient interaction. It often takes just a few moments to screen a patient for needs relating to the SDOHs. For example, healthcare providers could ask patients: "Do you currently have a place to stay/live?" "Are you worried that your food will run out before you have more to buy?" "Do you have refrigeration to keep your food fresh?" "Do you have money to pay for your medicine?" "Do you have transportation to/from your medical appointments?" and so forth. Some providers may feel reticence asking these questions because they do not want to embarrass patients, or worse, because they fear inadequacy addressing an identified need.

Integration of interactive social service reference tools such as NowPow into healthcare systems is one way to address these issues. NowPow is a powerful, web-based resource for social services and resources for SDOH needs (NowPow, 2018). For example, a provider can quickly search and find local resources for food insecurity, such as food pantries, or for exercise, such as fitness classes. There are several integrated tech solution options similar to NowPow, such as Healthify, Aunt Bertha, and Pieces (Cartier, Fichtenberg, & Gottlieb, 2019). Using technology to integrate SDOH screening and action plans has two distinct advantages. First, electronic health record (EHR) systems can prompt all healthcare providers to screen for SDOHs with standardized questions, thereby eliminating some of the reticence to asking. Second, the platforms like NowPow interface offers immediate referral information for local community services on topics related to identified need, thereby removing that fear of not being able to address the need(s) that arise(s).

While referral tools are very useful, it is our experience that sometimes a simple referral is not enough, particularly for more vulnerable individuals. In these cases, successful referral processes frequently include social needs care providers such as social workers who assess an individual's unique situation and needs, identify relevant resources and care providers, provide education on accessing that service, and update care plans accordingly to ensure the entire team is coordinated. EHRs and other tools described earlier can facilitate this process.

On a grander scale, developing and contributing to innovative care delivery models leveraging the built environment are other ways individuals can address SDOHs among patient populations. We present this example. Beginning in 2009, Rush University College of Nursing Faculty Practice partnered with a local Chicago business to design and implement an innovative primary care and wellness program for low-income workers at a foodservice industrial facility (Moss, 2017).

Foodservice workers represent one of the fastest growing groups within the service industry workforce (Bureau of Labor Statistics, 2019) and are among the lowest wage earners in the country with a median hourly wage of $9.04 (annual salary $18,803; National Employment Law Project, 2012). As outlined earlier in our SDOH discussion, lower income increases one's risk for disease and premature death (Woolf et al., 2015), as does lack of time for routine healthcare due to work schedule constraints and lack of affordable health insurance (Faghri, Kotejoshyer, Cherniack, Reeves, & Punnett, 2010; Wang, Chen, Hsu, & Wang, 2012). Low-income employees such as foodservice workers are therefore at a higher risk for chronic diseases such as hypertension, dyslipidemia, and diabetes, and even premature death (Harris, Huang, Hannon, & Williams, 2011; Woolf et al., 2015), suggesting additional resources beyond standard access to healthcare services are needed to address these health disparities and inequity.

The mission of the program is to provide quality, comprehensive, and cost-effective primary care and wellness services in a built environment, the worksite, to meet the needs of the diverse employee population. But in addition to providing primary care, the program staff partners with the employer to influence things that affect employee health, including the SDOHs. For example, most employees expressed difficulty obtaining nutritious food for themselves and their families. This was in part due to unpredictable shift schedules making it difficult to plan meals, but also due to lack of financial resources and the availability of grocery stores with healthy food options. Access to healthy food was addressed via the worksite clinic and employer by creating a nutritious, subsidized food program in the employee cafeteria.

In this example, program staff was able to inform employer policy to address an SDOH need, food insecurity, and the results have been striking. This small, microlevel policy change within the worksite, or the built environment, has influenced health outcomes such as improved blood pressure and diabetes control, decreased average waist circumference, and improved overall productivity. As a result, this program has been nationally recognized as an innovative nurse-led model of care and has been successfully replicated in similar built environments such as schools, housing communities, and other worksites. Within these new settings, the nurse-led care delivery model includes processes in place to assess and address the SDOHs in partnership with the built environment key stakeholders.

EDUCATION ON THE SDOHS FOR THE HEALTH PROFESSIONS

Social change to achieve health equity must happen across sectors—government, business and economics, community organizations, education, and healthcare systems. Healthcare professionals are ideal champions to engage in and lead these changes because they see firsthand the impact social policies have on their individual practice and on the health of the populations they serve. But in order to be effective, healthcare professionals must learn and maintain core competencies related to health policy, health disparities, and health equity.

Most core learning competencies for healthcare professions include principles relating to health equity, advocacy, and leadership. In nursing, educators look to the Quad Council Coalition (QCC) of Public Health Nursing Organizations' core competencies, which are as follows:

1. Monitor health status to identify and solve community health problems.
2. Diagnose and investigate health problems and health hazards in the community.
3. Inform, educate, and empower people about health issues.
4. Mobilize community partnerships and action to identify and solve health problems.
5. Develop policies and plans that support individual and community health efforts.
6. Enforce laws and regulations that protect health and ensure safety.
7. Link people to needed personal health services and ensure the provision of healthcare when otherwise unavailable.
8. Ensure competent public and personal healthcare workforce.
9. Evaluate effectiveness, accessibility, and quality of personal and population-based health services.
10. Research for new insights and innovative solutions to health problems
(Quad Council Coalition Competency Review Task Force, 2018).

These competencies are focused on nursing, but recognize most health professional education programs, such as for health administrators, physicians, and social work, address the link between health policy and improved health outcomes, and incorporate health policy leadership competencies into their programs (Heiman, Smith, McKool, Mitchell, & Bayer, 2015). At Rush University, an interprofessional elective titled "Health Equity and New Models of Care" aims to introduce students to concepts of health equity, social determinants, care coordination, and health policy. The first class begins with an article encompassing an interview with New York University professor and sociologist Eric Klinenberg regarding his book *Heat Wave* (Klinenberg, 2002). The interview provides students with an introduction to healthcare challenges specific to the city of Chicago—given many of the graduate students are new to the city proper—and in particular the disastrous 1995 Chicago heat wave in which over 700 individuals died. The Chicago heat wave is an example as to how a natural disaster became a social disaster, and how systemic health inequities led to disparities as to who was affected by the treacherous heat wave—those who were older, those who were socially isolated, those who were Black, and those who did not feel safe. In the end, Black older adults died at a rate 1.5 times greater than their White counterparts (Klinenberg, 2002).

Beginning in the first session, class discussion centers around the concept of natural disaster versus social disaster, and who bears the responsibility to ensure public health and well-being. Is it government, nonprofit, or corporate entities, for example, or does responsibility sit solely with individuals? The discussion begins with the simple question, Is housing healthcare? Just a few students' hands trickle into the air with an affirmative response, a bit unsure. The next question is posed, How about food—is food healthcare? A few more hands go into the air.

The class having generally acknowledged that housing and food are both integral to healthcare, the question is asked: Have you ever been asked by your healthcare provider about basic needs like this? Not one hand rises. Are healthcare institutions required to tackle these needs as components of overall health? The discussion begins, and a robust semester focused on health equity follows. The elective course serves as an introduction to health equity and is based around a community project, where the students are able to: apply their learnings about equity, disparities, and community health needs; implement tools such as a needs assessment, strengths, weaknesses, opportunities, and threats analysis; and provide a memo of recommendations for the organization. In a way, this is a method by which the students can see how health ought to be viewed broadly similarly to that of the WHO definition, and also see that health goes beyond the four walls of a hospital, and in some cases into community organizations or the built environment. This allows students to implement a health equity framework and think about how they can bring these concepts to their day-to-day lives. Some students have continued their projects as independent studies as well as doctoral projects, while others have helped to implement their recommendations with the aim of achieving better health equity.

RESEARCH

Healthcare researchers must construct research programs that develop and evaluate evidence-based solutions to health disparities caused by SDOH factors largely outside the traditional healthcare intervention scope (Srinivasan & Williams, 2014). This is a challenge because it may be difficult to investigate because of funding constraints or difficulty obtaining buy-in from key stakeholders such as community partners. On the corporate side, many hospitals have yet to routinely collect SDOH data, but it is evident that the concept of health equity is becoming the new normal. As examples, the American Hospital Association recently renamed the Institute for Diversity to the Institute for Diversity and Health Equity (American Hospital Association, 2018), and the Institute for Healthcare Improvement (IHI) created the Pursuing Equity Collaborative (IHI, 2018). At Rush University, the Office of Community Engagement was created and staffed with several high-level administrative personnel, all with the purpose of addressing the SDOHs (Rush, 2016). Naming a department with a presumed allocation of resources to fund it are steps in the right direction, and the justification for this allocation of resources is because research has demonstrated that connecting patients to community/social resources from the clinical setting can make a true, positive impact on health outcomes (Lindau et al., 2016).

From a different angle, consider this example of a study conducted that was not designed to explore SDOHs, but nevertheless stumbled upon them. A 2017 study explored the impact of worksite access to primary care on a low-income foodservice employee population. The first significant finding was that workers who had higher education, higher income, or who were White were the most likely to have better health-seeking behaviors (healthcare utilization and satisfaction) and health outcomes (workforce sustainability). Food production workers who were primarily minority and who had the lowest incomes compared to the other work categories were most likely to have poorer health-seeking behavior (healthcare utilization and satisfaction) and poorer health outcomes (health-related quality of life; see Moss, 2017).

These results support earlier findings about SDOHs, that access to healthcare services and inequity in health outcomes are interrelated factors in the equation (Flato & Zhang, 2016; Pincus et al., 1998; Rodney & Hill, 2014; Zogg et al., 2016). Further, it illustrates how research can contribute to the development of new questions relating to SDOHs. This in turn creates opportunity for improved approaches and standards of healthcare to address these disparities that otherwise might have continued unnoticed and unaddressed. Continually developing clinical questions and new data around the SDOHs is critical for continuing to make progress toward illuminating and addressing health disparities and health inequities.

POLICY ADVOCACY

Healthcare organizations and government agencies are increasingly focused on managing patient populations to improve population health outcomes (Meyer, 2017) and are more focused on using big data to do so (Schneeweiss, 2014). Using big data to track the intersection of care delivery and the SDOHs is important (Goar, 2017). Without this information, we are unable to determine whether our interventions are making a difference. Recently, individual providers advocated that the Medical Coding rule allow nurses and social workers, in addition to prescribers, to assign ICD-10 diagnosis codes to identifying the SDOHs. These are known as "Z codes" and cover issues such as illiteracy, unemployment, homelessness, inadequate housing, and lack of adequate food and safe drinking water (WHO, 2015).

Unfortunately, the use of the ICD-10 Z codes is not widely practiced, as their collection has not to date been incentivized. Some hospitals are beginning to use them to track information, but often this does not make up for capturing the data in the medical record to address a need at the point of care. However, this information can still be used to further inform policy makers interested in advocating for the social health needs of patients, or used by hospitals or health systems for quality improvement or program development purposes. Imagine the positive difference this policy change has made implementing an SDOH coding and tracking mechanism within the ICD-10 system.

■ Health Systems Evolving to Address SDOHs
....

The WHO defines health as a "state of complete physical, mental, and social well being and not merely the absence of disease or infirmity" (WHO, 2008, p. 33). While this definition is not new, it is evident that healthcare organizations have not routinely tackled this definition in full scope. The focus historically has been on the physical realm, leaving mental and social well-being interventions fragmented and disconnected (Lindau, 2016). However, healthcare organizations have a key role to play in addressing the SDOHs to achieve health equity, and are beginning to think about the care they provide with the WHO definition in mind, treating patients for social need, as many providers believe that social need leads to worse health outcomes (RWJF, 2011).

This has not been an overnight change, but rather has progressed slowly. One major indicator of this change is the shift from fee-for-service payment models to value-based care; and hospital systems are discovering that addressing SDOHs through value-based care decreased overall expenditures (Pruitt, Emechebe, Quast, Taylor, & Bryant, 2018). Government payers and private insurers also recognize a global approach to health equity saves money in the long run. This is because our traditional fee-for-service model encourages volume, but not always quality. It is without doubt that providers care about their patients' well-being. But all too often care management structures are not in place, and the incentives for payment are connected to productivity and how many people are seen, rather than quality of outcomes and what occurs during the said visit (Popescu, 2014). An example was in the development and implication of the Hospital Readmission Reduction Program, in which hospitals can be penalized for "excess" readmissions as per the Centers for Medicare and Medicaid Services (CMS; American Hospital Association, 2018).

This turn to quality, as the standard of the Patient Protection and Affordable Care Act (ACA) penalizes providers and healthcare institutions by limiting or eliminating financial reimbursements depending on health outcomes. Specifically, reimbursement is withheld for clinical situations that are deemed preventable. As per the American Hospital Association's stance on the Readmission Reduction program, there is much literature demonstrating connecting social determinants and readmissions such as income, insurance status, and access to pharmacies. In a recent Becker's Hospital Review article regarding a study from Connance, social determinants contributed to more than 50% of readmissions (Gooch, 2018). While this incentivizes hospitals with resources to invest in initiatives and community collaborations to identify and mitigate the impact of adverse SDOHs, the penalties have also reduced resources at some safety-net hospitals with high readmission rates potentially due to factors outside the hospitals' control (Castellucci & Caruso, 2019; Chaiyachati, Qi, & Werner, 2018).

Furthermore, since the adoption of the ACA or Obamacare, we are seeing more focus on keeping people well through new innovative models such as the rise of patient-centered medical homes (PCMHs), accountable care organizations (ACOs), medical neighborhoods, and most recently the federal Centers for Medicare and Medicaid Innovation (CMMI) Accountable Health Communities pilot. These shifts are beginning to tackle the WHO definition of health, in particular as we look at the fact that for far too long our institutions have not been well equipped to tackle SDOH needs.

In 2017, the IHI, a quality improvement think tank based out of Boston founded by former CMS administrator Don Berwick, created the Pursuing Equity Collaborative (IHI, 2018). The collaborative's main aim is to bring together representative organizations from across the United States to think about how to enhance equity within their respective organizations. The nine organizations in the program include Rush University Medical Center in Chicago, Brigham and Women's Hospital/South Jamaica Plains Health Center in Boston, Health Partners in Minnesota, Henry Ford Health System in Detroit, Kaiser Permanente in Northern California, Mainline Health in Philadelphia, Northwest Colorado Health, and Vidant Health in Greenville, South Carolina. These healthcare organizations have made health equity a strategic priority and have allocated resources accordingly to build structures and processes supporting the work.

With their successes, we see more organizations and associations committing to health equity initiatives, including most notably the American Hospital Association leading the #123forEquity Pledge as an extension of the National Call to Action to Eliminate Healthcare Disparities by the American Hospital Association, the American College of Healthcare Executives, the Association of American Medical Colleges, Catholic Health Association of the United States, and America's Essential Hospitals (American Hospital Association, 2019).

ORGANIZATIONAL NEEDS

To guide healthcare organizations in this work, the IHI has developed a five-component framework to guide organizations to impact health equity (Wyatt et al., 2016). These are: (a) make health equity a strategic priority; (b) develop structures and processes to support health equity work; (c) address determinants of health that healthcare organizations can directly impact; (d) decrease institutional racism within the organization; and (e) develop partnerships with community organizations (IHI, 2016). Furthermore, hospitals, as per the ACA, must conduct Triennial Community Health Needs Assessments (Internal Revenue Service [IRS], 2018). Through this process, the hospital determines the main health needs of the community it serves, and develops a Community Health Implementation Plan to address them. While the plan is particularly focused on the community, many hospitals are marrying their clinical care with the determined health needs of the population in a data-driven approach.

Evolving our existing health systems to address SDOHs requires significant culture change. While community health and population health have always been key tenets of community health centers, the majority of clinical care in the United States is provided from primary care practices, hospitals, and outpatient practices whose organizational strategy and culture are predominantly built on a foundation of episodic care and fee-for-service payment mechanisms (Parmelli et al., 2011; Wellman, Jeffries, & Hagan, 2017). The shift requires additional resources and an expansion of who is deemed a member of the care team, and who is involved in the planning and evaluation of initiatives. Ideally, these expanded teams include community stakeholders and enable meaningful collaboration across disciplines and sectors. By leveraging existing local coalitions and identifying meaningful ways to include community-based perspectives, clinicians and others within healthcare institutions can leverage their institution's power and assets while also efficiently building on progress.

While the payment changes described earlier (moving toward value-based care reimbursement models) do make it easier to create a business proposition for investing in such SDOH initiatives (Health Leads, 2019), these investments are often preventive in nature and are seeds leading to longer term impact, which is not always reflected in short-term reductions in ED visits or in healthcare costs. Because these outcome measures can be slow to change, it is important for program innovators to be creative in identifying other relevant outcomes (e.g., organizational pain points) and ways that SDOH initiatives influence them. For instance, universal screenings for transportation challenges may help prevent appointment no-shows, thereby easing clinic operations and maximizing revenue. Because of these sustainability challenges, it is critical for organizations to make institutional commitment to the work, which could manifest as anchor mission statements or reducing disparities in outcomes as part of the organization's strategic plan and Community Health Implementation Plan (Rush, 2016; Rush University Medical Center, 2017).

Applying change leadership principles to SDOH work suggests building a "guiding coalition" that includes diverse internal and external stakeholders (Pollack & Pollack, 2015; Weber & Joshi, 2000). Stakeholder diversity includes interprofessional healthcare providers as well as nonclinic staff, patients, and families. Global, diverse teams increase the likelihood the intervention will be relevant, feasible, and adopted. Engaging executive sponsors throughout the process helps ensure SDOH initiatives are aligned with institutional priorities and opportunities, such as fundraising campaigns or high-level strategic planning. Involving external healthcare, community-based, and governmental stakeholders ensures that the initiative does not duplicate existing services and can amplify the impact of your efforts by strengthening the community's role (Figure 8.3).

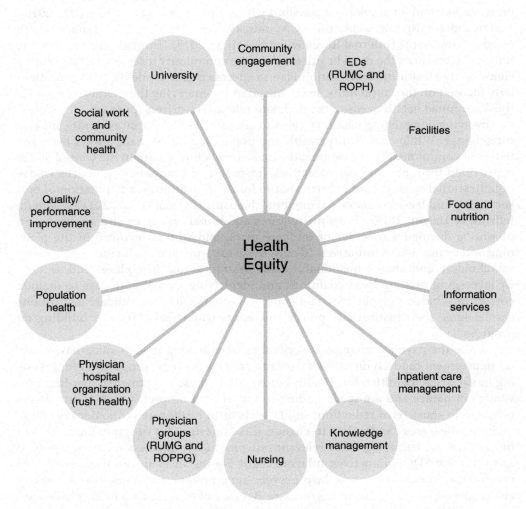

FIGURE 8.3 EXAMPLE FROM RUSH UNIVERSITY OF INTERNAL PARTNERSHIPS TO ADDRESS SDOHs.

ROPH, Rush Oak Park Hospital; ROPPG, Rush Oak Park Physicians Group; RUMC, Rush University Medical Center; RUMG, Rush University Medical Group; SDOHs, social determinants of health.

EXEMPLARS

In Exemplars 8.1, 8.2, and 8.3, we present a few examples of how healthcare organizations are incorporating SDOHs and health equity initiatives into their organizations.

Exemplar 8.1: Partnerships for Health

Partnerships are critical to improving health—no one organization can tackle this by itself. We offer this example. The Alliance for Health Equity (AHE), formerly the Health Impact Collaborative of Cook County, formed in 2015 as a reaction to the need for charitable hospitals and health systems to complete a community health needs assessment as per the ACA and IRS 501(r) guidelines (IRS, 2018). In the IRS guidelines, it is suggested that hospitals can complete a comprehensive needs assessment, and that led to the formation of what is now known as the AHE. In 2016, for the first time, 26 hospitals throughout Chicago and Cook County including Advocate Health (now Advocate Aurora Health), Loyola University Medical Center, Presence Health (now AMITA), and Rush University Medical Center all worked together to complete a needs assessment, settling on four main needs—social and structural determinants of health, chronic disease, access to care and community resources, and behavioral health (AHE, 2019).

This partnership was instrumental for these organizations, normally competitors, but they believe that there was power in partnership and collaboration. It was also very important to see social and structural determinants of health being acknowledged as the largest health need for their communities. This led to an even larger contingent for the 2019 Coummunity Health Needs Assessment (CHNA), as all major charitable hospitals and health systems are participating in the partnership. Other workgroups that formed as a result of the 2016 CHNA were focused on access, food, policy, social determinants, data, and mental health. Some successes of the AHE included widespread support for Illinois to pass Tobacco 21 legislation as well as helping the health systems and community partners come together around proposed changes to Public Charge legislation, a food insecurity scan, and trauma-informed guidelines.

Exemplar 8.2 Food Is Health

Rush, along with many other organizations in Chicago and Cook County, is committed to addressing food security for patients and community members. Rush is helping lead in this space in the region as a leadership member of the AHE as well as West Side United (WSU). WSU is a collaborative based in Chicago's West Side with an aim "to make their neighborhoods stronger, healthier and more vibrant places to live. It is comprised of healthcare institutions, residents, civic leaders, community-based organizations, businesses, and faith-based institutions" (WSU, 2019).

(*continued*)

Since its adoption of its Community Health Improvement Plan, Rush has taken a three-pronged approach to addressing food insecurity—thinking about patients, community members, and employees (Rush, 2016). In its internal efforts, Rush has begun questioning patients about food security through its Social Determinant of Health Screening tool. Rush is asking patients a tweaked version of the evidence-based Hunger Vital Signs questionnaire in partnership with the Greater Chicago Food Depository and West Side ConnectED.

Early results of the screener have demonstrated that food insecurity is the greatest social need for our primary care patients. Upon asking the questions, which for many health systems is a challenge in and of itself, patients can receive a direct referral to a food pantry such as the Oak Park River Forest Food Pantry, or a connection to an innovative nonprofit providing produce and proteins at lower costs for consumers in their own neighborhoods—Top Box Foods. The aim here is to think about food as health. How can one expect a patient to manage diabetes or heart failure without nutrition? Given this, Rush also recently partnered with AgeOptions in the western suburbs and was awarded a Federal Association for Community Living Grant to pursue a meal delivery program for higher risk older adults.

In addition to thinking about food needs of patients, Rush is committed to improving food security for our first community, our employees and students, as well as our surrounding communities. In 2016, Rush began a partnership with Top Box Foods to better address food insecurity with our employees and students. Top Box Foods is a nonprofit partner with a mission to make "healthy affordable food accessible to all" (Top Box Foods, 2018, "Our Goal"). In 2015, led by a nurse leader at Rush Oak Park Hospital, Rush began what is known as the Rush Surplus Project. This innovative program partners with the medical center and employee volunteers to pack all unused food from Rush's cafeterias and deliver the meals three times a week to the Oak Park River Forest Food Pantry and Franciscan Outreach, which is the second largest emergency shelter in the City of Chicago. In 2017, Rush provided just under 25,000 meals to community members in need.

Exemplar 8.3 Housing Is Health

The Camden Coalition was founded in 2002 by a family physician, Dr. Jeffrey Brenner, with the aim to address complex social needs of patients in partnership with other organizations. In 2015, the coalition launched its Housing First Program, which included 50 state-supplied vouchers to house individuals. Brenner has been quoted saying, "Housing is the best pill, the best scan, more powerful than surgery" (Camden Coalition, 2015).

A successful pilot housing program example can be found in a partnership between Rush and the Center for Housing and Health, a subsidiary of the AIDS Foundation of Chicago. Both organizations engage multidisciplinary teams to assess and place patients identified with high levels of low acuity needs. The

(continued)

hypothesis is that patients with low acuity needs but high levels of ED visits and/or inpatient admissions are more than likely experiencing a nonmedical challenge, most likely homelessness.

The pilot involves social workers from ambulatory settings and the ED conducting case reviews and specific assessments to determine potential appropriateness for the program.

Once assessed and identified as homeless, patients' profiles are presented before a panel consisting of medical providers (physicians, nurses, psychiatrists) for additional discussion and review. Following review, the team is joined by outreach workers, case managers, and others to provide intensive supportive services to ensure that patients are housed in temporary housing, working toward permanent supportive housing. At the time of writing (2019), there have been 38 proposed patients with five enrolled resulting in 13 ED visits and one hospital visit avoided. This has resulted in a total program saving of $231,084, but a program cost of only $50,000. The average referral time span to temporary housing is about 46 days and to permanent housing about 110 days. Much of this success is attributed to engaging an interdisciplinary group of healthcare professionals from diverse fields, thereby ensuring work is conducted in a coordinated fashion toward a common goal for the patient.

Health Is Well-Being

All of the exemplars described earlier view people's health as more than health status. Rather than being concerned only with reducing disparities in, say, diabetes A1C levels, a holistic view of health equity demands that we also look at disparities among other nonmedical indicators, such as having basic needs met, confidence in navigating the system and managing one's care plan, attainment of patient-identified goals, maintenance of functional status, or satisfaction with care. This holistic framing of health requires a broad, multipronged approach to promoting health equity: from models that identify and address needs through collaboration between interprofessional providers (e.g., nurses and social workers) in an effort to meet an individual's needs, to broader coalitions and partnerships to address systemic barriers to well-being in an effort to minimize the need for individual interventions in the first place.

◼ Conclusion

Public health experts generally agree that clinical care accounts for only 10% to 20% of the modifiable contributors to overall health outcomes (Hood et al., 2016). Individuals, institutions, and even our government see value in new commitment to social care in order to achieve health equity. Even the Secretary of the U.S. Department of Health and Human Services, Alex Azar, recently delivered remarks at the Hatch Foundation for Civility and Solutions and stated, "What if we provided solutions for the whole person, including addressing housing, nutrition and other social needs?" (2018, para. 30). Azar went on to talk about addressing multiple needs, not just one or an acute illness, and delivered similar remarks at the Commonwealth Foundation (Azar, 2018).

We can no longer conduct the business of healthcare in a vacuum, treating individuals only when they are sick and by addressing only physical health. Health inequities must be addressed by healthcare systems just as we would address any disease, and we must commit to connecting patients to resources addressing their social needs. The SDOHs are not just an abstract societal problem. Healthcare organizations and individuals should, and must, take responsibility for addressing them in order to achieve health equity for all. As one of the largest sectors of our economy (Sisko et al., 2019), if healthcare does not step up, who will?

■ Critical Thinking Exercises

1. You are the healthcare provider caring for a young child with asthma. His mother brought him to your clinic or hospital because his viral cold is lingering and exacerbating his asthma. You spend time educating the mother and young child on treatment recommendations, and equip her with a prescription for a nebulizer machine, pediatric mask, and medication. The nearest pharmacy to fill the prescription is about 2 miles away and the total cost is around $90.00.
   a. What questions relating to the SDOHs would be appropriate to ask the mother prior to her leaving your clinic?
   b. How can you, an individual, address the SDOHs identified?
   c. Describe two policy changes that might impact the SDOHs affecting this mother and child.
2. You are a nurse meeting for the first time Mr. A, a 42-year-old African American man interested in "getting healthier." He works the swing shift as a truck driver and often works five or six 12-hour shifts per week. He is divorced and is the primary care provider of three teenage children who live with him. He has eight children in total and two small grandchildren, and he financially supports all of them on his annual salary of $42,000. His medical history includes hypertension and type 2 diabetes, dyslipidemia, obesity, osteoarthritis, lumbar stenosis and disc displacement, and inguinal hernia. He has not seen a primary care provider regularly at any time in his adult life, and reports occasionally buying and taking blood pressure medicine "off the street" because he was told by a friend that "all Black people have high blood pressure and should take a pill for it."
   a. What SDOHs might be impacting Mr. A.'s health outcomes?
   b. As an individual healthcare provider, what could you do to address each SDOH identified in this scenario?
   c. Suggest two policy initiatives that might impact the SDOHs affecting Mr. A.
3. You are a hospital administrator and your hospital readmission rates have steadily increased over the past 6 months. A root cause investigation indicates a small patient population that is homeless as the core group of individuals driving the high readmission rates. List three ways you, the hospital administrator, can address SDOHs impacting this patient population. Explain your rationale for each strategy.

■ Discussion Questions

1. As a nursing professional, what have you seen with regard to the integration of the SDOHs into your clinical practice or health system setting? How would you champion the integration of the SDOHs into your clinical setting? Describe how your healthcare organization can (or could) change policies and procedures to impact these SDOHs.
2. What barriers or facilitators do you see with regard to integration of the SDOHs into the clinical setting? For example, what are the pros and cons of screening for the determinants of health in the clinical setting?
3. How can nurses gain a better understanding of how the SDOHs impact the health of individuals, families, and communities at large?
4. What is the role of nursing education, research, and policy advocacy with regard to advancing addressing the SDOHs in healthcare settings?

■ Resources

American Hospital Association: www.aha.org

Centers for Disease Control and Prevention: www.cdc.gov

Centers for Disease Control and Prevention. (2013). *The state of aging and health in America 2013*. Atlanta, GA: U.S. Department of Health and Human Services. Retrieved from https://www.cdc.gov/aging/pdf/State-Aging-Health-in-America-2013.pdf

Furunes, T., & Mykletun, R. (2010). Age discrimination in the workplace: Validation of the Nordic Age Discrimination Scale (NADS). *Scandanavian Journal of Psychology, 51*(1), 23–30. doi:10.1111/j.1467-9450.2009.00738.x

Healthy People 2020: www.healthypeople.gov

Institute for Healthcare Improvement: www.ihi.org

Integrated Benefits Institute. (2012). *Poor health costs U.S. economy $576 billion according to the Integrated Benefits Institute*. Retrieved from http://www.prnewswire.com/news-releases/poor-health-costs-us-economy-576-billion-according-to-the-integrated-benefits-institute-169460116.html

Lathrop, B. (2013). Nursing leadership in addressing the social determinants of health. *Policy, Politics, & Nursing Practice, 14*(1), 41–47. doi:10.1177/1527154413489887

Mahony, D., & Jones, E. (2013). Social determinants of health in nursing education, research, and health policy. *Nursing Science Quarterly, 26*(3), 280–284. doi:10.1177/0894318413489186

Moody's Analytics. (2017). *The Health of America report: Understanding health conditions across the U.S.* Retrieved from https://www.bcbs.com/sites/default/files/file-attachments/health-of-america-report/BCBS.HealthOfAmericaReport.Moodys_02.pdf

Persaud, S. (2018). Addressing social determinants of health through advocacy. *Nursing Administration Quarterly, 42*(2), 123–128. doi:10.1097/NAQ.0000000000000277

Quad Council Coalition of Public Health Nursing Organizations: www.quadcouncilphn.org

U.S. Department of Health and Human Services. (2010). *Healthy People 2020: An opportunity to address societal determinants of health in the US*. Retrieved from https://www.healthypeople.gov/sites/default/files/SocietalDeterminantsHealth.pdf

U.S. Department of Health and Human Services Office of Minority Health: www.minorityhealth.hhs.gov

World Health Organization: www.who.int
World Health Organization. (2015). *The international statistical classification of diseases and related health problems, 10th revision (ICD-10)*. Geneva, Switzerland: Author.

■ References

Alliance for Health Equity. (2019). *About Us*. Retrieved from https://www.allhealthequity .org/about-us

Amadeo, K. (2017). The rising cost of health care by year and its causes. *The Balance: U.S. Economy*. Retrieved from https://www.thebalance.com/causes-of-rising-healthcare -costs-4064878

American Hospital Association. (2018). *Introducing the New Institute for Diversity and Health Equity*. Retrieved from https://www.aha.org/news/insights-and -analysis/2018-02-12-introducing-new-institute-diversity-and-health-equity

American Hospital Association. (2019). *Equity of Care 123forEquity*. Retrieved from http://www.equityofcare.org/pledge/index.shtml

Ansell, D. (2017). *The death gap: How inequality kills*. Chicago, IL: The University of Chicago Press.

Azar, A. (2018). *The root of the problem: America's social determinants of health*. Retrieved from https://www.hhs.gov/about/leadership/secretary/speeches/2018-speeches/the -root-of-the-problem-americas-social-determinants-of-health.html

Bureau of Labor Statistics. (2019). *News release: Employment projections—2018–2028*. Retrieved from https://www.bls.gov/news.release/pdf/ecopro.pdf

Camden Coalition. (2015). *Camden Coalition launches Housing First program*. Retrieved from https://camdenhealth.org/camden-coalition-launches-housing- first-south-jersey

Cartier, Y., Fichtenberg, C., & Gottlieb, L. (2019). *Community resource referral platforms: A guide for health care organizations*. Retrieved from https://sirenetwork.ucsf.edu/ tools-resources/resources/community-resource-referral-platforms-a-guide-for -health-care-organizations

Castellucci, M., & Caruso, M. (2019). *Hospitals want readmissions program to account for social determinants*. Retrieved from https://www.modernhealthcare.com/safety -quality/hospitals-want-readmissions-program-account-social-determinants

Centers for Disease Control and Prevention. (2008). *Community Health and Program Services (CHAPS): Health disparities among racial/ethnic populations*. Atlanta, GA: U.S. Department of Health and Human Services.

Chaiyachati, K., Qi, M., & Werner, R. (2018). Changes to racial disparities in readmission rates after Medicare's hospital readmissions reduction program within safety-net and non-safety-net hospitals. *JAMA Network Open, 1*(7), e184154. Retrieved from https://www.ncbi.nlm.nih.gov/pmc/articles/PMC6324411

County Health Rankings & Roadmaps. (2016). County Health Rankings model [Image file]. Retrieved from https://www.countyhealthrankings.org/county-health-rankings-model

Donelan, K., DesRoches, C., Dittus, R., & Buerhaus, P. (2013). Perspectives of physicians and nurse practitioners on primary care practice. *The New England Journal of Medicine, 368*, 1898–1906. doi:10.1056/NEJMsa1212938

Dubay, L., & Lebrun, L. (2012). Health, behavior, and health care disparities: Disentangling the effects of income and race in the United States. *International Journal of Health Services, 42*(4), 607–625. doi:10.2190/HS.42.4.c

Faghri, P., Kotejoshyer, R., Cherniack, M., Reeves, D., & Punnett, L. (2010). Assessment of a worksite health promotion readiness checklist. *Journal of Occupational Environmental Medicine, 52*(9), 893–899. doi:10.1097/JOM.0b013e3181efb84d

Flato, H., & Zhang, H. (2016). Inequity in level of healthcare utilization before and after universal health coverage reforms in China: Evidence from household surveys in Sichuan Province. *International Journal of Equity in Health, 15*, 96. doi:10.1186/s12939-016-0385-x

Goar, E. (2017). Don't sleep on Z codes. *For The Record, 29*(5), 14. Retrieved from https://www.fortherecordmag.com/archives/0517p14.shtml

Gooch, K. (2018). *Social determinants of health contributed to half of hospital readmissions, study finds.* Retrieved from https://www.beckershospitalreview.com/population-health/social-determinants-of-health-contributed-to-half-of-hospital-readmissions-study-finds.html

Harris, J., Huang, Y., Hannon, P., & Williams, B. (2011). Low-socioeconomic status workers: Their health risks and how to reach them. *Journal of Occupational and Environmental Medicine, 53*(2), 132–138. doi:10.1097/JOM.0b013e3182045f2c

Health Leads. (2019). *Funding whole-person health: Opportunities to make essential needs initiatives more sustainable.* Retrieved from https://healthleadsusa.org/resources/funding-whole-person-health-opportunities-to-make-essential-needs-initiatives-more-sustainable

Heiman, H., Smith, L., McKool, M., Mitchell, D., & Bayer, C. (2015). Health policy training: A review of the literature. *International Journal of Environmental Research and Public Health, 13*(1), ijerph13010020. doi:10.3390/ijerph13010020

Hood, C., Gennuso, K., Swain, G., & Catlin, B. (2016). County health rankings: Relationships between determinant factors and health outcomes. *American Journal of Preventive Medicine, 50*(2), 129–135. doi:10.1016/j.amepre.2015.08.024

Institute for Healthcare Improvement. (2018). *Pursuing equity launch enhancement.* Retrieved from http://www.ihi.org/about/news/Pages/Pursuing-Equity-Launch-Announcement.aspx

Institute of Medicine. (2011). *The future of nursing: Leading change, advancing health.* Washington, DC: National Academies Press.

Internal Revenue Service. (2018). *Requirements for 501(c)(3) hospitals under the Affordable Care Act – Section 501(r).* Retrieved from https://www.irs.gov/charities-non-profits/charitable-organizations/requirements-for-501c3-hospitals-under-the-affordable-care-act-section-501r

Kindig, D. (2015). From health determinant benchmarks to health investment benchmarks. *Preventing Chronic Disease, 12.* Retrieved from https://www.cdc.gov/pcd/issues/2015/15_0010.htm

Kindig, D., & Stoddart, G. (2003). Models for population health: What is population health? *American Journal of Public Health, 93*(3), 380–383. doi:10.2105/AJPH.93.3.380

Klinenberg, E. (2002). *Heat wave: A social autopsy of disaster in Chicago.* Chicago, IL: University of Chicago Press.

Korda, R., Clements, M., & Kelman, C. (2009). Universal health care no guarantee of equity: Comparison of socioeconomic inequalities in the receipt of coronary procedures in patients with acute myocardial infarction and angina. *BMC Public Health, 14*(9), 460. doi:10.1186/1471-2458-9-460

Krieger, N., Barbeau, E., & Soobader, M. (2005). Class matters: U.S. versus U.K. measures of occupational disparities in access to health services and health status in the 2000 U.S. National Health Interview Survey. *International Journal of Health Services, 35*(2), 213–236. doi:10.2190/JKRE-AH92-EDV8-VHYC

Lindau, S., Makelarski, J., Abramsohn, E., Beiser, D., Escamilla, V., Jerome, J., . . . Miller, D. (2016). CommunityRx: A population health improvement innovation that connects clinics to communities. *Health Affairs, 35*(11), 2020–2029. doi:10.1377/hlthaff.2016.0694

Meyer, M. (2017). How HIEs use data to improve population health. *Journal of AHIMA.* Retrieved from http://journal.ahima.org/2017/04/19/how-hies-use-data-to-improve-population-health

Millman, M. (Ed.). (1993). *Access to health care in America.* Washington, DC: National Academies Press.

Moss, A. (2017). *The impact of worksite access to primary care services among low-income foodservice workers.* (Unpublished doctoral dissertation). Rush University College of Nursing, Chicago, IL.

MPH@GW Staff. (2018). *What's the difference between equity and equality?* Retrieved from https://publichealthonline.gwu.edu/blog/equity-vs-equality

National Employment Law Project. (2012). *Big business, corporate profits, and the minimum wage.* New York, NY: National Employment Law Project Data Brief, July 2012. Retrieved from https://s27147.pcdn.co/wp-content/uploads/2015/03/NELP-Big-Business-Corporate-Profits-Minimum-Wage.pdf

NowPow. (2018). *About NowPow.* Retrieved from https://nowpow.workable.com

Office of Disease Prevention and Health Promotion. (n.d.-a). *Access to health services.* Retrieved from https://www.healthypeople.gov/2020/topics-objectives/topic/Access-to-Health-Services

Office of Disease Prevention and Health Promotion. (n.d.-b). *Social determinants of health.* Retrieved from https://www.healthypeople.gov/2020/topics-objectives/topic/social-determinants-of-health

Parmelli, E., Flodgren, G., Beyer, F., Baillie, N., Schaafsma, M., & Eccles, M. (2011). The effectiveness of strategies to change organizational culture to improve healthcare performance: A systematic review. *Implementation Science, 6*(1), 33. doi:10.1186/1748-5908-6-33

Pincus, T., Esther, R., DeWalt, D., & Callahan, L. (1998). Social condition and self- management are more powerful determinants of health than access to care. *Annals of Internal Medicine, 129*(5), 406–411. doi:10.7326/0003-4819-129-5-199809010-00011

Pollack, J., & Pollack, R. (2015). Using Kotter's eight stage process to manage an organizational change program: Presentation and practice. *Systemic Practice and Action Research, 28*(1), 51–66. doi:10.1007/s11213-014-9317-0

Popescu, G. (2014). Economic aspects influencing the rising costs of health care in the United States. *American Journal of Medical Research, 1*(1), 47–52. Retrieved from https://addletonacademicpublishers.com/search-in-ajmr/2078-economic-aspects-influencing-the-rising-costs-of-health-care-in-the-united-states

Pruitt, Z., Emechebe, N., Quast, T., Taylor, P., & Bryant, K. (2018). Expenditure reductions associated with a social service referral program. *Population Health Management, 21*(6), 469–476. doi:10.1089/pop.2017.0199

Quad Council Coalition Competency Review Task Force. (2018). *Community/public health nursing competencies.* Retrieved from http://www.quadcouncilphn.org/documents-3/2018-qcc-competencies

Reblin, M., & Uchino, B. (2008). Social and emotional support and its implication for health. *Current Opinion in Psychiatry, 21*(2), 201–205. doi:10.1097/YCO.0b013e3282f3ad89

Robert Wood Johnson Foundation. (n.d.). Could where you live influence how long you live? Retrieved from https://www.rwjf.org/en/library/interactives/where youliveaffectshowlongyoulive.html

Robert Wood Johnson Foundation. (2011). *Health care's blind side: The overlooked connection between social needs and good health: Summary of findings from a survey of America's physicians.* Retrieved from http://www.rootcausecoalition.org/wp-content/uploads/2017/04/Health-Cares-Blind-Side.pdf

Rodney, A., & Hill, P. (2014). Achieving equity within universal health coverage: A narrative review of progress and resources for measuring success. *International Journal for Equity in Health, 10*(13), 72. doi:10.1186/s12939-014-0072-8

Rush. (2016). *Rush community health needs assessment.* Retrieved from https://www.rush.edu/sites/default/files/rush-chna-2016.pdf

Rush University Medical Center. (2017). *Anchor mission playbook.* Retrieved from https://www.rush.edu/sites/default/files/anchor-mission-playbook.pdf

Schneeweiss, S. (2014). Learning from big health care data. *New England Journal of Medicine, 370,* 2161–2163. doi:10.1056/NEJMp1401111

Sisko, A., Keehan, S., Poisal, J., Cuckler, G., Smith, S., Madison, A., . . . Hardesty, J. (2019). National health expenditure projections, 2018-27: Economic and demographic trends drive spending and enrollment growth. *Health Affairs, 38*(3). Retrieved from https://www.healthaffairs.org/doi/abs/10.1377/hlthaff.2018.05499

Srinivasan, S., & Williams, S. (2014). Transitioning from health disparities to a health equity research agenda: The time is now. *Public Health Reports, 129*(2), 71–76. doi:10.1177/00333549141291S213

Strout, K. (2012). Wellness promotion and the Institute of Medicine's *Future of Nursing* report: Are nurses ready? *Holistic Nursing Practice, 26*(3), 129–136. doi:10.1097/HNP.0b013e31824ef581

Top Box Foods. (2018). *Home.* Retrieved from https://www.topboxfoods.com/cook-county-chicago/home

University of Wisconsin Population Health Institute. (2018). *County Health Rankings & Roadmaps.* Retrieved from http://www.countyhealthrankings.org

U.S. Department of Health and Human Services Office of Minority Health. (2019). *About the Office of Minority Health.* Retrieved from https://minorityhealth.hhs.gov/omh/browse.aspx?lvl=1&lvlid=1

Wang, S., Chen, L., Hsu, S., & Wang, S. (2012). Health care utilization and health outcomes: A population study of Taiwan. *Health Policy Plan, 27*(7), 590–599. doi:10.1093/heapol/czr080

Weber, V., & Joshi, M. (2000). Effecting and leading change in health care organizations. *The Joint Commission Journal on Quality Improvement, 26*(7), 388–399. doi:10.1016/S1070-3241(00)26032-X

Wellman, J., Jeffries, H., & Hagan, P. (2017). *Leading the Lean healthcare journey: Driving culture change to increase value* (2nd ed.). Boca Raton, FL: CRC Press.

West Side United. (2019). *Our mission.* Retrieved from https://westsideunited.org/about-us/mission

Woolf, S., Aron, L., Dubay, L., Simon, S., Zimmerman, E., & Luk, K. (2015). *How are income and wealth linked to health and longevity?* Washington, DC and Richmond, VA: Urban Institute and Virginia Commonwealth University. Retrieved from http://www.urban.org/sites/default/files/publication/49116/2000178-How-are-Income-and-Wealth-Linked-to-Health-and-Longevity.pdf

World Health Organization. (2008). *Closing the gap in a generation: Health equity through action on the social determinants of health.* Geneva, Switzerland: Author.

World Health Organization. (2017). *10 facts on health inequities and their causes.* Retrieved from https://www.who.int/features/factfiles/health_inequities/en

World Health Organization. (2018). *Social determinants of health.* Retrieved from http://www.who.int/social_determinants/en

Wyatt, R., Laderman, M., Botwinick, L, Mate, K., & Whittington, J. (2016). *Achieving health equity: A guide for health care organizations* [IHI White Paper]. Cambridge, MA: Institute for Healthcare Improvement. Retrieved from http://www.ihi.org/resources/Pages/IHIWhitePapers/Achieving-Health-Equity.aspx

Zimmerman, E., Woolf, S., & Haley, A. (2015). *Understanding the relationship between education and health.* Rockville, MD: Agency for Healthcare Research and Quality. Retrieved from https://nam.edu/wp-content/uploads/2015/06/BPH-Understanding TheRelationship1.pdf

Zogg, C., Scott, J., Jiang, W., Wolf, L., & Haider, A. (2016). Differential access to care: The role of age, insurance and income on race/ethnicity-related disparities in adult perforated appendix admission rates. *Surgery, 16D*(5), 1145–1154. doi:10.1016/j.surg.2016.06.002

9

Structural Determinants of Health: An American Indian Exemplar

Margaret P. Moss

CHAPTER OBJECTIVES

- ⊙ Identify who are American Indian/Alaska Native people in the United States
- ⊙ Distinguish between social and structural determinants of health
- ⊙ Construct how historical, geopolitical, and cultural realities intersect in American Indian/Alaska Native people and can manifest in contemporaneous health issues/ health disparities

KEY CONCEPTS

Historical trauma   Medicine wheel
Seven generations

KEY TERMS

American Indians/Alaska Natives   Structural health disparities
Social determinants of health   Indigenize
Structural determinants of health

■ Introduction

Invasion is a Structure, not an Event.

—Wolfe, 1994

American Indians and Alaska Natives (AIAN) exhibit some of the most egregious health disparities not just in *Indian Country*, the United States, or North America, but also in the Western Hemisphere (Garrett, Baldridge, Benson, Crowder, & Aldrich, 2015; Kinghorn et al., 2018; Moss, 2015; Warne & Lajimodiere, 2015). Indian Country is an actual legal term denoting reservations, pueblo, and trust lands in and under the control of the United States as well as dependent communities (18 U.S.C. § 1151 1949). And yet, what does the nursing profession or health professions at large understand regarding the history, traumas, politics, policies, and funding issues encompassing this population? These spaces each affect the health of America's first peoples.

In the United States, there has been little focus on American Indian history and even less on current events in the K–12 educational system. Therefore, when students arrive in their health profession programs, they are largely ill-equipped to appropriately assess, treat, and evaluate care, especially care focused on issues unique to this population. These issues are rooted in targeted federal policies, born in the 1800s, that guide most of federal Indian law today. Some of these policy periods were the following (Moss, 2010):

- The *reservation era* in the 1800s, where AIAN were moved onto government reservations and their land was taken and sold. Usually, they were moved to lands unfarmable and barely livable. There are still just over 300 reservations in the United States.
- The *allotment and assimilation period (1887–1943)*, where boarding schools, and White adoption and fostering out of Indian children occurred by the tens of thousands, where children often died, were assaulted, ridiculed, were stripped of their clothes, hair, language, religion, and families. Some never saw their families again. Although the official period ended in 1947, these practices each continued into the late 1970s. Fostering out of culture still occurs at alarming rates.
- And, the *termination period and relocation period (1945–1960)*, where Congress decided to terminate legal government-to-government statuses for some tribes. This relationship is termed "Federal Recognition" as decided in the Marshall Trilogy accredited to Chief Justice Marshall. The terminations meant that 100 tribes were now no longer tribes in the eyes of Congress; therefore, the United States no longer "owed" them anything. This had implications for education, housing, healthcare, and other services afforded to tribal members of recognized tribes.

There were just fewer than 1,000 nursing baccalaureate programs in the United States (American Association of Colleges of Nursing [AACN], n.d.); very few have dedicated courses on AIAN health, and even fewer have *mandatory* coursework in this area. This author knows of only a handful, and usually west of the Mississippi River.

Through some powerful and recent examples, it is the purpose of this chapter to illustrate this unseeing of structures. Structures, and therefore structural determinants of health, are necessarily rooted in history. They are historical, and therefore accepted almost without question; they are political, and therefore often viewed as untouchable; and they are inextricably tied to funding/monies, again an uphill battle. This chapter illustrates some AIAN realities and concepts and provides a model focused on structural disparities in health for AIAN in the United States.

■ Nursing Education: What Does It (Not) Teach?

The knowledge gap in nursing education on structural determinants of health and in particular, how smaller populations are affected, is both wide and deep. In this case, historic to current information on the population AIAN is breathtakingly undertaught. There are thousands of prelicensure nursing programs in the United States. There are just fewer than 1,000 bachelor's degrees (AACN, n.d.), just more than 1,000 associate degrees in nursing (ADN; Nurse Journal, n.d.), and more than 1,000 second-degree or accelerated nursing programs (Registered Nursing.org, n.d.). Therefore, more than 165,000 RNs graduate each year in the first two categories alone (Department for Professional Employees [DPE], 2015); that is, 1.5 to 2 million, if held consistent every decennial.

Of this, the largest of the health professions rolling out these numbers, few nursing programs have mandatory courses either on structural health determinants or on

American Indian topics. We need to purposively add AIAN context and health perspective, that is, *indigenize* nursing and health curricula to include this first population of the Americas now lost in curricula and not coincidently, last in many health indicators. Otherwise, is nursing ready to care for AIAN patients on any individual or population health level as we move further into the 21st century?

Throughout this text, there have been several same or similar terms with slightly differing definitions. The fields encompassing health disparity, inequities, and diversity are not well settled, being fairly new spaces in American health. The definitions used in *this* chapter are specific to the ideas within it. As this chapter falls within the section on population health, the American Indian/Alaska Native term as the population of interest here will be defined first.

■ American Indians/Alaska Natives

AIAN ARE THE MOST REGULATED PEOPLE IN THE UNITED STATES

In the United States, who is and who is not an American Indian or Alaska Native is a matter of law, with both federal and tribal pieces. In this chapter, we specifically use the AIAN name as it aligns with U.S. law (the full name will be used for emphasis at times). "Indians" is actually the legal term in the United States and in Canada denoting the first or indigenous peoples of the Americas. Interestingly *"Indians" are the only named population in the U.S. Code.* The U.S. Code of Federal Regulations (CFR) "is the codification of the general and permanent rules published in the Federal Register by the departments and agencies of the Federal Government" (Government Publishing Office [GPO], 2019a, p. 1). Indians fall under Title 25.

In the law (U.S. perspective), the Congress designates which tribes have what is termed "federal recognition" (U.S. Bureau of Indian Affairs [BIA], n.d.). Federal recognition is a government-to-government relationship, born out of treaties and from the three cases of the Marshall Trilogy: *Johnson v. M'Intosh, Cherokee Nation v. Georgia,* and *Worcester v. Georgia* (Goetting, 2008). The Marshall Trilogy comprises three seminal rulings by Chief Justice John Marshall from the early 1800s, which in large part still guide federal Indian law today. "They continue to be the court's, and therefore the Constitution's, definitive statement on the personhood of tribal Indians" (Goetting, 2008, p. 211). Taking these statements together, one can surmise that perspectives on American Indians would be out of step (driven by the context of the 1800s) with more inclusive ideas of 2019. This is a *structural problem* for moving forward in federal Indian law and all aspects that it touches, including health and healthcare. Some definitions from the U.S. Code on Indians follow in Box 9.1.

The other "test" is a matter for the AIAN community itself to acknowledge the person claiming heritage or lineage as one of their own. Does that community know you, or can they place you or your relatives or ancestors as being from the community?

There is a seminal statement showcasing the Congress's power over AIAN identity, from the case United States *v.* Wheeler, 435 U.S. 313, 323 (1978): **"The sovereignty that the Indian tribes retain is of a unique and limited character. It exists only at the *sufferance of Congress* and is subject to complete defeasance."** This means the Congress designates who is a tribe in the United States, and therefore can terminate their status at any time. The tribes themselves designate who is a member.

BOX 9.1 Relevant Definitions in the U.S. Code of Federal Regulations, Title 25, Indians

Continental United States means the contiguous 48 states and Alaska.

Documented petition means the detailed arguments and supporting documentary evidence submitted by a petitioner claiming that it meets the Indian Entity Identification (§ 83.11(a)), Governing Document (§ 83.11(d)), Descent (§ 83.11(e)), Unique Membership (§ 83.11(f)), and Congressional Termination (§ 83.11(g)) Criteria and claiming that it:

(2) Meets the Community (§ 83.11(b)) and Political Authority (§ 83.11(c)) Criteria.

Federally recognized Indian tribe means an entity listed on the Department of the Interior's list under the Federally Recognized Indian Tribe List Act of 1994, which the Secretary currently acknowledges as an Indian tribe and with which the United States maintains a government-to-government relationship.

Indigenous means native to the continental United States in that at least part of the petitioner's territory at the time of first sustained contact extended into what is now the continental United States.

Member of a petitioner means an individual who is recognized by the petitioner as meeting its membership criteria and who consents to being listed as a member of the petitioner.

Office of Federal Acknowledgment or OFA means the Office of Federal Acknowledgment within the Office of the Assistant Secretary—Indian Affairs, Department of the Interior.

Petitioner means any entity that has submitted a documented petition to OFA requesting Federal acknowledgment as a federally recognized Indian tribe.

Previous Federal acknowledgment means action by the Federal government clearly premised on identification of a tribal political entity and indicating clearly the recognition of a relationship between that entity and the United States.

Roll means a list exclusively of those individuals who have been determined by the tribe to meet the tribe's membership requirements as set forth in its governing document. In the absence of such a document, a roll means a list of those recognized as members by the tribe's governing body. In either case, those individuals on a roll must have affirmatively demonstrated consent to being listed as members.

Secretary means the Secretary of the Interior within the Department of the Interior or that officer's authorized representative.

Tribe means any Indian tribe, band, nation, pueblo, village, or community.

Source: From Government Publishing Office. (2019b). Code of Federal Regulations: Title 25 - Indians. Retrieved from https://www.govinfo.gov/content/pkg/CFR-2019-title25-vol1/xml/CFR -2019-title25-vol1-sec83-1.xml

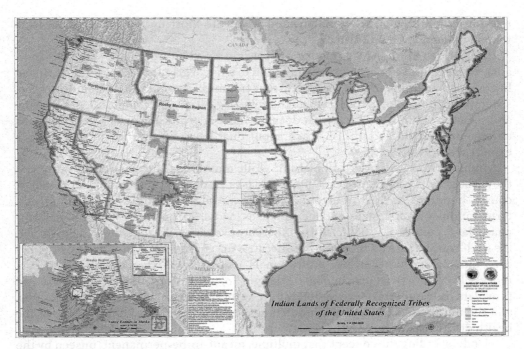

FIGURE 9.1 BUREAU OF INDIAN AFFAIRS REGIONS.

Source: From U.S. Bureau of Indian Affairs. (2016). *A Bureau of Indian Affairs map of Indian reservations in the contiguous United States.* Retrieved from https://www.bia.gov/sites/bia.gov/files/assets/bia/ots/webteam/pdf/idc1-028635.pdf

But, if the overarching tribal status is taken away, one is no longer an AIAN in the eyes of the government.

These Marshall Trilogy roots are *unseen* and unknown by most Americans including healthcare professionals. There are currently more than 300 reservations holding 573 federally recognized tribes in the United States (BIA, n.d.; see Figure 9.1). As a nurse, do you know in which region you practice? And what the implications may be?

Do you know what the implications are around whether the patient is from a federally recognized tribe? That is, are they AIAN in the eyes of the United States? If so, they are eligible for services out of the Indian Health Service (IHS). Is there one nearby? If they are not, they may be afforded some state programs. There are dozens more tribes that are state recognized only, with still others recognized by both levels of government (Moss, 2015). There are also descendants from derecognized/terminated or never recognized tribes, and ethnic AIAN with no discernable tribe-specific roots as they were either discarded or stolen as manifestations of federal policies. And, importantly, today about 78% of AIAN live off-reservation with 60% being urban (U.S. Census, 2012). Nurses in urban and other areas will be taking care of AIAN patients and will not know unless they become familiar with their catchment areas and/or ask all patients how they identify.

Each of these facts, terms, and concepts is key for nursing professionals to know. Yet, rarely are these facts taught in either K–12 or higher education unless students seek out specific programs or elective courses. Therefore, how will cultural competency, relevance, humility, or safety be ensured when the most underlying, seminal facts remain untaught and unlearned?

Disparities in the AIAN population, specifically, stem from legal status (as Indians), where they live or get care, and how and to what degree they experience/manifest historical, contemporaneous, or concurrent traumas. These traumas stem from persistent, intentional, long-standing, and targeted legal, economic, political, geographic, and social structures. And yet, what does the nursing profession or health professions at large understand about this? Teach about this? Research on this? In this author's experience, very little.

In his writing on settler colonialism, Wolfe makes clear the answer to: Why can't they just get over it? (American Indians/Alaska Natives, in this case). "It" being, of course, hundreds of years of extermination, removal, reservations, assimilation, and termination of federal, state, and local policies (Moss, 2010). The resulting loss of language, land, culture, way of life, full or inherent sovereignty, health, safety, religion, and life itself continues. And they continue because the structures continue to exist. However, nursing and other health professionals are largely unschooled in these occurrences. They have been unschooled by design. So, unless individual practitioners and providers have undertaken years-long study of these policies, the resulting structures, and the ultimate social and health outcomes, there will be little to no change in the health disparities in the AIAN population.

Understanding the concept that multiple, meant-to-be-permanent, unseen by the dominant culture, structures are in the way is seminal to an understanding of health disparities in the United States today vis-à-vis American Indians/Alaska Natives. Through some powerful and recent examples, it is the purpose of this chapter to illustrate this concept for nursing. Structures, and therefore structural determinants of health, are necessarily rooted in history, but allowed to continue, unseen and unexplicated today. The laws are historical, and therefore accepted almost without question; they are political, and therefore often viewed as untouchable; and they are inextricably tied to funding/monies, again an uphill battle.

AIAN FACTS

There are some facts every nurse (and, in fact, every American) should know. Pre-contact, that is pre-1492 as a generally accepted marker, there were estimates of several tens of millions of indigenous people across what is now Canada and the United States, the zenith of population (Moss, 2015). The nadir occurred at the 1990 census with about 90,000 (Moss; see Figure 9.2). What does this look like?

What if your "population" could be knocked out almost to extinction and that those remaining suffered removal, reservation, assimilation, and termination policies?

AIAN HEALTH

The outward signs of health and illness in the AIAN population are periodically recorded in the *Trends in Indian Health* publication put out by the U.S. Public Health Service, IHS. The last one was in 2014. The IHS provides direct healthcare to AIAN from federally recognized tribes free of charge (IHS, 2019). Services out of the scope of a particular facility are paid for or not on a case-by-case basis. However, one hears

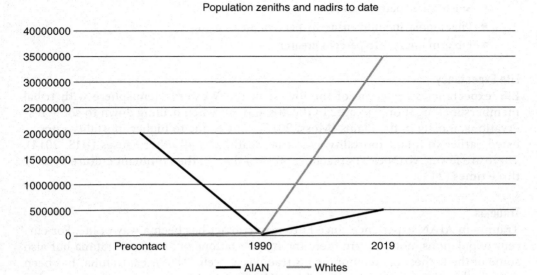

FIGURE 9.2 CENSUS COMPARISONS: AIAN AND WHITES IN THE UNITED STATES.

AIAN, American Indians and Alaska Natives.

statements like "life or limb only" as to what will be authorized for pay, or "better get sick by June" before the money runs out. IHS services arise out of treaties and public laws. However, funding has chronically and persistently been the lowest for any group per capita receiving any federal funding.

Mortality

From the IHS Trends report (2014, p. 5):

> In 2007–2009, the AI/AN (IHS service area) age adjusted death rates for the following causes were considerably higher than those for the U.S. all races population in 2008. These AI/AN rates have been adjusted to compensate for misreporting of AI/AN race on state death certificates. The following list is a comparison of [the] AI/AN age adjusted rate (using data that are also adjusted for misreporting of AI/AN race on the state death certificates) to the U.S. rate where there are substantial differences.
>
> Comparison of 2007–2009 AI/AN death rates to 2008 U.S. all races death rates.

- Alcohol related—520 percent greater;
- Tuberculosis—450 percent greater;
- Chronic liver disease and cirrhosis—368 percent greater
- Motor vehicle crashes—207 percent greater;
- Diabetes mellitus—177 percent greater;
- Unintentional injuries—141 percent greater;
- Poisoning— 118 percent greater;
- Homicide—86 percent greater;

- Suicide—60 percent greater;
- Pneumonia and influenza—37 percent greater; and
- Firearm injury—16 percent greater

Life Expectancy

Life expectancies are some of the lowest in the Western Hemisphere with tribal members making it only to ages in the 40s and 50s when drilling down to some reservations, mostly in the Plains (Moss, 2015). This is due to higher mortality rates as listed earlier in infant mortality, maternal death, and all other causes (IHS, 2014). There are fewer AIAN elders reaching 65 (7%) than in the dominant culture by over three times (24%).

Traumas

Trauma in AIAN experience since European contact has been a way of life. For current populations, not only are there the manifestations of historical trauma but also some of the highest contemporaneous traumas as well. "Historical trauma" has been described in the literature by Braveheart (1998). It is intergenerational trauma, that is, traumas visited on one's ancestors have manifestations in descendants today. It is unresolved grief and also referred to as a "soul wound" (Duran, Duran, Heart, Yellow Horse Brave Hearth, & Horse-Davis, 1998). All of the policies and histories since contact manifest today in lowered health for AIAN.

American Indian and Alaska Native women also suffer the most sexual assault (46%), rape (1 in 3), and murder (10 times higher on some reservations) than any other group (U.S. Department of Justice [DOJ], 2012). This is due in large part to laws still on the books referring to when a non-Indian comes on to Indian lands and commits a crime. Even if it were murder, a tribe can hold a nonmember for only 364 days maximum. The murder perpetrators are mostly non-Indian men. The reality is that they are rarely caught or prosecuted. It is in effect "open season" on AIAN women in some reservation areas (Moss, 2015). These are stunning statistics. Again, these laws are holdovers and are structural facilitators to harm in Indian Country. But, how many Americans are aware?

By comparison, AIAN people see the ramped-up and breaking national news 24-hour cycles when dominant culture women have been murdered or go missing. There has been a paucity of stories on the women who go missing the most.

■ Seven Generations

Seven generations is a concept that is a "structure" to many North American tribes. By this is meant a recognizable framework of identifiable parts. The parts consist of members, ancestors, future generations, thoughts, actions and, importantly, consequences. Yet, it is simple in its overarching theme: What you do today, you should make sure there will be good outcomes at least seven generations out. And, conversely, do not do something today that could have far-reaching negative consequences. What follows is an example of this concept with implications for health in AIAN people today.

A LITERAL STRUCTURAL EXEMPLAR: THE GALLOWS

The Dakota 38 execution was the largest mass execution in the United States and took place on December 26, 1862.

(Schilling, 2017, p. 10)

The "Dakota 38 +2" is significant U.S. history that is almost never taught in the United States (Wastvedt, 2017). But this author uses it for a variety of teachings. The Dakota 38 refers to the hanging of 38 (+2 more) American Indian men and boys, as ordered by President Abraham Lincoln in 1862, the day after Christmas (Beck, 2014; Laviolette, 1991; Schilling, 2017). It occurred in Mankato, Minnesota. This constitutes the largest mass execution ordered by a sitting president on U.S. lands (Beck, 2014; Schilling, 2017). There were little to no trials afforded to the men (Schilling, 2017). The men and boys largely spoke no English. American Indians broadly know about this travesty, especially the Dakota and other tribes in the region.

Broken treaties, starvation, and lack of promised annuities led to "uprisings" by the Upper and Lower Sioux Agencies (Beck, 2014; Laviolette, 1991; Schilling, 2017). The Upper Sioux with 400 to 800 warriors stormed the agency's warehouses. Capt. John Marsh, commander, allowed food distribution to the men to take back to their families and they left agreeing to wait for the annuities (Beck, 2014).

However, the Lower Sioux Agency was not able to hold off further attacks. Marsh was killed (Beck, 2014). Similar causes were behind the Lower Sioux uprisings: starvation, forced assimilation, loss of almost every aspect of the lives they had known, raping of their women, withholding money, and continual encroachment on the lands they held historically (Beck, 2014). The warriors did kill hundreds of settlers in these uprisings. Minnesotans wanted all of the Dakota either killed or marched out of the territory. Captured Sioux who were not executed were held in prisoner camps by the hundreds. Racism was rampant: "Let them eat grass," attributed to the settler sentiment of the time. An interesting context is that all this occurred 6 days before the Emancipation Proclamation, January 1, 1863 (National Archives, n.d.). Lincoln is widely known for the latter and almost never for the former, except by AIAN (see Figure 9.3).

SEVEN GENERATIONS LATER

In 2017, the Walker Art Museum in Minnesota commissioned a White artist to replicate the Gallows of 1862. This would have been 155 years later. Generations are often thought of as 20 to 25 years. This would be seven generations from the last gallows. The horror and evil of the previous mass execution are as real today for the AIAN people.

Neither the museum nor the artist consulted AIAN people, especially from the tribes involved, nor the elders. AIAN are so marginalized by the greater society that even in something as numbing as this, no one thought it important to speak with affected communities. During the same week in 2017, a single noose was found hanging near the National Museum of African American History and Culture (Boissoneault, 2017). It made national news. In the same week, Lebron James (a basketball player) had a racial slur written across his gate (Rogers, 2017). This also made national news.

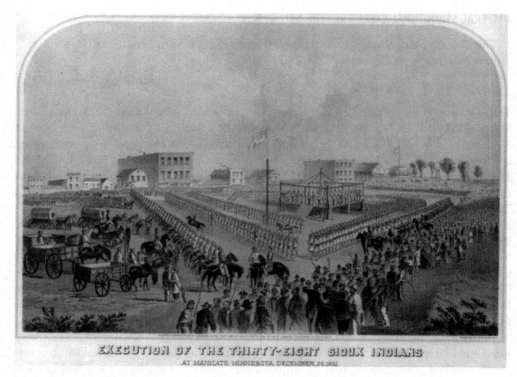

FIGURE 9.3 HANGING OF 38 + 2 SIOUX INDIANS AS ORDERED BY PRESIDENT LINCOLN IN 1862, MANKATO, MINNESOTA.

Note: This media file is in the public domain in the United States. This applies to U.S. works where the copyright has expired, often because its first publication occurred prior to January 1, 1924, and if not then due to lack of notice or renewal.

Source: From Childs, W. H. (1863). *Execution of 38 Sioux Indians* [Image file]. Retrieved from https://commons.wikimedia.org/wiki/File:MankatoMN38.JPG

However, a Gallows big enough to hang 40 AIAN did not appear on any national news (this author checked websites of Fox, CNN, and MSNBC at the time; see Figure 9.4). This illustrates the absolute invisibility of the American Indian population in news, media, and the minds of non-Indians.

INVISIBILITY, WHITE PRIVILEGE, AND HEALTH

There were quite wildly differing reactions to the Gallows by AIAN and non-Indians. The structure serves as a real-life metaphor for what the dominant culture sees versus what AIAN people see regarding traumatic structures. The AIAN observing and hearing about the Gallows were traumatized and retraumatized. They saw a stark reminder of their ancestors climbing the steps to their fates in 1862. They were crying as they observed in total disbelief that this structure was raised at all. There was no discussion with any AIAN persons or groups or tribes. No elders were consulted. They put up hundreds of posters and handmade signs in response (see Figures 9.5 and 9.6).

In stark contrast, people from the dominant culture were walking their dogs by the structure. Their kids were playing on it like a park feature. It is in fact built right

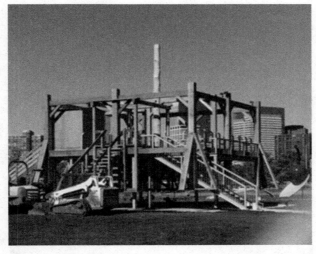

FIGURE 9.4 REPLICATED GALLOWS ON WHICH 40 DAKOTA MEN WERE HANGED, ERECTED IN THE TWIN CITIES, 2017.

Photo: Marique Moss, 2017, Minneapolis, MN.

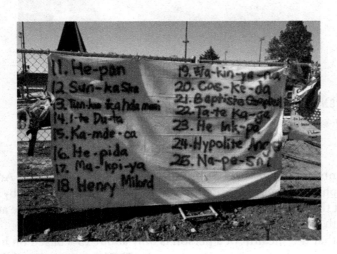

FIGURE 9.5 REMEMBER THEIR NAMES.

Photo: Marique Moss, 2017, Minneapolis, MN.

next to a slide as seen in one of the photos. Even if the structure is seen, it brings on only curiosity, not fear, terror, and trauma.

The health implications here are toxic stress and historical, intergenerational trauma felt instantly and viscerally by the AIAN people.

■ Structural Health Disparity Model

The Structural Health Disparity Model (Exhibit 9.1) demonstrates the need for health professionals to pay attention not only to health outcomes and health status but also to

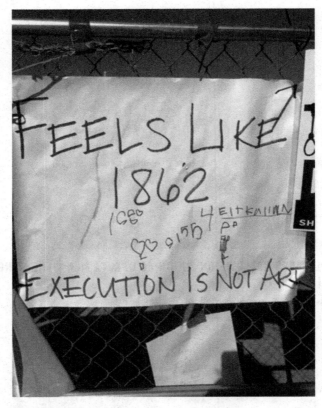

FIGURE 9.6 SIGN AT THE GALLOWS.

Photo: Marique Moss, 2017, Minneapolis, MN.

the determinants of the health of the person, here the AIAN patient. And the patient has domains: physical, mental, emotional, and spiritual, as depicted by the medicine wheel found at the center of the model. Each of these domains must be attended to for optimum health.

We know that the "health" of a person is only about 15% based on healthcare and 85% based on "other" determinants (Magnan, 2017). These are the *social* determinants of health. According to the World Health Organization (WHO), "The social determinants of health (SDH) are the conditions in which people are born, grow, work, live, and age, and the wider set of forces and systems shaping the conditions of daily life" (WHO, n.d.). These include contexts for the person around poverty, education, safety, employment, and housing to name a few.

Revisiting an earlier statement, AIAN within the healthcare space are the most regulated people in the United States in one of the most regulated industries. These are some of the *structural* determinants of health for AIAN. When healthcare for AIAN is regulated by the executive branch and funded (or not) by the Congress and the AIAN themselves are determined to be eligible or not by both their tribe (as a member) and the government as a member of a legitimate tribe, barrier after barrier is thrown up on the path to health. We can see health status outwardly through usual practice; social determinants are often ignored or partially hidden in this unseen

EXHIBIT 9.1 MOSS STRUCTURAL HEALTH DISPARITY MODEL FOR AMERICAN INDIAN/ALASKA NATIVE HEALTH

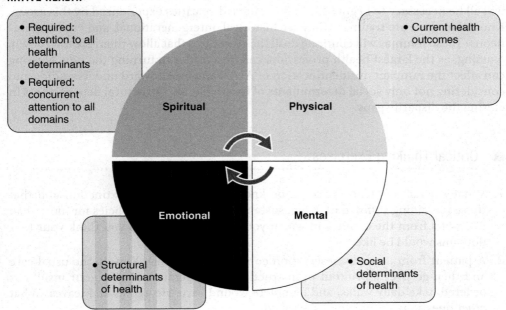

- Required: attention to all health determinants
- Required: concurrent attention to all domains

- Current health outcomes

Spiritual

Physical

Emotional

Mental

- Structural determinants of health

- Social determinants of health

VISIBILITY TO HEALTH PROFESSIONALS	LEVELS OF DETERMINANTS OF HEALTH	MANIFESTATIONS
Visible	Health outcomes	Diabetes, suicide, diseases of the heart and liver, poor mental health
Visible but obscured	Social determinants of health	Poverty, food insecurity, inadequate housing, safety, employment, education
Hidden	Structural determinants of health	Laws, history, policy, funding

population; and structural determinants are largely hidden as discussed due to lack of education. Health disparities then will persist until attention is paid to the ideas of funding, policy, and legal changes among others. Each of these feeds into the social determinants of health and, ultimately, to the health of the person.

■ Conclusion

In this chapter, we have discussed the definition of a population that is rarely understood. And yet, this population has been in North America for 10,000 to 15,000 years prior to all others. There is a legal determination as to who is an AIAN in the United States. That definition is being an enrolled member or identified citizen of a federally recognized tribe. This brings with it historical and cultural assaults and resilience (or not) against the hundreds of years of federal, state, and local policies such as, "Kill the Indian and save the child/man" used to justify the assimilation period. But, this knowledge *is necessary* for the health professional. Correct identity of AIAN patients, knowledge of services available, and understanding the social determinants of health will all be necessary to begin reducing the huge disparities experienced by this group. Know that there are traumas. They are historical, intergenerational, and contemporaneous. These traumas will continue until the structures that allow them are torn down. Nursing, as the largest health profession, can be a leader in turning the tide. Nursing can affect the rampant misidentification of AIAN and look toward understanding and considering not only social determinants of health but also structural determinants in closing the disparity gaps.

■ Critical Thinking Exercises

1. What if your "population" could be knocked out almost to extinction and that those remaining suffered targeted, sustained, and persistent policies for more than 200 years from the country in which you now live? What do you think your four domains would be like?
2. A patient from a nearby reservation comes to your clinic. You do the usual care and then go over a printout of instructions: Refrigerate and take your insulin as ordered, take daily walks, and complete wound care. He agrees and leaves. What *other* questions should you have asked?

■ Discussion Questions

1. What are the two ways in which a person can be identified as American Indian or Alaska Native? Why would making this determination be important for you to make?
2. Discuss the reasons that the AIAN patient may need extra time to trust you as the health provider.
3. Pick one structural determinant of health and discuss how it may lead to poor health outcomes.

■ Resources

Cascone, S. (2017). Walker Art Center's controversial gallows sculpture will be removed and ceremonially burned. Retrieved from https://news.artnet.com/art-world/walker-sculpture-garden-to-remove-sam-durant-scaffold-977447

Vincent, G. K., & Velkoff, V. A. (2010). *THE NEXT FOUR DECADES: The older population in the United States: 2010 to 2050*. Washington, DC: U.S. Census Bureau. Retrieved from https://www.census.gov/prod/2010pubs/p25-1138.pdf

Indian Health Service: https://www.ihs.gov

CFR. (1947). Title 25 of the Code of Federal Regulations, Federal acknowledgment of American Indian tribes. §83.10.

CFR. (1949). Title 25 of the Code of Federal Regulations, Indian country defined, 1151.

Wolfe, P. (2006). Settler colonialism and the elimination of the native. *Journal of Geno-cide Research, 8*(4), 387–409. doi:10.1080/14623520601056240

■ References

American Association of Colleges of Nursing. (n.d.). *Baccalaureate education.* Retrieved from   https://www.aacnnursing.org/Nursing-Education-Programs/Baccalaureate-Education

Beck, P. N. (2014). *Inkpaduta: Dakota leader.* Norman: University of Oklahoma Press.

Boissoneault, L. (2017). Noose found in National Museum of African American History and Culture. *Smithsonian.com.* Retrieved from https://www.smithsonianmag.com/smithsonian-institution/noose-found-national-museum-african-american-history-and-culture-180963519

Bureau of Indian Affairs. (n.d.). *About us.* Retrieved from https://www.bia.gov/about-us

Brave Heart, Maria Yellow Horse. (1998). The return to the sacred path: Healing the historical trauma and historical unresolved grief response among the Lakota through a psychoeducational group intervention. *Smith College Studies in Social Work, 68*(3), 287–305. doi:10.1080/00377319809517532

Childs, W. H. (1863). *Execution of 38 Sioux Indians* [Image file]. Retrieved from https://commons.wikimedia.org/wiki/File:MankatoMN38.JPG

Department for Professional Employees. (2015). *Nursing: A profile of the profession: Fact sheet 2015.* Retrieved from https://dpeaflcio.org/programs-publications/issue-fact-sheets/nursing-a-profile-of-the-profession

Duran, E., Duran, B., Heart, Yellow Horse Brave Heart, M., & Horse-Davis, S. Y. (1998). Healing the American Indian soul wound. In Y. Danieli (Ed.), *International handbook of multigenerational legacies of trauma* (pp. 341–354). New York, NY: Springer.

Garrett, M. D., Baldridge, D., Benson, W., Crowder, J., & Aldrich, N. (2015). Mental health disorders among an invisible minority: Depression and dementia among American Indian and Alaska Native elders. *The Gerontologist, 55*(2), 227–236. doi:10.1093/geront/gnu181

Goetting, N. (2008). The Marshall Trilogy and the Constitutional dehumanization of American Indians. *HeinOnline, 21,* 207–224. Retrieved from https://heinonline.org/HOL/LandingPage?handle=hein.journals/guild65&div=26&id=&page=

Government Publishing Office. (2019a). *Code of federal regulations (CFR), 1996 to present.* Retrieved from https://www.govinfo.gov/help/cfr

Government Publishing Office. (2019b). Code of Federal Regulations: Title 25 - Indians. Retrieved from https://www.govinfo.gov/content/pkg/CFR-2019-title25-vol1/xml/CFR-2019-title25-vol1-sec83-1.xml

Indian Health Service. (2014). *Trends in Indian health 2014 edition.* Retrieved from https://www.ihs.gov/sites/dps/themes/responsive2017/display_objects/documents/Trends2014Book508.pdf

Indian Health Service. (2019). *About IHS.* Retrieved from https://www.ihs.gov/aboutihs

Kinghorn, B., Fretts, A., Fretts, A., O'Leary, R., Karr, C., Rosenfeld, M., & Best, L. (2018). Social determinants of asthma in Cheyenne River Sioux American Indian children. *American Journal of Respiratory and Critical Care Medicine, 197,* A2038. Retrieved from https://www.atsjournals.org/doi/abs/10.1164/ajrccm-conference.2018.197.1_MeetingAbstracts.A2038

Laviolette, G. (1991). *The Dakota Sioux in Canada.* Winnipeg, MB, Canada: DLM Publications.

Magnan, S. (2017). Social determinants of health 101 for health care: Five plus five. *NAM Perspectives*. doi:10.31478/201710c

Moss, M. P. (2010). American Indian health disparities: By the sufferance of Congress? *Hamline Journal of Public Law & Policy, 32*, 259–261. Retrieved from https://heinonline.org/HOL/LandingPage?handle=hein.journals/hplp32&div=6&id=&page=

Moss, M. P. (2015). *American Indian health and nursing*. New York, NY: Springer Publishing Company.

National Archives. (n.d.). *The Emancipation Proclamation*. Retrieved from https://www.archives.gov/exhibits/featured-documents/emancipation-proclamation

Nurse Journal. (n.d.). *Associates degree in nursing (ADN)*. Retrieved from https://nurse-journal.org/adn-degree/associates-degree-nursing

Registered Nursing.org. (n.d.). *Accelerated nursing programs – BSN & MSN*. Retrieved from https://www.registerednursing.org/degree/accelerated-nursing-programs

Rogers, M. (2017). Lebron James focused on family, not NBA finals, after racist attack. *USA Today*. Retrieved from https://www.usatoday.com/story/sports/nba/2017/05/31/lebron-james-focused-family-not-nba-finals-after-racist-attack/102362612

Schilling, V. (2017). The traumatic true history and name list of the Dakota 38. *Indian Country Today*. Retrieved from https://newsmaven.io/indiancountrytoday/archive/the-traumatic-true-history-and-name-list-of-the-dakota-38-3awsx1BAdU2v_KWM81RomQ

U.S. Bureau of Indian Affairs. (2016). *A Bureau of Indian Affairs map of Indian reservations in the contiguous United States*. Retrieved from https://www.bia.gov/sites/bia.gov/files/assets/bia/ots/webteam/pdf/idc1-028635.pdf

U.S. Census Bureau. (2012). *The American Indian and Alaska Native population: 2010*. Retrieved from http://www.census.gov/prod/cen2010/briefs/c2010br-10.pdf

U.S. Department of Justice. (2012). *Protecting Native American and Alaska Native women from violence: November is Native American heritage month*. Retrieved from https://www.justice.gov/archives/ovw/blog/protecting-native-american-and-alaska-native-women-violence-november-native-american

United States v. Wheeler, 435 U.S. 313, 323 (1978).

Warne, D., & Lajimodiere, D. (2015). American Indian health disparities: Psychosocial influences. *Social and Personality Psychology Compass, 9*(10), 567–579. doi:10.1111/spc3.12198

Wastvedt, S. (2017). *History we don't teach: Mankato hangings an uneasy topic for MN schools*. Retrieved from https://www.mprnews.org/story/2017/06/08/mankato-hangings-an-uneasy-topic-for-minnesota-schools

World Health Organization. (n.d.). *Social determinants of health*. Retrieved from https://www.who.int/social_determinants/en

Wolfe, P. (1994). Nation and miscegenation: Discursive continuity in the post-Mabo era. *Social Analysis: The International Journal of Social and Cultural Practice, 36*, 93–152. Retrieved from https://www.jstor.org/stable/23171805

10

Global Health Equity for LGBTQ People and Populations

William E. Rosa, Patricia J. Moreland, and Tonda L. Hughes

CHAPTER OBJECTIVES

- ⊙ Explain inequalities faced by lesbian, gay, bisexual, transgender, queer or questioning (LGBTQ) people and populations in healthcare and in society
- ⊙ Identify opportunities for policy advancement related to the current global health agenda that will promote equity for all people
- ⊙ Discuss the role of cultural humility and self-reflection in a healthcare system afflicted by implicit bias and health disparities that disproportionately impact sexual and gender minorities (SGMs)

KEY CONCEPTS

Cultural humility	LGBTQ health
Global health	Self-reflection
Health equity	Social determinants of health
Policy and advocacy	Social justice
Health disparities	

KEY TERMS

Culture	SDGs: Sustainable Development Goals
Discrimination	SGM: sexual and gender minority
Equity	Transgender woman/man: refers to
LGBTQ: lesbian, gay, bisexual,	individuals whose current sexual iden-
transgender, queer or questioning	tity does not match their sex at birth

■ Introduction

On June 2, 2018, Kai Schultz published a story in *The New York Times* glimpsing the raw and painful edges of what it means to be gay in India. Schultz (2018) was reporting on those impacted by the myriad implications of India's Section 377, the law that identifies SGM citizens as criminals and legally allows a host of injustices to be perpetrated upon them. The article describes a brief account of the risks associated with being SGM in a country where marginalization and violence is protected by institutionalized prejudice. These include secrecy, family shame, and abandonment; social stigma and bullying; a range of mental and physical abuses; rape; fiscal and professional extortion; intense fear of harm or being "outed"; harassment by neighbors and police; and mistreatment by employers. Unfortunately, it is not only India where one can be arrested or legally victimized due to SGM status in the absence of crimes committed—or incur mental cruelty or bodily injury made permissible by discriminatory policies. Such inequities faced by LGBTQ communities can be found worldwide (Abaver & Cishe, 2018; Charlton et al., 2018; Elliott et al., 2015; Hughes, Wilsnack, & Kantor, 2016; Hunt, Bristowe, Chidyamatare, & Harding, 2017; Lanham et al., 2019: Muller & Hughes, 2016; Qiao, Zhou, & Li, 2018; Sandfort, Frazer, Matebeni, Reddy, Southey-Swartz, 2015; Taylor, Dhingra, Dickson, & McDermott, 2018). In settings where social and environmental determinants of health include criminalization of same-sex relationships, and mistreatment and misunderstanding is embedded at both interpersonal and system levels, good health and well-being become not merely elusive but nearly impossible. For example, there are approximately 72 countries in the world where same-sex relationships are illegal, and in eight of these, people who participate in such relationships can be given a death sentence (Amnesty International, n.d.). LGBTQ persons come from every walk of life, social class, race, ethnicity, religion, and age group. Multiple health organizations acknowledge widespread disparities in the care of LGBTQ people and highlight their unique needs at the individual, group, and population levels as well as make recommendations aimed at promoting mental and physical health and well-being, reducing healthcare costs, and advancing respect and safety in the healthcare milieu (Centers for Disease Control and Prevention [CDC], 2018a; Office of Disease Prevention and Health Promotion, 2014; World Health Organization, 2016).

In this chapter, the authors seek to emphasize salience of health equity for LGBTQ people on a global scale and raise awareness of readers about the health needs of the LGBTQ population related to safety, well-being, inclusion, holistic welfare, and human dignity. Nurses in fields of practice, research, education, and policy are optimally positioned to ensure equitable services to all people, particularly those historically disenfranchised from the benefits of appropriate and respectful healthcare.

■ Background and Significance

An emerging body of evidence points to substantial sexual orientation–related health disparities related to systemic discrimination and an historical pathologizing of sexual minority identities and behaviors (Drescher, 2015; Institute of Medicine [IOM], 2011). Globally, LGBTQ individuals experience both overt and covert demonstrations of discrimination as well as unconscious bias during interactions within society and the healthcare system (IOM, 2011). Understanding the inequities faced by LGBTQ individuals as a social injustice issue is central to reducing these disparities.

INEQUALITIES IN HEALTH

A growing body of research conducted in Australia, Europe, and the United States has found LGBTQ individuals to be at higher risk for psychological distress (Elliott et al., 2015; Graugaard, Giraldi, Frisch, Falgaard, & Davidsen, 2015), depression, anxiety, and suicidal ideation (Bostwick, Boyd, Hughes, & McCabe, 2010; Chakraborty, McManus,

Brugha, Bebbington, & King, 2011; di Giacomo, Krausz, Colmegna, Aspesi, & Clerici, 2018; King et al. 2008; Steele et al., 2017; Taylor et al., 2018), alcohol and other drug abuse (Coulter et al., 2015; Hughes, Szalacha, & McNair, 2010; Hughes et al., 2016; McCabe, Hughes, Bostwick, West, & Boyd, 2009), cardiovascular disease (Caceres et al., 2017; Farmer, Bucholz, Flick, Burroughs, & Bowen, 2013), diabetes (Beach, Elasy, & Gonzales, 2018), some forms of cancer (e.g., breast, uterine, cervical, anal, colorectal, lung; Boehmer, Miao, & Ozonoff, 2011; Machalek et al., 2012; Meads & Moore, 2013; Quinn et al., 2015), physical disability (Fredriksen-Goldsen, Kim, Barkan, Muraco, & Hoy-Ellis, 2013), and asthma (Heck & Jacobson, 2006; Landers, Mimiaga, & Conron, 2011; Veldhuis, Bruzzese, Hughes, & George, 2019) than their heterosexual counterparts. Globally, men who have sex with men (MSM) and transgender women are disproportionately burdened by HIV infection (Castro et al., 2016; CDC, 2018b; De Boni, Veloso, & Grinsztein, 2014; Poteat, Reisner, & Radix, 2014; Seekaew et al., 2018). In 2017, the CDC reported that gay and bisexual men accounted for 66% of the diagnoses of HIV among males 13 years of age and older in the United States (CDC, 2019).

DISCRIMINATION AND VIOLENCE

Despite an urgent call from the United Nations (UN; UN Human Rights Council, 2011) to end violence and discrimination against LGBTQ individuals worldwide, a pervasive pattern of homicidal and hate-motivated violence and sexual assault continues to be reported (Abaver & Cishe, 2018; Juarez-Chavez, Cooney, Hidalgo, Sanchez, & Poteat, 2018; Muller & Hughes, 2016; Ritterbusch, Salazar, & Correa, 2018; Sandfort et al., 2015; Yi et al., 2018). Across continents, lesbian, bisexual, and transgender women are at higher risk for sexual violence and victimization compared to their heterosexual counterparts (Muller & Hughes, 2016; Rothman, Exner, & Baughman, 2011; Sandfort et al., 2015; Szalacha, Hughes, McNair, & Loxton, 2017). A study conducted in the United States found transgender women to have more than four times the risk of homicide than women in the general population (Human Rights Campaign, 2015). Similarly, in a recent review of literature, lesbian and bisexual women in the United States were found to have a 43% median lifetime rate of sexual assault victimization (Rothman et al., 2011). Some research, particularly research conducted in Southern Africa, has found high rates of sexual violence among lesbian and bisexual women (Muller & Hughes, 2016; Sandfort et al., 2015). Homophobic sexual violence, sometimes referred to as "corrective rape," appears to be particularly prevalent in South Africa (Muller & Hughes, 2016). This form of sexual violence is perpetrated against women who identify as sexual minority (SMW) (or are presumed to be lesbian or bisexual) by men in an effort to "correct" their sexual orientation (Koraan & Geduld, 2015). The ideological justification for corrective rape is that the rape will "cure" the woman of her lesbianism and put her on the "right" path to being "straight" (Koraan & Geduld, 2015). Although most recent reports of homophobic rape have been reported in Southern Africa, it is believed to occur in all regions of the world (Blondeel et al., 2018). It is notable that corrective rape appears to be a growing problem in South Africa, given that South Africa's postapartheid constitution explicitly prohibits discrimination based on sexual orientation (Koraan & Geduld, 2015). The social marginalization of SMW in South Africa and elsewhere increases their risk of HIV and other sexually transmitted diseases, alcohol and other drug abuse, and mental distress (Sandfort et al., 2015).

INEQUALITIES AND DISPARITIES IN HEALTHCARE ACCESS

Inequalities in access to healthcare negatively impact health outcomes of LGBTQ individuals (IOM, 2011). Access barriers include lack of health insurance, discriminatory attitudes of healthcare providers, and healthcare providers' lack of knowledge of LGBTQ healthcare issues (Albuquerque et al., 2016; IOM, 2011; Jackman, Bosse, Eliason, & Hughes, 2019).

Health Insurance

Lack of health insurance has been identified as a structural barrier to healthcare access for LGBTQ people, particularly in the United States (Baker & Durso, 2017; IOM, 2011). Research indicates that SGMs are more likely than their heterosexual counterparts to be unemployed, uninsured, and unable to afford health services (Baker & Dorso, 2017; Charlton et al., 2018; Kates, Ranji, Beamesderfer, Salganicoff, & Dawson, 2014). Employment discrimination has been found to contribute to LGBT unemployment and lack of insurance (Pew Research Center, 2013; Sears & Mallory, 2011). In a national survey conducted in 2013 by the Pew Research Center, 21% of LGBT respondents reported being treated unfairly in relation to hiring, pay, or promotions (Pew Research Center, 2013). A similar survey by the Williams Institute (Sears & Mallory, 2011) found that among LGBT individuals who were open about their sexual orientation in the workplace, 38% reported harassment in the past 5 years and 7% felt they had lost a job because of their sexual orientation. The failure of the United States to enact legislation that protects LGBT individuals from employment discrimination illustrates one of the barriers to healthcare access for this vulnerable population. At the time of writing, 28 states have no employment nondiscrimination law covering sexual orientation or gender identity. In 29 states, employers can legally fire transgender people (Human Rights Campaign, 2019).

Provider Discrimination

Prejudicial and discriminatory attitudes of healthcare providers have been reported by LGBTQ people worldwide. In a survey of 93,078 LGBT people in 28 European countries, 10% reported feeling personally discriminated against by healthcare personnel in the 12 months prior to the survey (European Union Agency for Fundamental Rights, 2013). To avoid discriminatory or stigmatizing treatment, LGBTQ people often conceal their sexual orientation or gender identity, thereby reducing the ability of providers to understand and address SGM-specific health needs (Qiao et al., 2018). Research in Central and Southern Africa has found high levels of healthcare provider stigma and discrimination against LGBT individuals (Hunt et al., 2017; Muller & Hughes, 2016). In Muller and Hughes's (2016) systematic review of the literature on SMW's health in Southern Africa, lesbian and bisexual women were reluctant to use health services, including preventive care, due to healthcare provider discrimination. In Zimbabwe, lesbian, gay, bisexual, transgender, and intersex people, as well as sex workers, reported enduring disrespectful and humiliating comments from healthcare providers when they disclosed their sexual orientation (Hunt et al., 2017). Conforming to heterosexual norms and nondisclosure of sexual orientation was believed to be conditional to accessing healthcare. Research by Poteat, Logie, et al. (2014) in Lesotho found that SMW were more likely to disclose their sexual identity to family members than to healthcare providers (45% vs. 25%). SMW described discriminatory care and perceptions that healthcare providers were often unprepared to address their sexual health needs. Although they expressed concerns about HIV and sexually transmitted infections (STIs), limited access to appropriate safer-sex materials influenced SMW's ability to protect themselves from sexually transmitted diseases.

Extant literature suggests that transgender people are particularly susceptible to stigma and discrimination within society and in healthcare settings (Aparicio-García, Díaz-Ramiro, Rubio-Valdehita, López-Núñez, & García-Nieto, 2018; Li et al., 2017; Rodriguez-Madera et al., 2017; Silva et al., 2016; Walters, Paterson, Brown, & McDonnell, 2017; Yi et al., 2018). Societal resistance to or intolerance of gender-nonconforming presentation and behavior is believed to explain, in large part, the higher rates of discrimination and violence that trans people experience (Wilson et al., 2019). The 2015 U.S. Transgender Survey (James et al., 2016) found that one-third of transgender persons who saw a healthcare provider in the year prior to completing the survey reported at least one negative healthcare experience related to their gender identity, such as being verbally harassed or refused treatment. Prior negative experiences with healthcare providers contribute to delays in seeking healthcare and can result in more serious illnesses or conditions that are more difficult to treat.

In the Latin American and Caribbean countries of El Salvador, Trinidad and Tobago, Barbados, and Haiti, transgender women reported experiences of pervasive stigma and discrimination in the healthcare setting (Lanham et al., 2019). They were frequently denied health services or given a lower priority than other patients. Some healthcare providers refused to use their chosen name or to recognize their identity as a woman because their identity card had a male name. Threats of physical abuse because of their gender identity or sexual preference were reported by participants in all countries.

Provider Knowledge and Cultural Competence

In the United States, the IOM (2011) identified inadequate LGBT health education in medical and nursing curricula as a structural barrier to SGMs obtaining high-quality, culturally sensitive care. Several published studies and literature reviews support this (Carabez, Pellegrini, Mankovitz, Eliason, & Dariotis, 2014; De Guzman, Moukouloub, Scott, & Zerwic, 2018; Lim, Johnson, & Eliason, 2015; Stewart & O'Reilly, 2017). The Lim et al. (2015) study with faculty in baccalaureate nursing programs in the United States found limited knowledge, experience, and readiness for teaching LGBT health. Of the 1,231 faculty members surveyed, 43% reported limited or somewhat limited knowledge of LGBT health–related issues. Topics most frequently taught included HIV and STIs, homophobia, LGBT youth issues, violence, and hate crimes. The topics least taught included minority stress, issues related to health insurance, and tobacco, alcohol, and drug use. The median time spent teaching LGBT health content was approximately 2 hours (Lim et al., 2015). In a survey of nursing students' knowledge of LGBT issues, almost 40% of the 122 participants felt unprepared to provide LGBT care, and 85% said their nursing education did not prepare them to care for LGBT people (Carabez et al., 2014). In addition to the lack of LGBT health–related content in nursing curricula, research indicates that access to educational materials relevant to caring for LGBT persons is limited (De Guzman et al., 2018). These authors conducted a content analysis of two commonly used health assessment textbooks and found limited and sometimes inaccurate information about LGBT health concerns. Existing content focused primarily on HIV and STIs (De Guzman et al., 2018). Coverage of LGBT health in nursing journals is also limited (Eliason, Dibble, & DeJoseph, 2010). These authors reviewed articles published in the top 10 nursing journals from 2005 to 2009 and found that only 0.16% of articles directly addressed LGBTQ health issues (Eliason et al., 2010). This study was recently updated and extended by Jackman et al. (2019), with results showing only slight improvement in coverage of LGBT health issues. Lack of understanding about LGBT-specific health concerns can affect a nurse's ability to provide sensitive, culturally competent care to LGBT people. Carabez et al. (2015) surveyed 268 nurses in the San Francisco Bay Area and found that 80% had no education or training on LGBT issues; those who received some training had only a single lecture in nursing school or a broader diversity training that briefly mentioned LGBT issues. In a systematic review of the literature that explored the knowledge, beliefs, and attitudes of nurses and midwives related to the healthcare needs of LGBTQ patients, inadequate care was often related to a culture of heteronormativity (Stewart & O'Reilly, 2017). "Heteronormativity" is a systemic bias that recognizes heterosexuality as normal and natural and assumes that the majority of sexual relationships are heterosexual (McCabe, Dragowski, & Rubinson, 2013). The assumption of heteronormativity can influence a nurse's language and behavior and result in LGBTQ individuals remaining silent about important health issues for fear that disclosure may lead to stigmatization and discrimination (Fisher, Fried, Desmond, Macapagal, & Mustanski, 2018). Nondisclosure of sexual orientation and gender identity decreases the likelihood that appropriate health education and counseling will be provided—which can negatively impact the health outcomes of LGBTQ individuals.

■ The UN 2030 Agenda for Sustainable Development

Health equity for LGBTQ people is not possible without a strategic focus on improving social, economic, biological, and environmental determinants of health that threaten the welfare of these populations. On January 1, 2016, the UN put into motion the single most ambitious and determined agenda in its history focused on equity and inclusion for all. Affirmatively adopted by all 193 Member States of the UN General Assembly in September 2015, the 2030 Agenda for Sustainable Development seeks to eradicate poverty; promote planetary, environmental, and animal health; and take strategic steps toward peace and prosperity for all human beings worldwide (UN, 2016). The agenda includes 17 Sustainable Development Goals (SDGs) that are further divided into 169 targets. The 17 SDGs are listed in Box 10.1.

Most relevant to a discussion on health equity from a global perspective, these SDGs seek to "leave no one behind" while focusing on five primary themes: People, Planet, Peace, Prosperity, and Partnership. The SDGs were created as a humanitarian action plan and replaced the eight Millennium Development Goals (UN, n.d.) that were in place from 2000 to 2015. They provide a holistic framework to drive local and transnational policies aimed at identifying and narrowing disparities, achieving universal health coverage, and creating long-term global safety in precarious and unjust systems. The SDGs reflect the values and efforts of Florence Nightingale and the ethos of modern nursing, a profession committed to social justice and equitable care for all, including those who are marginalized and invisible (Dossey, Rosa, & Beck, 2019; Rosa, Dossey, Watson, Beck, & Upvall, 2019). Nurses and the nursing profession have vital roles in attaining each of the SDGs through leadership, advocacy, and integration of

Box 10.1: The 17 SDGs

SDG 1. End poverty in all its forms everywhere.

SDG 2. End hunger, achieve food security and improved nutrition, and promote sustainable agriculture.

SDG 3. Ensure healthy lives and promote well-being for all at all ages.

SDG 4. Ensure inclusive and equitable quality education and promote lifelong learning opportunities for all.

SDG 5. Achieve gender equality and empower all women and girls.

SDG 6. Ensure availability and sustainable management of water and sanitation for all.

SDG 7. Ensure access to affordable, reliable, sustainable, and modern energy for all.

SDG 8. Promote sustained, inclusive, and sustainable economic growth, full and productive employment, and decent work for all.

SDG 9. Build resilient infrastructure, promote inclusive and sustainable industrialization, and foster innovation.

SDG 10. Reduce inequality within and among countries.

SDG 11. Make cities and human settlements inclusive, safe, resilient, and sustainable.

SDG 12. Ensure sustainable consumption and production patterns.

SDG 13. Take urgent action to combat climate change and its impacts.

SDG 14. Conserve and sustainably use the oceans, seas, and marine resources for sustainable development.

SDG 15. Protect, restore, and promote sustainable use of terrestrial ecosystems, sustainably manage forests, combat desertification, and halt and reverse land degradation and halt biodiversity loss.

SDG 16. Promote peaceful and inclusive societies for sustainable development, provide access to justice for all, and build effective, accountable, and inclusive institutions at all levels.

SDG 17. Strengthen the means of implementation and revitalize the Global Partnership for Sustainable Development.

SDG, Sustainable Development Goal.

Source: From United Nations. (2016). *Transforming our world: The 2030 Agenda for Ssustainable Development.* Retrieved from https://sustainabledevelopment.un.org/content/documents/21252030%20Agenda%20for%20Sustainable%20Development%20web.pdf

the UN 2030 Agenda through local national and international initiatives related to practice, education, research, and policy (Rosa, 2017a; Rosa, Upvall, Beck, & Dossey, 2019).

Unfortunately, the SDGs do not explicitly address protection of the rights of LGBTQ people. Even SDG 5, which seeks to Achieve Gender Equality and Empower All Women and Girls, overlooks the welfare of transgender and gender-nonconforming persons and obscures the need for concerted efforts that protect and preserve the lives and well-being of LGBTQ people (Rosa, 2017b). Stonewall International (Dorey, 2016) acknowledges that although the SDGs represent positive advancement for civil society, the agenda could and should have taken the next step in addressing systemic inequities that disproportionately affect LGBTQ people and result in higher poverty levels and poorer health among these populations. Stonewall International (Dorey, 2016) provides recommendations to include LGBTQ protections throughout the enactment of specific SDGs. In Table 10.1, the left-hand column lists the relevant SDGs and associated targets, the middle column describes the need and rationale, and the right-hand column includes corresponding action items.

Stonewall International (Dorey, 2016) makes final recommendations to advance the inclusion of LGBTQ human rights in alignment with SDG attainment by promoting the following:

- Fund and support for local LGBTQ organizations and their initiatives to meet the needs of their communities.
- Collaborate with all policy stakeholders across disciplines about "no one left behind"; advocate for the appropriate training, support, and education needed to ensure LGBTQ people are a part of SDG advancement every step of the way.
- Employ LGBTQ-specific indicators; collect and evaluate data that is relevant to the LGBTQ context.
- Institute LGBTQ-inclusive policies for staff and beneficiaries and promote the same for all collaborating partners and colleagues.
- Hold governments and service providers accountable for equitable and sensitive inclusion of LGBTQ persons.
- Invite LGBTQ groups to participate and contribute to the development, implementation, and evaluation of all support programs to meet needs and avoid harm.

Health equity is a central component of the SDGs. Without including LGBTQ considerations in the 2030 Agenda and the policies it influences, it remains inadequate and inherently exclusive. In fact, continued global silence regarding the needs and vulnerabilities of LGBTQ populations leaves behind the very people who most need the respect and protections central to the vision of the SDGs.

◼ Cultural Humility: Health Equity's Essential Thread

To provide safe and inclusive environments for LGBTQ individuals, many U.S. initiatives have sought to foster inclusive practices and to promote patient-/family-centered care through effective communication (The Joint Commission, 2011) and to identify healthcare allies that promote equity for LGBTQ patients, families, visitors, and

TABLE 10.1 THE SDGS AND LGBTQ EQUITY: RELEVANT GAPS AND RECOMMENDED ACTION ITEMS

SDGS/TARGETS	RELEVANT GAPS	RECOMMENDED ACTION ITEMS
Goal 1. End poverty in all its forms everywhere. ■ Target 1.3: Implement nationally appropriate social protection systems and measures for all ■ Target 1.4: By 2030, ensure that all men and women have equal rights to economic resources, as well as access to basic services, ownership and control over land and other forms of property	■ Discrimination complicates the abilities of LGBTQ persons to earn income, remain safe, and achieve goals ■ Discrimination can be a predictor of poverty; increased poverty can incur further exclusion ■ International development projects disproportionately attend to the needs of opposite-sex couples	■ Conduct additional research to identify economic discrimination of LGBTQ people ■ Advocate LGBTQ inclusion in private sector development projects ■ Include LGBTQ needs in social assistance programs, particularly for the poorest to strengthen communities ■ Empower LGBTQ people to establish their own businesses
Goal 3. Ensure healthy lives and promote well-being for all at all ages. ■ Target 3.7: By 2030, ensure universal access to sexual and reproductive services ■ Target 3.8: Achieve universal health coverage for all	■ Clinics in uninformed settings may refuse care to LGBTQ people; education may omit LGBTQ sexual and reproductive considerations ■ LGBTQ people frequently receive poor health services due to lack of healthcare worker awareness or inappropriate services ■ Those LGBTQ people impacted by exclusion and stigma may experience greater mental health challenges and receive limited support	■ Promote LGBTQ antidiscrimination policies ■ Train healthcare workers to understand LGBTQ needs ■ Create outreach health services for LGBTQ persons and communities ■ Develop improved, accessible services that meet the needs of HIV and other sexually transmitted infection care and supports the well-being of LGBTQ persons ■ Foster safe spaces and services that meet wider needs of the population ■ Provide services for trans people to move through their transitions safely
Goal 4. Ensure inclusive and equitable quality education and promote lifelong learning opportunities for all. ■ Target 4.5: By 2030, ensure equal access to all levels of education and vocational training for children in vulnerable situations. ■ Target 4.7: By 2030, ensure education for human rights [and] promotion of a culture of peace and non-violence	■ LGBTQ young people worldwide are often bullied due to their sexuality, excluded by peers and teachers ■ Some LGBTQ students leave prematurely secondary to poor treatment; others receive poor grades that impact future opportunities ■ Lifelong mental health is impacted by the student years and experiences	■ Offer guidance and training for teachers/counselors that inform sensitive and inclusive LGBTQ education ■ Adopt zero-tolerance policies regarding bullying ■ Ensure curricula are LGBTQ-inclusive and profile positive images and role models ■ Integrate sexual and reproductive education appropriate for students questioning sexual orientation or gender identity ■ Promote a culture of nondiscrimination and acceptance

(continued)

TABLE 10.1 THE SDGS AND LGBTQ EQUITY: RELEVANT GAPS AND RECOMMENDED ACTION ITEMS (*CONTINUED*)

SDGS/TARGETS	RELEVANT GAPS	RECOMMENDED ACTION ITEMS
Goal 5. Achieve gender equality and empower all women and girls. ■ Target 5.1: End all forms of discrimination against all women and girls everywhere. ■ Target 5.2: Eliminate all forms of violence against all women and girls	■ Lesbian, bisexual, and trans women may experience multiple forms of discrimination and violence due to intersectionality of LGBTQ identity and gender ■ International development projects disproportionately attend to the needs of opposite-sex couples ■ Harmful gender stereotypes limit people from being themselves; gender-based violence often seeks to punish those who do not conform to such norms	■ Programs should address issues faced by lesbian, bisexual, and trans women ■ Prioritize organizations led by LGBTQ women through funding and grant opportunities ■ Expand the definition of "gender" employed by policies and programs to role-model inclusivity ■ Promote programs that challenge the harm perpetrated by gender norms
Goal 10. Reduce inequality within and among countries. ■ Target 10.2: By 2030, empower and promote the inclusion of all, irrespective of age, sex, disability, race, ethnicity, origin, religion or economic or other status ■ Target 10.3: Ensure equal opportunity including by eliminating discriminatory laws, policies, and practices	■ Discrimination against LGBTQ people is often reinforced by laws, policies, and practices that fail to meet the needs of LGBTQ people or intentionally exclude them; examples include forced sterilization of trans people; disallowing trans people to change legal gender; illegalizing same-sex marriage; prohibiting LGBTQ nongovernmental organizations or public campaigning; excluding LGBTQ people from accessing social services	■ Fund LGBTQ groups working toward equality and the end of discriminatory laws, policies, and practices ■ Support LGBTQ-led campaigns that promote social justice ■ Educate that the "other status" of Target 10.2 includes LGBTQ people ■ Make sure personal and professional partners do not discriminate, honoring the Target 10.2 call for equality

Goal 11. Make cities and human settlements inclusive, safe, resilient, and sustainable. ■ Target 11.1: By 2030, ensure access for all to adequate, safe, and affordable housing and basic services	■ High rates of LGBTQ homeless can result from discrimination (e.g., rejection/abuse by family, mistreatment/bullying by friends, prejudice from landlords) ■ LGBTQ homeless people are vulnerable to higher likelihood of violence, sexual abuse, and a host of physical/mental health problems ■ Support services and poor education regarding LGBTQ needs may cause continued exclusion from necessary support systems	■ Educate local government and housing authorities to attend to the needs of LGBTQ youth ■ Provide safe houses and other specialist services for at-risk LGBTQ persons vulnerable to homelessness, such as young people and older adults ■ Advocate affordable and nondiscriminatory housing ■ Attend to the needs of LGBTQ communities regarding safe housing
Goal 16. Promote peaceful and inclusive societies for sustainable development, provide access to justice for all and build effective, accountable, and inclusive institutions at all levels. ■ Target 16.1: Significantly reduce all forms of violence and related death threats. ■ Target 16.3: Ensure equal access to justice for all.	■ Police and security in many countries refuse to take LGBTQ reports of violence seriously ■ Police and security in many countries are part of the attack and harassment on LGBTQ people, often considered justified by discriminatory laws ■ LGBTQ people may underreport violence or death threats in settings where they do not believe they will be protected ■ Homophobic, transphobic, and biphobic attitudes exacerbate vulnerability of LGBTQ people to human rights abuses	■ Ensure programs that support policing, criminal justice, and/or civil society are active in addressing hate crimes ■ Provide sensitivity training for police, security, and those in the criminal justice system to empower them to mitigate LGBTQ hate crimes and discrimination ■ Foster abilities and willingness of authorities to document hate crimes against LGBTQ persons

LGBTQ, lesbian, gay, bisexual, transgender, queer or questioning; SDG, Sustainable Development Goal.
Source: Data from Dorey, K. (2016). *The sustainable development goals and LGBT inclusion.* London, England: Stonewall. Retrieved from https://www.stonewall.org.uk/system/files/sdg-guide2.pdf

employees (Human Rights Campaign, 2018). As a result, many healthcare workers are trained in cultural awareness and sensitivity as a means to ensure whole-person inclusive care. "Cultural humility" was coined by Tervalon and Murray-Garcia (1998) when working with medical residents in a multicultural institution and may be a helpful tool for creating reflective and equitable environments. The authors identified three main pillars of cultural humility: (a) self-reflection and lifelong learning in order to accept, understand, and incorporate differing beliefs and health practices; (b) patient-focused interviewing and care that replace power imbalances seen in paternalistic provider–patient dyads; and (c) community-based care and advocacy that leads to mutually beneficial partnerships for both providers and recipients of healthcare services (Tervalon & Murray-Garcia, 1998).

Cultural humility is quite different from cultural competence. According to Soulé (2016), cultural competence is rooted in active volition, in a way of *doing* that emphasizes expert clinical skill and acumen. Conversely, cultural humility is based on passive volition and focuses on creating a new way of *being* that stresses human wholeness, engagement, and a continual process of deepening relationships with self and others. Cultural humility maintains particular defining attributes, such as openness, self-awareness, being egoless, a focus on supportive interactions, and a commitment to self-reflection and self-critique (Foronda, Baptiste, Reinholdt, & Ousman, 2016). Self-reflection is a substantial component of promoting cultural humility and culturally humble practices in the healthcare of LGBTQ people. The attributes of cultural humility identified by Foronda et al. (2016), accompanied by reflective questions for the reader that relate to LGBTQ health equity, can be found in Table 10.2.

In the global sphere, health inequities for LGBTQ people occur at individual, community, and societal levels. Translating the concepts of cultural humility into logical steps that promote the welfare of individuals and populations is vital. Acquaviva (2017) used the pneumonic CAMPERS to aid in the creation of safe and nonjudgmental healthcare environments for LGBTQ patients, offering concrete steps to improve self-awareness. CAMPERS represents seven steps: Clear purpose, Attitudes, Mitigation plan, Patient, Emotions, Reactions, and Strategy. While originally created for LGBTQ patients in hospice and palliative care settings, CAMPERS can also be used to advance health equity for LGBTQ persons at the community level across global healthcare venues. Each of the CAMPERS steps accompanied by Acquaviva's (2017) identified actions and considerations for developing community-based care for LGBTQ people is presented in Table 10.3. Community-based considerations may be particularly helpful for nurses who wish to contribute to public health initiatives and to the development of programs—both locally and globally—that advance health equity for LGBTQ people.

■ Conclusion

During the writing of this chapter, a major policy victory was won. In September 2018, India's Supreme Court justices unanimously voted to decriminalize homosexuality with the repeal of the country's Section 377 (Sommerlad, 2018). Since the law went into effect in 1861, LGBTQ persons in India have systematically been oppressed and at risk of imprisonment, loss of employment, and a host of other socioeconomic inequalities. Although this ruling represents a significant step forward, LGBTQ people and

TABLE 10.2 THE ATTRIBUTES OF CULTURAL HUMILITY AND CARE OF LGBTQ PERSONS: QUESTIONS FOR SELF-REFLECTION

ATTRIBUTES OF CULTURAL HUMILITY (IDENTIFIED BY FORONDA ET AL., 2016)	QUESTIONS FOR SELF-REFLECTION
Openness	■ Is the act of being open to the life experiences of LGBTQ patients essential to my delivery of whole-person care? ■ Am I willing to invite all aspects of the health narrative of LGBTQ patients despite my own personal judgment or discomfort? ■ How can I develop new habits and practices of remaining open to the needs of LGBTQ patients and their families amid systemic time and resource constraints?
Self-awareness	■ Do I harbor misconceptions or prejudice regarding the health of LGBTQ patients? ■ In what ways could my own nursing practice improve to ensure more equitable and respectful environments for LGBTQ communities? ■ How does my need to complete health assessments and clinical tasks interfere with my ability to remain fully present and available to the evolving health experience of LGBTQ persons in my care?
Egoless	■ What intentional actions can I take to ensure I engage LGBTQ patients as equals deserving respect and dignity? ■ Am I conscious to surrender any airs of superiority that prevent me from being approachable and of service? ■ What are the steps I can take to promote a humble attitude and a welcoming environment for LGBTQ patients and their loved ones?
Supportive interactions	■ How do I actively take accountability for the quality of my relationships with LGBTQ patients, families, and communities? ■ Does my nursing care promote positive human exchanges throughout its delivery? ■ Do I elicit unmet needs from LGBTQ patients in my care to ensure timely and equitable allocation of resources?
Self-reflection and critique	■ What personal practices do I maintain to foster my own accountability in delivering equitable nursing care? ■ How do I grow in awareness of any implicit or unconscious biases that may deter health equity for LGBTQ people and negatively impact associated health outcomes? ■ In what ways do I strive to make peace between my beliefs and preferences as a person as it relates to LGBTQ people and my moral/ethical obligation to provide safe, respectful, inclusive, and culturally humble care?

LGBTQ, lesbian, gay, bisexual, transgender, queer or questioning.

populations in India and across the world continue to face inequities in healthcare and throughout society. Policy changes are needed at local, regional, national, and international levels to protect against discrimination and violence. A focus on integrating LGBTQ health priorities into global health initiatives, such as the UN 2030 Sustainable Development Agenda, and educating healthcare providers in cultural humility at

TABLE 10.3 CAMPERS: ACTIONS AND COMMUNITY CONSIDERATIONS

CAMPERS (ACQUAVIVA, 2017)	ACTIONS (ADAPTED FROM ACQUAVIVA, 2017)	COMMUNITY CONSIDERATIONS
Step 1. Know your clear purpose.	■ Identify the purpose of the interaction. ■ Understand the purpose may shift over time based on need and abilities of the nurse.	■ Research the history and policy influences of the LGBTQ community in this context. ■ Resolve discrepancies between the goals of your initiative and the needs of the community. ■ Use multiple sources to identify and hone purpose, including personal insight from community members, identified leadership, and empirical findings.
Step 2. Know your attitudes and beliefs.	■ Consider inherent assumptions present entering into, throughout, and after leaving encounter. ■ Identify biases, prejudices, learned social norms, and ways they injure patient welfare.	■ Elicit objective assistance to ensure personal attitudes and beliefs do not detract from advancement of project goals. ■ Collaborate with community members to ensure adequate representation and to avoid the delivery of contextually irrelevant care.
Step 3. Know your mitigation plan.	■ Rectify power imbalances by inviting mutual partnership throughout the process. ■ Reframe alienating language.	■ Invite the community voice through the inception, development, implementation, and evaluation of the initiative. ■ Ensure language is respectful and used in accordance with community preferences.
Step 4. Know the patient.	■ Assess vital health information: gender identity, gender pronouns used, support systems, short- and long-term goals, etc.	■ Consider this community to be the patient or client; use markers of identity that are respectful and community-identified. ■ Understand how the LGBTQ community at hand exists within and is treated by related powers within the health, legal, and socioeconomic systems.

Step 5. Know your emotions.	■ Acknowledge human emotions, build mechanisms to process them, and avoid allowing them to interfere with care.	■ Build alliances within the community to translate unproductive feelings into strategic actions for health equity and advancement. ■ Promote environments of respectful communication to healthily process feelings across the spectrum of emotions.
Step 6. Know your reactions.	■ Understand personal reactions to frustration, anger, or impatience in order to remain available and responsive to the needs at hand.	■ Study the reactions of partners and community leaders to promote understanding relationships throughout the program. ■ Invite transparency and accountability to ensure program goals are not hindered by unforeseen reactions.
Step 7. Know your strategy.	■ Review interactions with all patients to improve service and consider what could be done differently in the future.	■ Create opportunities for frequent team- and trust-building to invite ongoing improvement. ■ Promote frequent evaluations to ensure program action items are in alignment with program goals and increased LGBTQ equity.

CAMPERS, Clear purpose, Attitudes, Mitigation plan, Patient, Emotions, Reactions, and Strategy; LGBTQ, lesbian, gay, bisexual, transgender, queer or questioning.

all levels and across settings to narrow health disparities, are critically important steps that need to be taken to reduce health disparities arising from sexual and/or gender minority status.

■ Discussion Questions

1. In what ways have I observed healthcare inequities for LGBTQ persons at local, regional, national, or international levels?
2. What implicit biases or misconceptions regarding LGBTQ people or their health do I hold?
3. What improvements can I make to my practice and how can I advocate to ensure the provision of environments that are safe and supportive of LGBTQ people and their health needs?
4. What are my opportunities, personally and professionally, to advance equity for all healthcare recipients including LGBTQ and other marginalized groups?

■ Resources

Human Rights Campaign. (n.d.). Glossary of terms. Retrieved from https://www.hrc.org/resources/glossary-of-terms

Hansen, H., Riano, N. S., Meadows, T., & Mangurian, C. (2018). Alleviating the mental health burden of structural discrimination and hate crimes: The role of psychiatrists. *American Journal of Psychiatry, 175*(10), 929–933. doi:10.1176/appi.ajp.2018.17080891

It Gets Better Project: Global initiative to uplift, empower, and connect LGBTQ youth. https://itgetsbetter.org

National Resource Center on LGBT Aging: https://lgbtagingcenter.org

Project Implicit*: Self-assessment of implicit biases. https://www.projectimplicit.net/index.html

Self-assessment tests: https://implicit.harvard.edu/implicit/takeatest.html

The Trevor Project: Crisis and suicide prevention services for LGBTQ young adults under 25. https://www.thetrevorproject.org/get-help-now/#sm.00000bhifegyr2eeqqyu8qlz4h2el

■ References

Abaver, D. T. & Cishe, E. N. (2018). Violence, abuse and discrimination: Key factors militating against control of HIV/AIDS among the LGBTI sector. *Sahara Journal, 15*(1), 60–70. doi:10.1080/17290376.2018.1492960

Acquaviva, K. D. (2017). *LGBTQ-inclusive hospice and palliative care: A practice guide to transforming professional practice.* New York, NY: Harrington Park Press.

Albuquerque, G. A., Garcia, C. D., Quirino, G. D., Alves, M. J., Belém, J. M., Figueiredo, F. W., . . . Adami, F. (2016). Access to health services by lesbian, gay, bisexual, and transgender persons: Systemic literature review. *BMC International Health and Human Rights, 16*(2), 1–10. doi:10.1186/s12914-015-0072-9

Amnesty International. (n.d.). *LGBTI rights.* Retrieved from https://www.amnesty.org/en/what-we-do/discrimination/lgbt-rights

Aparicio-García, M. E., Díaz-Ramiro, E. M., Rubio-Valdehita, S., López-Núñez, M. I., & García-Nieto, I. (2018). Health and well-being of cisgender, transgender and non-binary young people. *International Journal of Environmental Research and Public Health, 15*(10), 1–11. doi:10.3390/ijerph15102133

Baker, K., & Durso, L. E. (2017). *Why repealing the Affordable Care Act is bad medicine for LGBT communities.* Washington, DC: Center for American Progress.

Beach, L. B., Elasy, T. A., Gonzales, G. (2018). Prevalence of self-reported diabetes by sexual orientation: Results from the 2014 Behavioral Risk Factor Surveillance System. *LGBT Health, 5*(2), 121–130. doi:10.1089/lgbt.2017.0091

Blondeel, K., de Vasconcelos, S., García-Moreno, C., Stephenson, R., Temmerman, M., & Toskin, I. (2018). Violence motivated by perception of sexual orientation and gender identity: A systematic review. *Bull World Health Organ, 96*, 29–41. doi:10.2471/BLT.17.197251

Boehmer, U., Miao, X., & Ozonoff, A. (2011). Cancer survivorship and sexual orientation. *Cancer, 117*(16), 3796–3804. doi:10.1002/cncr.25950

Bostwick, W. B., Boyd, C. J., Hughes, T. L., & McCabe, S. E. (2010). Dimensions of sexual orientation and the prevalence of mood and anxiety disorders in the United States. *American Journal of Public Health, 100*(3), 468–475. doi:10.2105/AJPH.2008.152942

Caceres, B. A., Brody, A., Luscombe, R. E., Primiano, J. E., Marusca, P., Sitts, E. M., & Chyun, D. (2017). A systematic review of cardiovascular disease in sexual minorities. *American Journal of Public Health, 107*(4), e13–e21. doi:10.2105/AJPH.2016.303630a

Carabez, R., Pellegrini, M., Mankovitz, A., Eliason, M., Ciano, M., & Scott, M. (2015). "Never in all my years. . .": Nurses' education about LGBT health. *Journal of Professional Nursing, 31*(4), 323–329. doi:10.1016/j.profnurs.2015.01.003

Carabez, R., Pellegrini, M., Mankovitz, A., Eliason, M., & Dariotis, W. (2014). Nursing students' perceptions of their knowledge of lesbian, gay, bisexual, and transgender issues: Effectiveness of a multi-purpose assignment in a public health nursing class. *Journal of Nursing Education, 54*(1), 50–53. doi:10.3928/01484834-20141228-03

Castro, R., Ribeiro-Alves, M., Correa, R. G., Derrico, M., Lemos, K., Grangeiro, J. R., . . . Grinsztein, B. (2016). The men who have sex with men: HIV Care Cascade in Rio de Janeiro, Brazil. *PLoS One, 11*(6), 1–11. doi:10.1371/journal.pone.0157309

Centers for Disease Control and Prevention. (2018a). *Lesbian, gay, bisexual, and transgender health.* Retrieved from https://www.cdc.gov/lgbthealth/index.htm

Centers for Disease Control and Prevention. (2018b). *HIV and gay and bisexual men.* Retrieved from https://www.cdc.gov/hiv/group/msm/index.html

Centers for Disease Control and Prevention. (2019). *HIV in the United States and dependent areas.* Retrieved from https://www.cdc.gov/hiv/pdf/statistics/overview/cdc-hiv-us-ataglance.pdf

Chakraborty, A., McManus, S., Brugha, T. S., Bebbington, P., & King, M. (2011). Mental health of the non-heterosexual population of England. *British Journal of Psychiatry, 198*(2), 143–148. doi:10.1192/bjp.bp.110.082271

Charlton, B. M., Gordan, A. R., Reisner, S. L., Sarda, V., Samnaliev, M., Austin, S. B. (2018). Sexual orientation–related disparities in employment, health insurance, healthcare access and health-related quality of life: A cohort study of US male and female adolescents and young adults. *BMJ Open, 8*(6), 1–9. doi:10.1136/bmjopen-2017-020418

Coulter, R. W., Blosnich, J. R., Bukowski, L. A., Herrick, A. L., Siconolfi, D. E., & Stall, R. D. (2015). Differences in alcohol use and alcohol-related problems between transgender- and nontransgender-identified young adults. *Drug Alcohol Dependence, 154*, 251–259. doi:10.1016/j.drugalcdep.2015.07.006

De Boni, R., Veloso, V. G., & Grinsztein, B. (2014). Epidemiology of HIV in Latin America and the Caribbean. *Current Opinion in HIV and AIDS, 9*(2), 192–198. doi:10.1097/COH.0000000000000031

De Guzman, F. L. M., Moukouloub, L. N. N., Scott, L. D., & Zerwic, J. J. (2018). LGBT inclusivity in health assessment textbooks. *Journal of Professional Nursing, 34*(6), 483–487. doi:10.1016/j.profnurs.2018.03.001

di Giacomo, E., Krausz, M., Colmegna, F., Aspesi, F., & Clerici, M. (2018). Estimating the risk of attempted suicide among sexual minority youths: A systematic review and meta-analysis. *JAMA Pediatrics, 172*(12), 1145. doi:10.1001/jamapediatrics.2018 .2731

Dorey, K. (2016). *The sustainable development goals and LGBT inclusion*. London, UK: Stonewall. Retrieved from https://www.stonewall.org.uk/system/files/sdg-guide.pdf

Dossey, B. M., Rosa, W. E., & Beck, D. M. (2019). Nursing and the Sustainable Development Goals (SDGs): From Nightingale to now. *American Journal of Nursing, 119*(5), 44–49. doi:10.1097/01.NAJ.0000557912.35398.8f

Drescher, J. (2015). Out of DSM: Depathologizing homosexuality. *Behavioral Sciences, 5*(4), 565–575. doi:10.3390/bs5040565

Eliason, M. J., Dibble, S. L., & DeJoseph, J. (2010). Nursing's silence on lesbian, gay, bisexual, and transgender issues. *Advances in Nursing Science, 33*(3), 206–218. doi:10.1097/ANS.0b013e3181e63e49

Elliott, M. N., Kanouse, D. E., Burkhart, Q., Abel, G. A., Lyratzopoulos, G., Beckett, M. K., . . . Roland, M. (2015). Sexual minorities in England have poorer health and worse health care experiences: A national survey. *Journal of General Internal Medicine, 30*(1), 9–16. doi:10.1007/s11606-014-2905-y

European Union Agency for Fundamental Rights. (2013). *European Union Lesbian, Gay, Bisexual and Transgender Survey*. Retrieved from http://fra.europa.eu/en/publication/ 2014/eu-lgbt-survey-european-union-lesbian-gay-bisexual-and-transgender-survey -main

Farmer, G. W., Bucholz, K. K., Flick, L. H., Burroughs, T. E., & Bowen, D. J. (2013). CVD risk among men participating in the National Health and Nutrition Examination Survey (NHANES) from 2001 to 2010: Differences by sexual minority status. *Journal of Epidemiology and Community Health, 67*(9), 772–778. doi:10.1136/jech-2013-202658

Fisher, C. B., Fried, A. L., Desmond, M., Macapagal, K., & Mustanski, B. (2018). Perceived barriers to HIV prevention services for transgender youth. *LGBT Health, 5*(6), 350–358. doi:10.1089/lgbt.2017.0098

Foronda, C., Baptiste, D. L., Reinholdt, M. M., & Ousman, K. (2016). Cultural humility: A concept analysis. *Journal of Transcultural Nursing, 27*(3), 210–217. doi:10.1177/1043659615592677

Fredriksen-Goldsen, K. I., Kim, H. J., Barkan, S. E., Muraco, A., & Hoy-Ellis, C. P. (2013). Health disparities among lesbian, gay, and bisexual older adults: Results from a population-based study. *American Journal of Public Health, 103*(10), 1802–1809. doi:10.2105/AJPH.2012.301110

Graugaard, C., Giraldi, A., Frisch, M., Falgaard, E., & Davidsen, M. (2015). Self-reported sexual and psychosocial health among non-heterosexual Danes. *Scandinavian Journal of Public Health, 43*(3), 309–314. doi:10.1177/1403494814563371

Heck, J. E., & Jacobson, J. S. (2006). Asthma diagnosis among individuals in same-sex relationships. *Journal of Asthma, 43*(8), 579–584. doi:10.1080/02770900600878289

Hughes, T. L., Szalacha, L. A., & McNair, R. P. (2010). Substance use and mental health disparities: Comparisons across sexual identity groups in a national sample of young Australian women. *Social Science & Medicine, 71*, 824–831. doi:10.1016/j.socscimed.2010.05.009

Hughes, T. L., Wilsnack, S. C., & Kantor, L. (2016). The influence of gender and sexual orientation on alcohol use and alcohol-related problems: Toward a global perspective. *Alcohol Research: Current Reviews, 38*(1), 121–132. Retrieved from https:// www.ncbi.nlm.nih.gov/pmc/articles/PMC4872607

Human Rights Campaign. (2015). *Addressing anti-transgender violence: Exploring realities, challenges, and solutions for policymakers and community advocates.* Retrieved from https://assets2.hrc.org/files/assets/resources/HRC-AntiTransgenderViolence-0519.pdf

Human Rights Campaign. (2018). *Healthcare equality index 2018: Rising to the new standard of promoting equitable and inclusive care for lesbian, gay, bisexual, transgender & queer patients and their families.* Retrieved from https://assets2.hrc.org/files/assets/resources/HEI-2018-FinalReport.pdf?_ga=2.50764521.1798512725.1535207653-628098703.1535207653

Human Rights Campaign. (2019). *An important step toward workplace equality: An executive order on federal contractors.* Retrieved from https://www.hrc.org/resources/an-important-step-toward-workplace-equality-an-executive-order-on-federal-c

Hunt, J., Bristowe, K., Chidyamatare, S., & Harding, R. (2017). 'They will be afraid to touch you': LGBTI people and sex workers' experiences of accessing healthcare in Zimbabwe: An in-depth qualitative study. *BMJ Global Health, 2*, e000168. doi:10.1136/bmjgh-2016-000168

Institute of Medicine. (2011). *The health of lesbian, gay, bisexual, and transgender people: Building a foundation for better understanding.* Washington, DC: National Academies Press. Retrieved from http://www.nationalacademies.org/hmd/Reports/2011/The-Health-of-Lesbian-Gay-Bisexual-and-Transgender-People.aspx

Jackman, K., Bosse, J., Eliason, M. J., & Hughes, T. L. (2019). Sexual and gender minority health research in nursing. *Nursing Outlook, 67*(1), 21–38. doi:10.1016/j.outlook.2018.10.006

James, S. E., Herman, J. L., Rankin, S., Keisling, M., Mottet, L., & Anafi, M. (2016). *The report of the 2015 U.S. Transgender Survey.* Washington, DC: National Center for Transgender Equality.

The Joint Commission. (2011). *Advancing effective communication, cultural competence, and patient- and family-centered care for the lesbian, gay, bisexual, and transgender (LGBT) community: A field guide.* Retrieved from https://www.jointcommission.org/assets/1/18/LGBTFieldGuide_WEB_LINKED_VER.pdf

Juarez-Chavez, E., Cooney, E. E., Hidalgo, A., Sanchez, J., & Poteat, T. (2018). Violence experiences in childhood and adolescence among gay men and transgender women living in Perú: A qualitative exploration. *Journal Interpersonal Violence.* doi:10.1177/0886260518787811

Kates, J., Ranji, U., Beamesderfer, A., Salganicoff, A., & Dawson, L. (2014). *Health and access to care and coverage for lesbian, gay, bisexual, and transgender individuals in the U.S.* San Francisco, CA: Henry J. Kaiser Family Foundation. Retrieved from http://files.kff.org/attachment/Issue-Brief-Health-and-Access-to-Care-and-Coverage-for-LGBT-Individuals-in-the-US

King, M., Semlyen, J., Tai, S. S., Killaspy, H., Osborn, D., Popelyuk, D., . . . Nazareth, I. (2008). A systematic review of mental disorder, suicide, and deliberate self-harm in lesbian, gay and bisexual people. *BMC Psychiatry, 8*(70), 1–17. doi:10.1186/1471-244X-8-70

Koraan, R., & Geduld, A. (2015). "Corrective rape" of lesbians in the era of transformative constitutionalism in South Africa. *18*(5). 1931-1952. *ScieLO, South Africa.* Retrieved from http://www.scielo.org.za/scielo.php?script=sci_arttext&pid=S1727-37812015000500024

Landers, S. J., Mimiaga, M. J., & Conron, K. J. (2011). Sexual orientation differences in asthma correlates in a population-based sample of adults. *American Journal of Public Health, 101*(12), 2238–2241. doi:10.2105/AJPH.2011.300305

Lanham, M., Ridgeway, K., Dayton, R., Castillo, B. M., Brennan, C., Davis, D. A., . . . Evens, E. (2019) "We're going to leave you for last, because of how you are": Transgender women's experiences of gender-based violence in healthcare, education, and police encounters in Latin America and the Caribbean. *Violence and Gender Violence, 6*(1), 37–46. doi:10.1089/vio.2018.0015

Li, D. H., Rawat, S., Rhoton, J., Patankar, P., Ekstrand, M. L., Rosser, S. . . . Wilkerson, J. M. (2017). Harassment and violence among men who have sex with men (MSM) and Hijras after reinstatement of India's "Sodomy Law". *Sexuality, Research and Social Policy, 14*(3), 324–330. doi:10.1007/s13178-016-0270-9

Lim, F., Johnson, M., & Eliason, M. (2015) A national survey of faculty knowledge, experience, and readiness for teaching lesbian, gay, bisexual and transgender health in baccalaureate nursing programs. *Nursing Education Perspectives, 36*(3), 144–152. Retrieved from https://insights.ovid.com/crossref?an=00024776-201505000-00003

Machalek, D. A., Poynten, M., Jin, F., Fairley, C. K., Famsworth, A., Garland, S. M., . . . Grulich, A. E. (2012). Anal human papillomavirus infection and associated neoplastic lesions in men who have sex with men: A systematic review and meta-analysis. *Lancet Oncology, 13*(5), 487–500. doi:10.1016/S1470-2045(12)70080-3

McCabe, P. C., Dragowski, E. A., & Rubinson, F. (2013). What is homophobic bias anyway? Defining and recognizing microaggressions and harassment of LGBTQ youth. *Journal of School Violence, 12*(1), 7–26. doi:10.1080/15388220.2012.731664

McCabe, S. E., Hughes, T. L., Bostwick, W. B., West, B. T., & Boyd, C. J. (2009). Sexual orientation, substance use behaviors and substance dependence in the United States. *Addiction, 104*(8), 1333–1345. doi:10.1111/j.1360-0443.2009.02596.x

Meads, C., & Moore, D. (2013). Breast cancer in lesbians and bisexual women: Systematic review of incidence, prevalence and risk studies. *BMC Public Health, 13*, 1127. doi:10.1186/1471-2458-13-1127

Moreland, P., White, R., Riggle, E., Gishoma, D., & Hughes, T. L. (2019). Experiences of minority stress among lesbian and bisexual women in Rwanda. *International Perspectives in Psychology: Research, Practice, Consultation, 8*(4), 196–211. doi:10.1037/ipp0000114

Muller, A., & Hughes, T. L. (2016). Making the invisible visible: A systematic review of research on sexual minority women's health in southern Africa. *BMC Public Health, 16*, 307. doi:10.1186/s12889-016-2980-6

Office of Disease Prevention and Health Promotion. (2014). *Lesbian, gay, bisexual, and transgender health.* Retrieved from https://www.healthypeople.gov/2020/topics-objectives/topic/lesbian-gay-bisexual-and-transgender-health

Pew Research Center. (2013). A survey of LGBT Americans: Attitudes, experiences and values in changing times. Retrieved from http://www.pewsocialtrends.org/2013/06/13/a-survey-of-lgbt-americans

Poteat, T., Logie, C., Adams, D., Lebona, J., Letsie, P., Beyrer, C., & Baral, S. (2014) Sexual practices, identities and health among women who have sex with women in Lesotho: A mixed-methods study. *Culture, Health & Sexuality, 16*(2), 120–135. doi:10.1080/13691058.2013.841291

Poteat, T., Reisner, S. L., & Radix, A. (2014). HIV epidemics among transgender women. *Current Opinion in HIV and AIDS, 9*(2), 166–173. doi:10.1097/COH.0000000000000030

Qiao, S., Zhou, G., & Li, X. (2018). Disclosure of same-sex behaviors to health care providers and uptake of HIV testing for men who have sex with men: A systematic review. *American Journal of Health, 12*(5), 1197–1214. doi:10.1177/1557988318784149

Quinn, G. P., Sanchez, J. A., Sutton, S. K., Vadaparampil, S. T., Nguyen, G. T., Green, B. L., . . . Schabath, M. B. (2015). Cancer and lesbian, gay, bisexual, transgender/transsexual, and queer/questioning (LGBTQ) populations. *CA: A Cancer Journal for Clinicians, 65*(5), 384–400. doi:10.3322/caac.21288

Ritterbusch, A. E., Salazar, C., & Correa, A. (2018). Stigma-related access barriers and violence against trans women in the Colombian healthcare system. *Global Public Health, 13*(12), 1831–1845. doi:10.1080/17441692.2018.1455887

Rodriguez-Madera, S. L., Padilla, M., Varas-Diaz, N., Neilands, T., Guzzi, A. C., Florenciani, E. J., . . . Ramos-Pibemus, A. (2017). Experiences of violence among transgender women in Puerto Rico: An underestimated problem. *Journal of Homosexuality, 64*(2), 209–217. doi:10.1080/00918369.2016.1174026

Rosa, W. (2017a). *A new era in global health: Nursing and the United Nations 2030 Agenda for Sustainable Development.* New York, NY: Springer Publishing Company.

Rosa, W. (2017b). Goal 5. Achieve gender equality and empower all women and girls. In W. Rosa (Ed.), *A new era in global health: Nursing and the United Nations 2030 Agenda for Sustainable Development* (pp. 301-307). New York, NY: Springer Publishing Company.

Rosa, W. E., Dossey, B. M., Watson, J., Beck, D. M., & Upvall, M. J. (2019). The United Nations Sustainable Development Goals: The ethic and ethos of holistic nursing. *Journal of Holistic Nursing, 37*(4), 381–393. doi: 10.1177/0898010119841723

Rosa, W. E., Upvall, M. J., Beck, D. M., & Dossey, B. M. (2019). Nursing and sustainable development: Furthering the global agenda in uncertain times. *Online Journal of Issues in Nursing, 24*(2), Manuscript 1. doi:10.3912/OJIN.Vol24No02Man01

Rothman, E. F., Exner, D., & Baughman, A. (2011). The prevalence of sexual assault against people who identify as gay, lesbian or bisexual in the United States: A systematic review. *Trauma, Violence, & Abuse, 12*(2), 55–66. doi:10.1177/1524838010390707

Sandfort, T., Frazer, M. S., Matebeni, Z., Reddy, V., & Southey-Swartz, I. (2015). Histories of forced sex and health outcomes among southern African lesbian and bisexual women: A cross-sectional study. *BMC Women's Health, 15*, 22. doi:10.1186/s12905-015-0181-6

Schultz, K. (2018, June 2). Gay in India, where progress has come with only risk. *New York Times.* Retrieved from https://www.nytimes.com/2018/06/02/world/asia/gay-in-india-where-progress-has-come-only-with-risk.html

Sears, B., & Mallory, C. (2011). Documented evidence of employment discrimination and it's effects on LGBT people. Retrieved from https://williamsinstitute.law.ucla.edu/research/discrimination/documented-evidence-of-employment-discrimination-its-effects-on-lgbt-people

Seekaew, P., Pengnonyang, S., Jantarapakde, J., Sunsing, T., Rodbumrung, P., Trachunthong, P., . . . Phanuphak, N. (2018). Characteristics and HIV epidemiologic profiles of men who have sex with men and transgender women in key population-led test and treat cohorts in Thailand. *PLoS One, 13*(8), 1–13. doi:10.1371/journal.pone.0203294

Silva, G. W., Souza, E. F. L., Sena, R. C. F., Moura, I. B. L., Sobreira, M. V. S., & Miranda, F. A. N. (2016). Cases of violence involving transvestites and transsexuals in a northeastern Brazilian city. *Revista Gaúcha Enfermagem, 37*(2), 1–7. doi:10.1590/1983-1447.2016.02.56407

Sommerlad, J. (2018, September 6). Section 377: How India brought an end to the criminalisation of its LGBT+ community. *The Independent.* Retrieved from https://www.independent.co.uk/news/world/asia/section-377-india-gay-sex-crime-lgbt-supreme-court-dipak-misra-a8525116.html

Soulé, I. (2016). Flexible and responsive: Applying the wisdom of 'it depends'. In W. Rosa (Ed.), *Nurses as leaders: Evolutionary visions of leadership* (pp. 417–430). New York, NY: Springer Publishing Company.

Steele, L. S., Daley, A., Curling, D., Gibson, M. F., Green, D. C., Williams, C. C., . . . Ross, L. E. (2017). LGBT identity, untreated depression, and unmet need for mental health services by sexual minority women and trans-identified people. *Journal of Women's Health, 26*(2), 116–127. doi:10.1089/jwh.2015.5677

Stewart, K., & O'Reilly, P. (2017). Attitudes, knowledge and beliefs of nurses and midwives of the healthcare needs of the LGBTQ population: An integrative review. *Nurse Education Today, 53*, 67–77. doi:10.1016/j.nedt.2017.04.008

Szalacha, L., Hughes, T. L., McNair, R., & Loxton, D. (2017). Mental health as predicted by sexual identity and violence: Findings from the Australian Longitudinal Women's Health Study. *BMC Women's Health, 17*(1), 94. doi:10.1186/s12905-017 -0452-5

Taylor, P. J., Dhingra, K., Dickson, J., & McDermott, E. (2018). Psychological correlates of self-harm within gay, lesbian and bisexual UK university students. *Archives of Suicide Research.* doi:10.1080/13811118.2018.1515136

Tervalon, M., & Murray-Garcia, J. (1998). Cultural humility versus cultural competence: A critical distinction in defining physician training outcomes in multicultural education. *Journal of Health Care for the Poor & Underserved, 9*(2), 117–125. doi:10.1353/ hpu.2010.0233

United Nations. (n.d.). *Millennium development goals and beyond 2015.* Retrieved from http://www.un.org/millenniumgoals

United Nations. (2016). *Transforming our world: The 2030 Agenda for Sustainable Development.* Retrieved from https://sustainabledevelopment.un.org/content/ documents/21252030%20Agenda%20for%20Sustainable%20Development%20 web.pdf

United Nations Human Rights Council. (2011). *Discrimination and violence against individuals based on their sexual orientation and gender identity.* Retrieved from https:// www.ohchr.org/Documents/Issues/Discrimination/LGBT/A_HRC_29_23_One_ pager_en.pdf

Veldhuis, C. B., Bruzzese, J-M., Hughes, T. L., & George, M. (2019). Scoping review of risk factors for asthma in sexual and gender minority youth and adults. *Annals of Allergy, Asthma & Immunology, 122*(5):535.e1–536.e1. doi:10.1016/j.anai.2019.01.021

Walters, M. A., Paterson, J., Brown, R., & McDonnell, L. (2017). Hate crimes against trans people: Assessing emotions, behaviors, and attitudes toward criminal justice agencies. *Journal of Interpersonal Violence.* doi:10.1177/0886260517715026

Wilson, B. D., Choi, S. K., Augustaitis, L., Jadwin-Cakmak, L., Neubauer, L. C., & Harper, G. W. (2019). Sexual and gender minorities in Western Kenya. *Williams Institute.* Retrieved from https://williamsinstitute.law.ucla.edu/research/sex-gender-minority -kenya

World Health Organization. (2016). *Gender, Equity and Human Rights (GER): FAQ on health and sexual diversity: An introduction to key concepts.* Retrieved from http:// www.who.int/gender-equity-rights/news/20170329-health-and-sexual-diversity -faq.pdf?ua=1

Yi, S., Tuot, S., Chhim, S., Chhoun, P., Mun, P., & Mburu, G. (2018). Exposure to gender-based violence and depressive symptoms among transgender women in Cambodia: Findings from the National Integrated Biological and Behavioral Survey 2016. *International Journal of Mental Health Systems, 12*(24), 1–11. doi:10.1186/s13033-018 -0206-2

11   Veterans and Health Equity

Linda Spoonster Schwartz

CHAPTER OBJECTIVES

- Recognize the juxtaposition of health equity and the unhealthy practice of war
- Discuss how Veterans may carry the "wounds of war throughout their entire lives"
- Distinguish health/mental issues for Veterans between major conflicts

KEY CONCEPTS

Serving in a time of war   Posttraumatic stress disorder

KEY TERMS

Citizen soldiers   Service-connected benefits

Veterans   Agent Orange

Department of Veterans Affairs

■ Introduction

It's about how we treat our veterans every single day of the year. It's about making sure they have the care they need and the benefits that they've earned when they come home. It's about serving all of you as well as you've served the United States of America.

—Barack Obama (2010, para. 13)

"FOR THOSE WHO FAITHFULLY SERVED"

There are some important differences in considering the topic of "health equity" and the unhealthy practice of waging war. A great deal of time and study has centered on identifying and quantifying barriers to achieving the highest levels of health for individuals and communities. Most of these activities have focused on linking social and demographic determinants such as race, gender, age, income, education, and geographic location as benchmarks to assess barriers or protective effects to achieving and maintaining a healthy life. More recently, the emphasis has broadened to "defining health equity as 'social justice in health' with the identification of health disparities as the metric used to measure progress toward equity" (Braverman & Gottlieb, 2014, p. 19).

Throughout America's history, war and revolution have been major forces in shaping the nation's traditions, identity, and status in the international community. The United

States has been officially engaged in war for 141 years of the 232 years since the founding of this nation. In the course of these military operations, over 43.2 million men and women have served in America's armed forces and militias. Of this number, an estimated 20,234,000 (47%) are living today with a majority 16,962,000 (84%) serving in a time of war (U.S. Department of Veterans Affairs, 2017).

■ The Department of Veterans Affairs (VA)

Historically, services evolved as a response to the perceived and demonstrated needs of Veterans and the expectations of the American people. In the wake of World War I, the numbers of casualties and variations in needs prompted President Wilson to realign a variety of Veterans specific programs and benefits under the aegis of a Veterans Bureau. However, the burgeoning needs of Veterans and their survivors resulted in the 1930 creation of the Veterans Administration (VA) to consolidate and coordinate all government activities affecting war Veterans. Eligibility for a range of services, compensation, levels of care, and benefits were all prescribed by Congress in Title 38 U.S. Code and supporting regulations. For decades, the VA was essentially a closed system with immense powers and very little accountability, questionable impartiality, and no legal recourse to challenge level of care decisions or compensation determinations. With over 26 million living Veterans, the inequities in treatment, benefits, and access to programs required more oversight. In 1988, Congress enacted Public Law 100-527, which changed the Veterans Administration, an independent government agency, to Cabinet-level status renamed the U.S. Department of Veterans Affairs (USDVA).

Over time, the VA has evolved into three major divisions of services: Veterans Health Administration (VHA), Veterans Benefits Administration (VBA), and National Cemetery Administration (NCA). The agency's 2019 Budget and 2020 Advance Appropriations request totals $198.6 billion, an increase of $12.1 billion over 2018. This budget request is second only to the Department of Defense (DOD). The majority of this funding, $109.7 billion in mandatory funding, is used for Veteran benefits with the remaining $76.5 billion in discretionary funding for Veteran healthcare programs (Shane, 2018).

The NCA, also known as "Memorial Affairs," is tasked with oversight of the National Cemetery System, which consists of 135 national cemeteries, 130 state Veteran cemeteries, and 33 soldiers' lots (U.S. Department of Veterans Affairs, 2018b, p. 61). The VBA, through 56 Regional Benefit Offices, administers the determination of levels of service-connected disabilities, disbursement of compensation payments and pensions, educational benefits, vocational rehabilitation programs, and home loan programs. The best known is the Health Care Administration, which is responsible for the largest integrated health network in America with over 1,868 points of service, which includes 1,234 outpatient sites; 143 hospitals; telehealth systems; readjustment counseling centers; research facilities; and academic affiliations (National Center for Veterans Analysis and Statistics [NCVAS], 2018; see Figure 11.1). Additionally, there are specific "Centers," such as the Center for Women Veterans (CWV) and Center for Minority Veterans (CMV), which focus their efforts on specific groups of Veterans who may need special assistance or present specific health needs. The Office of Public Affairs (OPA), Mental Health (OMH) and Policy and Planning (OPP) and Readjustment Counseling Services (RCS) provide specific expertise and support to a clinical line and/or provide administrative and research support to the entire agency.

Department of Veterans Affairs
Organizational snapshot*

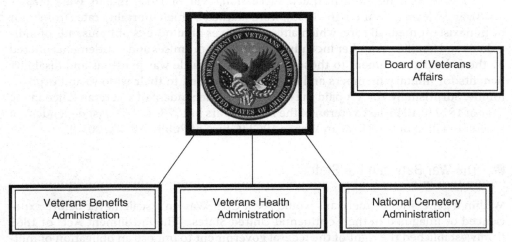

Board of Veterans Affairs

Veterans Benefits Administration

Veterans Health Administration

National Cemetery Administration

FIGURE 11.1 UNITED STATES DEPARTMENT OF VETERANS AFFAIRS ORGANIZATION DEPARTMENTS.

*This chart includes only the main VA branches.

Veterans of military service have not always received the respect and honor of their nation. However, over time, they have been vested with special status, privileges, and entitlements by generations of presidents, Congress, governors, and their fellow citizens. On the surface, these advantages seem to be expressions of gratitude and honor and reasonable repayment for loss of wages, health, and opportunities forfeited by serving in defense of our nation. However, these entitlements have not always been forthcoming. For generations, there has not been a more honorable, steadfast, or impassioned struggle than the decades of fighting to achieve justice and health equity for the men and women who have fought for centuries to win and sustain the freedoms we all enjoy. Just how this vast system has become a multi–billion-dollar investment has been one of the longest and most turbulent sagas in America's history.

■ Citizen Soldiers

America, unlike many societies, has not been committed to maintaining a large "standing military force." From the beginning of our nation, there has been heavy reliance on the patriotism of "citizen soldiers" called to action in defense of country and freedom. The founding fathers and their successors recognized that patriotism alone would not sustain a heart for soldiering in times of crisis. The "summer soldier and the sunshine patriot" needed more than rhetoric and political conjuring to persuade troops to serve the duration of the war. In the absence of "Conscription" or "Draft" and considering that the success of the fledgling nation depended on the success of the Army and Navy,

Congress authorized pensions of varying amounts and duration for disabled Veterans, widows, or orphaned children of those who served until the end of the war (Veterans Administration, 1967, p. 30).

Conflicts that followed in quick succession, War of 1812, Indian Wars (1817–1898), and Mexican War (1846–1848), were marked by high mortality rates from poor or nonexistent medical care, which altered the lives of hundreds of thousands of individuals and families. Another incentive added to the promises and entitlements offered by the federal government to those who served in battle was pensions and disability benefits for military members and eventually extended to their widows and orphans for life. Surprisingly, the VA paid the last surviving dependent of a Veteran killed in the War of 1812 in 1946, last Veteran of the Indian Wars in 1973, and the last dependent of a Veteran killed in the Mexican War in 1962 (Office of Public Affairs, 2018).

■ The War Between the States

Within a generation, Americans would see a Civil War on a scale never before experienced or imagined in the Continental United States. "The Enrollment Act" of 1863 firmly established the right of the federal government to impose an obligation of military service on every citizen, better known as a "Draft." Civic and patriotic organizations in the north and south rallied to support their troops. Pioneering efforts by Clara Barton, founder of the American Red Cross, and Dorothea Dix, Superintendent of Army Nurses, mirrored the work of Florence Nightingale and brought nursing and care of troops to the fields of battle for the first time. This active involvement of noncombatants became an important factor in the evolution of care and support for those who bore the brunt of the fighting and dying on both sides.

The Civil War marked a new attitude about the human cost of war and the residual problems Veterans on both sides of the struggle suffered. The "wounds of war" also encompassed the many readjustment needs of those who had served, including Veterans suffering from "soldier's heart," now known as posttraumatic stress disorder (PTSD), confusion, and mental disorders from repeated blasts and cannonades, very similar to traumatic brain injuries, alcoholism and substance abuse, unemployment, and homelessness, which are still experienced by Veterans today.

When Congress authorized the first pensions for Revolutionary War soldiers, the precedent established the government as the responsible entity to help and support those who served in America's armed forces. However, the post–Civil War period not only enhanced that reputation, but it also reaffirmed the belief that Congress would be the guardian, benefactor, and protector of the casualties of war-disabled Veterans, widows, and orphans. With this, the dye was cast that future generations could rely on Congress to provide the care and assistance needed to make them "whole" again. The attempt to balance the generosity of the authorized entitlements and benefits with the ever-growing demands and needs of ensuing generations of Veterans created a financial enigma.

■ Veterans Organizations

Within months of the end of the Civil War, groups of Veterans banded together for the purposes of mutual support and fraternal and patriotic activities in towns and cities across the North. The tradition gained great popularity when various divisions and units, including the Union Army, Navy, Marines, and U.S. Revenue Cutter Service, merged to create the Grand Army of the Republic (GAR) in 1866. The idea quickly gained momentum, growing to include hundreds of local posts in communities across the nation predominately in the North and West. Without really realizing the importance of this organization and the friendships that emerged, the GAR became the first organized Veterans advocates in American politics, supporting voting rights for Black Veterans, promoting patriotic education, helping to make Memorial Day a national holiday, lobbying the Congress to establish regular Veterans' pensions, and supporting Republican political candidates (Beath, 1899). The GAR set the tone and foundation for succeeding generations of Veterans to support each other, enrich their communities, and "step up" when Veterans were victimized by their own government. Veteran service organizations (VSOs), like the Disabled American Veterans, American Legion, and Vietnam Veterans of America, would play pivotal roles in the evolution of how America cared for their military members and Veterans.

■ World at War

When war was declared on December 8, 1941, President Roosevelt, Congress, and the entire country realized the fate of the world was at stake. The nation came together as never before to defeat the unbridled chaos, treachery, and butchery of the Axis powers. For the first time, war touched every town and city in America, and the entire civilian population was engaged to support the "war effort," with victory gardens, rationing, and war bond drives. "Freeing a man to fight" required women in the workforce, women in the military, and women on the assembly lines creating the weapons of war. By the war's end, over 16 million Americans had served in the military, which was the largest mobilization in the history of the nation. There were over 400,000 combat deaths and a steady string of over 670,000 casualties (Office of Public Affairs, 2018). These numbers underscored the meaning of the real hardships, dangers, and sacrifices made by those serving to "protect" the nation. At the end of the hostilities, Congress in the name of a "grateful nation" authorized legislation equalizing existing benefits to all generations of Veterans. Most importantly, the landmark "Servicemen's Readjustment Act of 1944," otherwise known as the "G.I. Bill," granted generous educational and training benefits, small business and home loans, and unemployment benefits to all Veterans of all military services.

With 100,000 troops being discharged from the military every month, and battle casualties in need of treatment arriving home at a rate of 1,200 per day, and approximately 5 million Veterans in need of hospitalization, the VA was hard-pressed to keep up with resources and manpower needed for this mission (Veterans Administration, 1967, p. 198). All of this coming at a time when the best physicians and nurses were still in military service, most of them in overseas areas, President Harry Truman, a World War I combat Veteran, was quick to appoint General Omar Bradley to be the new VA Administrator. In the first 6 months of his tenure, the massive demobilization of troops increased the population of 6.8 million Veterans to 13.5 million. Physicians and nurses were detailed from the active duty military to staff the existing and new facilities being constructed.

DISABILITY SELF-REPORT

By law, the mandatory criteria for rating a "service-connected disability" required facts supported by evidence that the "injury, disability or illness was incurred or aggravated during a period of active military service" (USDVA, 2018a, p. 13). Because of the overwhelming demand, VA opted to expedite the process by waiving the past system of requiring extensive documentation for claims of disabilities. Individual Veterans were able to apply for disability compensation and care, based solely on their own "self-reports" with a signed sworn affidavit. *No other documentation, exams, or inquiry were required for the claims to be accepted and approved.* Additionally, access to VA Health Care for any Veteran who declared he or she was unable to pay for care was immediately available (Veterans Administration, 1967, p. 240). It is important to remember that health insurance, as we know it, did not exist and it would be decades before Medicare and Medicaid would be available. *This unchecked access to healthcare for all Veterans was a prized advantage, which would hobble the VA for decades.*

Tapping into his organizational strengths and command skills, General Bradley reorganized the entire VA. He decentralized the benefits programs to the local levels and instituted a "fee-for-service" program, which paid VA-approved healthcare providers to care for disabled Veterans in their own communities, and realigned health services along service lines. With a great deal of forethought, General Bradley also sought affiliations with university medical schools (Veterans Administration, 1967, p. 193).

■ Benefit Disparity

American military members who served during the Korean War were much less fortunate than the Veterans of World War II (WWII). The technicality that Korea was a "police action," not a war, prevented these Veterans from being eligible for the entitlements that had been extended to the previous generations of Veterans. Although they were involuntarily "drafted" and pressed into service, these Veterans were not authorized to receive the "G.I. Bill," ineligible for non–service-connected pensions, barred from receiving healthcare from VA, and not entitled to burial benefits (Veterans Administration, 1967, p. 263). There were over 33,739 combat deaths and 103,284 battle casualties in Korea (DeBruyne, 2018). Where did these casualties go for care if not the VA? Who would bury them if not the country they served? It was not until 18 months after mobilization that this gross neglect reached the hallowed halls of Congress when Korean combat Veterans were denied treatment for their wounds at VA Hospitals. Stunningly, halfway through the war, Congress finally acted to extend the wartime benefits to all Korean Veterans.

VA was already reeling and overextended by the "open door" policy created by the financial need stipulation and the "self-reported service-connected disabilities" in addition to the casualties of WWII. The agency floundered under the burden of budget cuts and a cumbersome, disorganized, and unwieldy bureaucracy. *One of the major problems was the waiting list of 22,613 seeking admissions to VA Hospitals* (Veterans Administration, 1967, p. 250). The budget cuts accentuated the drain that services to these Veterans made on the system at the expense of Veterans who had sustained injuries and disabilities as a direct result of their military service. In the postwar era, Veterans and VSOs had come to regard the VA as their unlimited reward for winning the war. These dynamics converged to create a system of compensation and care that had become distorted with many receiving benefits to which they were not entitled.

President Eisenhower, once again, called on General Omar Bradley to conduct a review of the entire system. In November 1954, a review of the census of all VA patients yielded some startling facts. From the census at that time, 8.3% had been hospitalized for more than 20 years, another 33% had been hospitalized for more than 5 years, and 49% more than a year. Recommendations were made that service-connected disabled should be given the highest priority and treated generously (Veterans Administration, 1967, p. 263).

■ Vietnam

Although Vietnam was never officially declared a war, the 1964 "Gulf of Tonkin Resolution" gave President Johnson the green light to escalate the war. The uncertainty of a Selective Service Lottery prompted many "draft-eligible" men to enlist in the service of their choice rather than risk being forced into the Army. Several nuances in the Draft Board policies' system would taint the induction process.

The first policy of "channeling" authorized deferments to young men enrolled in higher education; professionals and certain skilled technicians were particularly popular. The second, designed to reduce unemployment of inner-city youth, granted 100,000 waivers per year to minority males who did not meet required mental health or physical criteria to enter the armed forces. Better known as "Project 100,000," it is conceivable that after 10 years of war, more than 1 million service members, who never met the enlistment criteria and should have been deferred, had served in the military (Greenhill, 2006). In essence, *the method of "channeling" and "Project 100,000" harvested a generation of young, poor, disadvantaged, lower- and middle-class men for service in time of war*. These social inequities would play a considerable role in the readjustment needs of returning Vietnam Veterans.

From the first arrival of "U.S. military advisors" in 1954 until the 1975 Mayaguez incident, 9.4 million men and women would serve in the U.S. Armed Forces; over 3.4 million Americans would be stationed in Vietnam (U.S. Department of Veterans Affairs, 2017). The average age of the combat soldier in Vietnam was 18 years (Keib, 1982). The sophistication of battlefield trauma care and medical evacuation systems saved more critically wounded and disabled men and women than in any previous wars.

More wounded survived, there was a 98% "save rate" but they returned home with extensive injuries and wounds, the likes of which had never been seen before. (Starr, 1972, p. 32)

Data from VA indicated that the rate of leg amputations in Vietnam was 70% higher than during the Korean War and 300% greater than WWII. In cases of paraplegia or paralysis of the lower extremities, the rate was 50% higher than during the Korean War and 1,000% greater than during WWII (Starr, 1972, p. 32). The rates of multiple amputations of two or more extremities were more than 300% higher than those who survived in WWII (Keib, 1982).

■ Never Again Will One Generation of Veterans Turn Their Backs on Another

After the decided victories of WWII, the stalemates in Korea and Vietnam had a bitter taste for the proud nation. The unpopularity of the Draft ultimately spawned an antiwar movement, which focused on the soldiers fighting and dying in a foreign land, instead of the policy makers who created the war. The "Fall of Saigon," *widespread reports of drug problems* in the ranks of the military, daily broadcasts of shocking images of dying young Americans, wartime atrocities, and body counts left most Americans resentful, cynical, and in many cases hostile to the continued U.S. involvement in a protracted and costly foreign engagement.

For the first time in the history of the nation, the men who fought the war marched to demand its end. In 1967, a group of combat Veterans, who had experienced the corruption, incompetence, and futility of the fighting, organized Vietnam Veterans Against the War (VVAW) to bring an end to the war. Along with demands for proper care and services for all Veterans in VA Hospitals, employment rights, and educational benefits, they declared their intent to change the "establishment" that caused and continued the war in Indo-China (Helmer, 1974, p. 94). Although the Vietnam era was significantly longer, and Veterans were younger than during WWII, there *were no new benefit packages authorized by the VA*. Despite the influx of 7 million new Veterans, increased wages, and costs, VA's FY1975 and FY1976 budget authority was below that of FY1947, which made resources scarce for the returning Veterans (Scott, 2012). In 1972, Congress attempted to respond to these demands by passing the "Veterans Health Care Expansion Act" for VA to handle the increased needs of over 6 million Veterans of the Vietnam War. President Nixon promptly vetoed the measure because he felt it was fiscally irresponsible and inflationary. And the war played on.

INDIFFERENCE

Even the traditional VSOs, always steadfast in their support of the men in uniform, were distant and in some cases stridently aloof. Unable to understand the antiwar, antiestablishment attitudes of these new Veterans, the VSOs refused to accept them in their membership, calling them "crybabies" and "losers." The political power of these organizations was firmly behind the VA, the DOD, and the war. Vietnam Veterans saw this as yet another piece of the hollow machinery that fueled the war, sent them into combat, and abandoned them to fight. These factors created an atmosphere charged with disdain for the military, *indifference for the needs of Veterans,* and distrust of the establishment, which would fester for decades and isolate the men and women who served during the Vietnam War.

■ Healing the Wounds of War

At first it had no name; psychiatrists thought the symptoms and behaviors described by Vietnam Veterans were attributable to substance abuse, adjustment disorders, or schizophrenia. Clinicians had noted, early in the return of these Veterans, psychological trauma manifested in this population was a curious reflection of the unorthodox and turbulent unrest of the times.

> While there was a deep sense of distrust, bitterness, and suspicion, there was also strong evidence of pain, suffering, and a search for justice from a system most of them despised. Much like the camaraderie they had experienced in the jungle, VVAW chapters formed "rap groups" and started Psychological Information Services to help each other heal the wounds of their war. (Lifton, 1973, p. 84)

POSTTRAUMATIC STRESS DISORDER

Prior to 1980, a variety of terms such as "traumatic neurosis," "gross stress neurosis," or "transient situational neuroses" were used to describe the characteristic symptoms we now simply refer to as "posttraumatic stress disorder" and in more recent years, in an effort to destigmatize the condition, "posttraumatic stress" (PTS). Characteristic symptoms can include disturbing thoughts, feelings, or dreams related to the events, mental or physical distress, flashbacks, difficulty sleeping, and changes in how a person thinks and feels. PTSD can develop after a person is exposed to a traumatic event or recognizable stressor that would evoke significant symptoms of distress in almost everyone (Basu, 2014). And although similar disorders had been identified in warriors and war fighters throughout history, acknowledging this condition in the Vietnam Veterans somehow conveyed the idea that they were weaker and less courageous than Americans in past wars.

The intensity of the symptoms, experienced by Veterans, was frightening and for the most part unknown and poorly understood. Ultimately, research in the private sector, on the dynamics of stressors and responses, validated the diagnosis and opened the doors to improved understanding of the emotional responses to natural and man-made disasters, sexual assaults, and loss of loved ones, which freed individuals confronted by these situations to actively seek help in understanding their responses.

With the end of hostilities in Vietnam, Veterans who had organized VVAW saw the agenda of caring for each other was not ended and would take up more activism. In 1978, leaders from VVAW focused their efforts on supporting another fledgling group, Vietnam Veterans of America, Inc. (VVA), which ultimately emerged to be a formidable force in advocating for all Veterans. VVA would be the first VSO to include women Veterans as full members, and adopted "Never again will one generation of Veterans turn their backs on another" as their battle cry. VVA was successful in garnering Congressional support for recognizing PTSD as a natural consequence of war and authorization to create 136 Readjustment Counseling (more commonly known as Vet) Centers dedicated to providing holistic care and counseling for Vietnam Veterans and their families. One of the most important legacies of the Vietnam War was the creation of the Vet Centers Program, which has continued to expand and serve generations of Veterans for over 35 years and is still growing.

AGENT ORANGE

Agent Orange is a defoliant that contains high levels of dioxin, a known carcinogen, used extensively in Vietnam to deprive the enemy of cover from the thick jungle canopy and underbrush. Thought to be "safe" at the time, some Veterans suspected that their high rates of cancers, Hodgkin's disease, and birth defects in their children were related to their exposure to this toxic hazard. Because dioxin has a half-life of 30 years, the lag time from exposure to the appearance of symptoms or disease could take decades. In 1979, Veterans brought a "class action" lawsuit against the chemical companies, mainly Monsanto, that had produced the defoliant. The lawsuit was eventually settled by the companies in 1984 with a $180 million payout. Sadly, the Veterans who had "won" their case received an average of only $3,000 from their lawsuit (Stout, 2018). At the same time, Veterans continued to file claims with VA for care and compensation. VA refused to even look at the claims or treat their health problems, citing the lack of scientific evidence that Agent Orange was linked to the problems claimed by Veterans. Admiral Elmo Zumwalt, who had actually ordered the use of Agent Orange when he was Commander of Naval Forces Vietnam, stepped up to lead, coach, and mentor Vietnam Veterans fighting for justice for the dead and disabled victims of Agent Orange. Eventually VVA would propose legislation to have an independent scientific body review all dioxin-related studies and inform VA of their findings on a regular basis. In 1990, the House Veterans Affairs Committee took up HR 565, which outlined VVA's Agent Orange agenda. However, Congressional leaders baulked at the idea and the original proposal died in committee. Undaunted, the Veterans persisted and found advocates who used parliamentary sleight of hand and old-time backroom politics to see the "Agent Orange Act of 1991" become law (Stout, 2018).

Congress later tasked the Institute of Medicine (IOM) to review all studies on Veterans and exposure to Agent Orange for any scientific evidence to support additional conditions that could be linked to these toxic substances. This process has also paved the way to formalize the procedures for identifying conditions associated with Gulf War illness (GWI) and exposure to burn pits encountered by Iraq and Afghan Veterans. Presently, there are over 50 individual health conditions considered presumptive disabilities and 20 birth defects recognized by VA as being associated with exposure to Agent Orange (VVA, 2017, p. 4). To date, over 650,000 Veterans and their survivors have received compensation and care (Stout, 2018). This triumph also stands as a legacy of the Vietnam War. These protocols and processes for determining exposures and their consequences continue for investigating toxic exposures and health problems encountered by Iraq and Afghan Veterans and their families.

■ Invisible Veterans

Prior to 1980, very little was ever said about military women and even less was known about them. It was not until the 1980 U.S. Census that women were asked if they served in the military. To the surprise of many, 1.2 million women were identified as Veterans. This startling discovery prompted Congress and the VA to begin concerted efforts to reach out to this unknown population. Congress immediately commissioned a "Survey of Women Veterans" to determine the needs and experiences of these missing patriots. Interestingly, the study found that 57% of these women did not even know they were eligible for services from the VA (Harris, 1985). Although women had served honorably in every major American war since the founding of the nation, their mostly unofficial and inconspicuous roles contributed to their anonymity. Even before the ban on women in combat was lifted in 2013, thousands of women had served in combat areas and situations in every war (Vogt, 2015). Because the number of women serving in the military had been restricted by law to be no more than 2% of the active duty force, women were not always prominently noticed. With the advent of the "All Volunteer Force" in the 1970s, participation and opportunities in the military substantially improved. At the start of the Gulf War in 1991, almost 11% of the military were women and in 2018, over 18% of the forces were women (Center for Women Veterans, 2014).

These women had paid a high price for their service. For example, women did not receive pay and allowances commensurate with men of equal rank. Married women were ineligible to join the Nurse Corps. In fact, being married was grounds for a dishonorable discharge from the corps—a punishment usually reserved for grave crimes and convicted criminals. When marriage was finally permitted, women were not authorized to be stationed with their husbands. Although marriage for women in the enlisted ranks was permitted, pregnancy was unthinkable. For women married or unmarried, pregnancy was also grounds for a dishonorable discharge and immediate dismissal (Holm, 1982, p. 290). Despite these limitations, more than 384,000 women served in the military in WWII. The "Women's Armed Services Act" of 1948 finally gave women a permanent place in the military. Despite lingering inequities with regard to rank, occupational specialty, and restricted assignments, this landmark legislation bestowed official recognition to over two centuries of military service women had given to the nation.

When President Harry S. Truman ordered U.S. forces into Korea in 1950, the entire complement of women in the armed services numbered just 22,000, of which nearly 7,000 served in the healthcare professions (Leipold, 2012). In contrast, over 265,000 women served in the military during Vietnam. Neither the DOD nor the VA can provide reliable data on the number of women who actually served in Vietnam. Best estimates range from 7,500 to 10,000. Most of these women were nurses although others served in administrative support positions. For 60% of the nurses who were assigned to Vietnam, it was their first job in nursing (Schwartz, 1987). Many Americans did not even know women were actually stationed in the combat areas until years after the war.

For all the stresses of the Vietnam Era, there were improvements in the conditions such as equal pay and lifting the ceiling on the number of women who could serve and the rank they could attain. Marriage was also sanctioned. In 1976, pregnant women were permitted to stay in the military, though curiously their condition was termed "a service-connected disability." By 1980, one of the last bastions of exclusion for women fell to progress when women were authorized to attend the U.S. military service academies.

■ Coming Home

Soon after the 1980 Census, the discovery that women who had served in the military never knew they were Veterans prompted a review by Congress. Returning women who had served in Vietnam took note and resolved they would not be treated unfairly. One out of five women who served in Vietnam left with a permanent service-connected disability. Although these disabilities qualified them for care at the VA, when they attempted to access the system, they were either turned away or received substandard care (IOM, 1977). In 1983 during Senate Veteran Affairs Committee Hearings, Lynda Van Devanter, Army Nurse Corps, Vietnam Veteran and National Women's Director for VVA, noted that "In most cases, women cannot receive gynecological care from the VA, although this is the most elemental healthcare need of a woman veteran." She pushed the issue more by noting that some of the women complained they had been examined "in full view of men passing through the exam area" and that there was a general lack of privacy and lack of qualified gynecologists in VA hospitals. Van Devanter further suggested that the government had never really cared to find out what the stresses of war had been on women who had served in battle zones by calling attention to the 65 women who were held prisoners of war by the Japanese on Corregidor for the duration of WWII. She questioned, "Where are studies of those women?" (Severo & Milford, 1989, p. 303).

Thus began a new era of equity and recognition for women Veterans and all they had earned by their military service. A 1982 Government Accounting Office (GAO) report "Actions Needed to Ensure that Female Veterans Have Equal Access to VA Benefits" found "serious deficiencies with inadequate treatment facilities for women Veterans; unequal access to treatment and medical services; insufficient provisions for privacy; incomplete physical exams; little or no gynecological care and no systematic effort to inform women about their entitlements" (GAO, 1982, p. 6). The findings were further substantiated by personal accounts from women during Congressional hearings held later that year. Rising interest in women Veterans prompted yet another study by VA in 1985 which, after 5 years, again confirmed that more than half of the women were still unaware of their benefits. More importantly, results indicated that women Veterans had twice the rates of cancers than women in the general female population. Especially disturbing were the high rates of cervical, uterine, and ovarian cancers (45%; Buckley, 1990). This proved to be more disconcerting to women Veterans than to their VA health providers (Harris, 1991). Congress actually had to include language in the Veterans Health Act of 1992 "requiring VA to provide complete physicals including gynecological exams for all women veterans."

Equally troubling was the struggle to substantiate a diagnosis of PTSD for women who served in Vietnam. At that time, VA did not consider that a Veteran was eligible for a diagnosis of PTSD unless he or she had earned a "Combat Infantryman Badge," which is awarded to individuals "who fought in active ground combat while assigned as a member of Infantry, Ranger, or Special Forces unit" (Issacs, 2013). In fact, the first question on the VA assessment for PTSD was: Do you have a Combat Infantryman Badge?; if not, no matter what your symptoms or circumstances, you were not eligible for a VA diagnosis of PTSD. Women with the sentinel symptoms of PTSD were diagnosed as schizophrenic, bipolar, and as having adjustment disorder (Norman, 1988). The 1988 Vietnam Veterans Readjustment Study revealed that the nurses in Vietnam saw more death and dying in their care of casualties than combat soldiers with Infantryman Badges (Schwartz, 1998). This dramatically changed VA thinking about PTSD and eligibility for women and other noncombat personnel for treatment of PTSD. Thankfully, this struggle broadened our understanding of traumatic experiences to include all military members, first responders, and others who experience profound episodes of traumatic events.

GULF WAR: DESERT SHIELD/DESERT STORM (1990–1991)

From start to finish, Desert Storm lasted only 43 days and is sometimes called the "100-hour ground war" because that was how long the fighting actually lasted. At that time, there were 694,550 Americans serving in the combat area with 148 battle deaths and 467 nonfatal casualties (DeBruyne, 2018, p. 42). Within 100 days of the end of the hostilities, a military parade billed as the largest since WWII was held to honor the U.S. troops who participated in Operation Desert Storm. The parade, reviewed by President Bush, featured 10,500 personnel from every branch of the service and every unit that took part in the liberation of Kuwait (Gonzalez, 1991). While this was a stunning victory, this was the first "Welcome Home" for America's "All Volunteer Force." The parade and the honors showered on all who participated would set the standard and expectation for future engagements. More importantly, the full meaning of what the nation would and would not owe these volunteers would shape the debate about the future care and benefits offered to our military Veterans.

The war might have been over, but the battle for thousands of Gulf War Veterans was just beginning. Although the war was brief with relatively few injuries and deaths, a substantial number of returning Veterans began experiencing and reporting a variety of health problems that have persisted over time. Considered to be the signature health problem of this deployment, GWI is defined as a cluster of medically unexplained chronic symptoms that can include fatigue, headaches, joint and back pain, indigestion, respiratory disorders, sleep problems, and cognitive dysfunction (Gordon, 2018, p. 45). Eventually, over a third of the 700,000 military and civilians including coalition forces who served in the combat areas reported these symptoms. Service members who were deployed were exposed to many hazardous agents and situations, both known and unknown (Lang, 2016). These exposures included chemical and biological agents, burn-pit residue, depleted uranium, mandatory vaccines, oil-well fire smoke, dust, high ambient temperatures, heat stress, pesticides, and pyridostigmine bromide (PB), a prophylactic agent against potential nerve agent exposure. These toxic exposures are thought to be the cause of these symptoms (IOM, 2013).

Because these "soft symptoms" had no identifiable diagnostic test or treatment, there have been many skeptics who challenge the validity of the claims. In 1998, Congress tasked the IOM through the work of the Committee on Gulf War and Health to study the issue. After 10 years of study, the committee produced very few conclusive findings, which offered little more than the original symptoms first reported (IOM, 2010). As a result of this review and their own research, VA now accepts 10 functional disorders and 5 tropical diseases as compensable conditions associated with the service of deployed Gulf War Veterans. Perhaps the most controversial recommendation in the 2016 IOM report was the recommendation that there be no further research on the effects of Gulf War exposures and suggested it was time to "move forward and focus on the interconnectedness of the brain and body" (Veterans for Common Sense, 2016). This recommendation brought intense criticism from Veterans and their supporters, as it was very reminiscent of the Agent Orange debacle. Military and Veteran organizations rallied to seek justice and procure legislation to award benefits and care to the afflicted Veterans.

AFGHANISTAN: OPERATION ENDURING FREEDOM (OEF); IRAQ: OPERATION IRAQI FREEDOM (OIF)

The attacks of 9/11 plunged the entire nation into a new "defense" mode and the realities that war was no longer oceans away. Since 2001, about 2.5 million U.S. troops have been deployed to Iraq or Afghanistan. More than 6,000 men and women have lost their lives and over 48,000 have been injured (DeBruyne, 2018, pp. 9–16). America's heavy reliance on Reserve and Guard Units to serve in combat, multiple deployments of the same personnel with no end in sight, military families living in communities, and the severity of wounds sustained all mark this engagement as particularly challenging.

As soon as the first casualties started to return from Iraq and Afghanistan, America began to hear how advances in battlefield medicine, medevac, and the sophistication of trauma care were resulting in exceptional care and high "save" rates unequaled in previous wars. As heartening as this news was, the realities that casualties who did survive would have catastrophic injuries and need comprehensive support systems and constant care for their entire life sometimes got lost in the patriotic fervor of "Thank You for Your Service." Injured casualties, horrific burns, multiple wounds, and multiple amputations said more about the wars than any news reports. The term "blast concussion" seemed to minimize the extent of the cerebral damage, loss of function, and disabilities that ensued. While a new diagnosis, traumatic brain injury (TBI), was deemed the "signature wound of modern warfare," there was also a misconception that the treatment and rehabilitation plans existed and were effective. With no visible wounds to explain the subtle symptoms of cognitive difficulties, memory deficits, problems with balance, slurred words, and personality changes experienced by the casualties, military families struggled with the daunting and challenging realities of caring for these Veterans at home (Schwartz, 2008). Military and VA physicians began to speculate that these symptoms were fabricated disorders presented by soldiers who wanted to avoid further deployments or "score" disability compensation and care. This attitude, although familiar, was particularly demeaning to the battle-hardened Veterans (Lee, Sanders, & Cox, 2014).

Almost from the start of the war, there was concern about the poor condition of the protective metal armaments and quality of body armor issued to troops. The problems of blunt force trauma, closed head injuries, and repeated exposures to improvised explosive devices (IEDs) contributed to a mounting body of evidence that TBI was indeed a factor that needed to be addressed in modern battlefield medicine. Explaining the differences between PTSD, as psychological reaction to an abnormal event, and TBI, associated with actual trauma to the brain, was problematic because symptoms often overlapped and were hard to distinguish without diagnostic testing and clinical interviews. Initial screenings on troops returning from combat areas often missed subtle symptoms, which could be masked or concealed.

As a new approach to military mission readiness evolves, it has become apparent that America will not return to the past tradition of creating and maintaining large bases and instillations. In reality, military and Veteran healthcare will not be as accessible as it was in the past. We have yet to know the full consequences and long-term effects of multiple deployments in relationship to family stability, successful return to the community, and future recruitment potential. An entire "superstructure" of support systems has steadily developed to ease the problems associated with deployments and family needs. This has powered another transformation on how healthcare, programs, and services are being provided to military families and Veterans of the engagements in Iraq and Afghanistan.

■ VA Reinventing Itself

In the post-Vietnam period, a great deal has changed in the composition and needs of America's military and the nation's expectations for the quality of life and support for "America's All Volunteer Forces." With the end of the "Draft" in 1973, women now comprise more than 15% of the military; 93% or career military are married with children. (CWV, 2018). The support of family and significant others has emerged as a vital dynamic in successful recruitment, retention, and reintegration of our returning military from combat and deployment to civilian life. The shift away from the large DOD infrastructure also challenges the resources of state and local governments to meet these needs. Although Congress, the DOD, and VA may identify a problem and derive solutions to these needs, the process of enacting legislation and implementing programs is years in the making. In the age of text messaging, the response time is considered by many to be out of touch and negligent compared to what this generation of returning "wounded warriors" has come to expect in exchange for their service to the country.

As an example, VA touted the fact that the national average to process an initial disability claim for a Veteran was only 136 days; 4 months and 16 days is a long time to wait for a paycheck when you have no other income. Another disappointment can be a real lack of financial relief because disability benefits provide barely enough to live on. In 2018, a Veteran with a spouse and one child rated 100%, which is unemployable, permanent, and total disability, receives $36,685.56 per year. For each additional child, the VA will pay $1,013.88 per year (USDVA, 2018c).

The strategy of scaling back the size of the Active Duty Military and using "Citizen Soldiers of the Guard and Reserve," and repeated and prolonged deployments to combat and "hot" areas have also precipitated health issues, which have not been addressed in previous conflicts. Reserve and National Guard Units, returning to their communities directly from the combat areas, have brought their readjustment problems to the neighborhoods, schools, and workplaces of America. Issues that were not previously in the "public eye," such as mental health conditions, suicide, and military sexual trauma, have become headline news. Perhaps most troubling was the finding that 18 to 22 Veterans a day were taking their own lives. Equally concerning were the reports that the high rates of suicide in women Veterans were linked to sexual trauma and assaults they survived while on active duty (Burke, 2015).

The Suicide Data Report published in 2012 was an initial attempt to assess risk factors and incidence of suicide in the Veteran population *but was limited because the study used only Veterans enrolled in VA programs.* Although this was not a research-based analysis, it did provide important information for further action. Among the findings that quickly garnered attention, "22 veterans a day die from suicide" was a specific note that this number had "remained relatively stable over the past 12 years" (Kemp & Bossarte, 2012, p. 20). The finding that this stunning number had been "relatively stable" for 12 years brought intense scrutiny on VA and the needs of young Veterans returning from "harm's way" only to take their own lives. The most recent Suicide Data Report, released in 2018, provided evidence of dramatic changes in some previously noted trends. Veteran specific counts of suicide declined, overall to an average of 20 Veterans per day (OMH, 2018, p. 6). Even more disturbing was the finding that women Veterans were 1.8 times greater to take their own lives when compared to civilian women. Researchers also reported that this was an improvement from the previous 2014 finding that women Veterans were 2.5 times more likely to take their own lives than their civilian counterparts (VAOMH, 2018). The 2016 findings were a stunning indictment of VA for neglecting to address this glowing omission. In an effort to make better sense of the staggering discrepancy between male and female Veteran suicide rates, the Research and Development (RAND) Corporation began to closely study a crisis in the making.

Findings indicated that there was a link in dramatic rise in suicide among women in the military and sexual trauma, particularly incidences of harassment, domestic violence, and sexual assault while stationed overseas (Gorin, 2018). According to the VA, one in four women in the military reports sexual assaults or trauma. Many speculate that this number is likely low because of the stigma and possible consequences associated with reporting these crimes (Gordon, 2018, p. 47). In addition to the stressors of combat areas and conditions, the feelings of hopelessness and helplessness, which often occur after a sexual assault, are overwhelming and contribute to a sense of loss of self, despair, and suicidal ideation. Sexual trauma is a significant risk factor for suicide in a military setting because it also adds a sense of betrayal and insecurity when lives are at risk. Women Veterans are known to conceal their feelings, which can affect their duty performance and cause additional disciplinary actions against them. Researchers now identify military sexual trauma (MST) as one of the factors that increases risks of suicide, PTSD, unfavorable ratings, and ultimately dismissal from the military. Although DOD has implemented training programs, confidential reporting, and interventions for treatment, the process is often a quagmire for women who are suffering in a closed nonjudicial system that minimizes these events and often does not even investigate the reports that are made.

CARE IN THE COMMUNITY

During the 2010 debate on the Affordable Care Act (ACA), many comparisons about the proposed overhaul of medical care also raised the interest and scrutiny of America's largest integrated health system. Heavy criticism and fear of "socialized medicine" or rationing of healthcare opened the door for opponents to use VA as an example of how wrong things can get. As the 2014 ACA implementation date approached, reports of negligence, misdiagnosis, and ill-treatment of Veterans using the system escalated. While some of these complaints were superfluous, a legitimate scandal at the Phoenix Arizona VA Medical Center became a major factor in the future of care for America's Veterans.

Local news media reported a pervasive pattern of neglect and staff falsifying appointments or keeping double sets of records to escape complaints; 35 Veterans had died while waiting to be seen for care. The VA Office of the Inspector General (VAOIG) also found systematic problems involving delayed medical care for Veterans across the country; problems with scheduling cover-ups were also widespread. Data revealed that 120,000 Veterans were still waiting for an appointment or never receiving care (Griffin, 2014, pp. i–v). The Congress, the Federal Bureau of Investigation, and the White House launched additional probes.

CHOICE PROGRAM

The Veterans Access, Choice, and Accountability Act of 2014 (VACAA) required the VA to establish "the Choice Program" to improve Veterans' access to healthcare by authorizing eligible Veterans to use non-VA community providers. Criteria for this authorization included Veterans living more than 40 miles from a VA facility or unable to schedule an appointment within 30 days or having significant travel hardships. In 2018, the Choice Program was replaced by the VA Maintaining Internal Systems and Strengthening Integrated Outside Networks Act (VA MISSION Act), which used the same eligibility criteria and aimed to improve VA's ability to contract with healthcare providers, consolidate and improve VA community care programs, and expand caregiver benefits to all Veterans. While many saw this legislation to be pragmatic, given the expectations of healthcare systems in the 21st century, Veterans saw this as the beginning of the end for Veteran-focused care, preliminary efforts to dismantle the VA, and ultimately privatization of all VA Health Care. Key was the cost of $55 billion with a 5-year commitment to expedite Veterans' access to non-VA–preapproved community care at VA expense.

The utilization of VA Health Care services is often equated to the number of living Veterans in America. Mistakenly, most believe that every Veteran uses VA health programs. However, data indicate that of the estimated 20 million living U.S. Veterans, only 31% (6.2 million) actually use VA Health Care. Even more striking, only 68% of disabled Veterans choose VA for their care. Additionally, a minority, only 19% (3.8 million) of America's Veterans, rely exclusively on VA for their healthcare needs (U.S. Department of Veterans Affairs, 2017).

◾ Conclusion

NURSING IMPLICATIONS

The "Choice Option" and "VA Mission Act" provisions for community care programs have accelerated and elevated the need for healthcare providers at every echelon to understand their Veteran patients. Particularly significant, VA reported in 2017 alone, they processed 19 million claims for care by non-VA community providers. Far from the popular notion that all Veterans receive their care in the VA, the vast majority of Veterans with special experiences, increased risk factors to diseases, and complex needs actually receive their care in the community. Over time it has become apparent that military service in and of itself is an occupational hazard, fraught with stressors, toxic exposures, hazards, and safety risks not commonly encountered in the civilian population (American Academy of Nursing, 2013). There are real concerns about the possible shortfall in the comprehensive and appropriate diagnosis, care, and treatment of Veterans who use community healthcare providers. Very few healthcare providers actually include the simple question "Have you ever served in the military?" on their intakes, assessments, or health histories. This single question can be the key to timely assessments, diagnosis, and treatment of an individual. Because of the nature of military service, healthcare providers and their Veteran patients may not know the full effects and complexities of the occupational and environmental risks encountered in the military and the consequences these risks pose to health and future well-being.

In 2013, Vietnam Veterans of America, Inc., the American Academy of Nursing, and the National Association of State Directors of Veterans Affairs began a collaborative

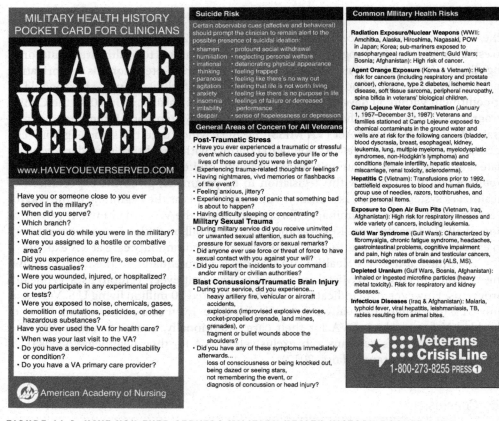

FIGURE 11.2 HAVE YOU EVER SERVED? MILITARY HEALTH HISTORY POCKET CARD FOR CLINICIANS.

Source: From Have You Ever Served. (n.d.). Clinician pocket card. Retrieved from http://www.haveyou-verserved.com/pocket-card--posters.html

effort to champion the program, Have You Ever Served? The purpose of the effort is to increase the awareness of nursing and allied professionals about the unique health exposures, stresses, and risks associated with serving in the armed forces of the United States and health conditions eventually borne by Veterans and family members. To facilitate this process, a clinical assessment tool was developed for clinicians designed to identify Veteran patients and conduct an interview that included military service history, "Common Military Health Risks," "General Areas of Concern for All Veterans," and health conditions linked to exposures (see Figure 11.2).

Nursing has a vital role to play in this campaign to educate providers about the multifaceted and complex needs of this growing population. Conditions such as PTS, exposures to toxins, head trauma, and blast concussions present challenges to Veterans and their families every day. These conditions may be misdiagnosed, undiagnosed, or untreated for years because clinicians have not asked their patients about service in the armed forces. The involvement of nursing, as a profession, in incorporating the question Have you ever served in the military? will provide valuable information to expand and better inform our practice and care for military members, Veterans, and their families.

REFLECTIONS

America's egalitarian roots, traditions, and belief in the common good have evolved into a system of caring for Veterans and their families, which is much envied by other nations. For those who have served and worn the uniform, there is a determination that they will "keep faith" with those who "faithfully serve" to ensure America matches the patriotic rhetoric with actions that ensure "those who have borne the battle" receive the care and support they have earned and deserve. This struggle is as fierce, and at times as protracted, as any of the battles and wars endured in the process. The democracy so hard-won and protected by our military and Veterans has become the greatest power they have in their struggles for justice. The lodestar for this effort must always be to ensure that America's service to Veterans is equal to and commensurate with the services they rendered to their country.

■ Critical Thinking Exercise

1. Does the United States have a responsibility to provide healthcare and services to military Veterans and their families? Explain.
2. How would you rate America's support for Veterans? Why?

■ Discussion Questions

1. In the news, what are some of the issues around Veterans' care of which you think nursing should be aware, and how can nursing contribute positively in the identified problem area?
2. You find that your patient is a woman Veteran. What resources can you identify that she may need? What resources are available?

■ Resources

Collins, E., Wilmoth, M., & Schwartz, L. (2013). "Have You Ever Served in the Military?" campaign in partnership with the Joining Forces Initiative. *Nursing Outlook, 61*(5), 375–376. doi:10.1016/j.outlook.2013.07.004

Gosoroski, D. M. (1996). For those who 'faithfully serve.' *Veterans of Foreign Wars Magazine, 84*(4), 13–16.

Gostin, L., & Wiley, L. (2016). *Public health law: Power, duty, restraint* (3rd ed.). Oakland, CA: University of California Press.

Harris, L. (1985). *Office of Information Management and Statistics, Research Division*. Washington, DC: Veterans Administration.

Holiday, L. F., Bell, G., Klein, R. E., & Wells, M. R. (2006). *American Indian and Alaska Native Veterans: Lasting contributions*. Washington, DC: Department of Veterans Affairs. Retrieved from https://www.va.gov/vetdata/docs/specialreports/aianpaper9-12-06final.pdf

Institute of Medicine. (1977). *Report to Senate Committee on Veterans Affairs: Study of Health Care for American Veterans*. Washington, DC: National Academy of Health Sciences US Government Printing Office.

Institute of Medicine. (2016). Update on health effects of serving in the gulf war. In *Gulf War and Health* (Vol. 10). Washington, DC: National Academy Press.

Issacs, C. (2013, April). Why the Combat Infantryman Badge counts. *Time Magazine*. Retrieved from http://nation.time.com/2013/04/05/to-cib-or-not-to-cib-that-is-the-question/print

Krepenvich, A. F. (1986). *The Army and Vietnam*. Baltimore, MD: Johns Hopkins University Press.

Mellon, A. W. (1922). *Statistics of income. US Treasury, Government Accountability Office*. Washington, DC. Government Printing Office.

Newport, F (2012). In U.S., 24% of Men, 2% of Women Are Veterans. *Gallop Politics*. Retrieved from https://news.gallup.com/poll/158729/men-women-veterans.aspx

Ortiz, S. (2006). The new deal for veterans: The economy act, the VFW and the origins of the New Deal dissent. *Journal of Military History, 70*(2), 415–438. doi:10.1353/jmh.2006.0119

Schwartz, L. (1992). *Our unknown warriors emerge from the shadows*. New Haven, CT: Yale School of Medicine.

Soucy, J. (2016). *National Guard remains a vital component of the war fight*. Retrieved from https://www.army.mil/article/164663/National_Guard_remains_a_vital_component_of_the_war_fight/

Title 38 US Code Chapter 11. (2013). *Veterans benefits: Compensation for service-connected disabilities or death*. Washington, DC: Government Printing Office.

U.S. Department of Defense. (2013). *"Armed Forces Strengths" Statistical Information Analysis Division*. Washington, DC: Department of Defense.

U.S. Department of Veteran Affairs. *Center for Women Veterans*. Retrieved from https://www.va.gov/womenvet

U.S. Department of Veterans Affairs: https://www.va.gov

Vietnam Veterans of America: https://www.vva.org

Women in Military Service to America: https://www.womensmemorial.org

References

Agent Orange Act of 1991, HR 556, 102nd Congress. (1991-1992). Retrieved from www.congress.gov/bill/102nd-congress/house-bill/556

American Academy of Nursing. (2013). *Have You Ever Served*. Clinician pocket card. Retrieved from http://www.haveyoueverserved.com/about.html

Basu, S. (2014). Complexities, lack of approved therapies challenge PTSD, TBI treatment. *US. Medicine Newsletter*.

Beath, R. B. (1899). *History of the Grand Army of the Republic*. New York, NY: Bryan Taylor Publishing. Retrieved from archive.org/details/historyofgrandar00beat

Braverman, P., & Gottlieb, L. (2014). Th e social determinants of health: It's time to consider the causes of the causes. *Public Health Reports, 129*(Suppl. 2), 19–31. doi:10.1177/00333549141291S206

Buckley, F. S. (1990). *Women Veterans: A decade of progress*. VA Advisory Committee on Women Veterans. Washington, DC: Veterans Administration.

Center for Women Veterans. (2014). *Women Veterans: A historical perspective*. Washington, DC: U.S. Department of Veteran Affairs.

DeBruyne, N. F. (2018). *American war and military operations casualties: Lists and statistics*. Washington, DC: Congressional Research Service.

Gonzalez, D. (1991, March 4). Gulf veterans to be honored in May parade. *New York Times*. Retrieved from https://www.nytimes.com/1991/03/04/nyregion/gulf-veterans -to-be-honored-in-may-parade.html

Gordon, S. (2018). *Wounds of war: How VA delivers health, healing and hope to the nation's Veterans*. Ithaca, NY: Cornell University Press.

Gorin, D. (2018). *Why so many military women think about suicide*. Veterans in America, RAND Corporation. Retrieved from https://www.rand.org/multimedia/podcasts/ veterans-in-america/why-so-many-military-women-think-about-suicide.html

Government Accountability Office. (1982). *Actions needed to ensure that Female Veterans have equal access to VA Benefits*. Washington, DC: Government Printing Office.

Greenhill, K. M. (2006, February 17). Don't dumb down the Army. *New York Times Opinion*. Retrieved from https://www.nytimes.com/2006/02/17/opinion/dont-dumb-down-the-army.html

Griffin, R. L. (2014). *Review of alleged patient deaths, patient waiting times and scheduling practices of VA health care systems*. Washington, DC: Department of Veteran Affairs

Harris, L. (1991). *The Commonwealth Fund: Survey of women veterans' health*. New York, NY: Commonwealth Fund.

Helmer, J. (1974). *The American soldier in Vietnam and after*. New York, NY: The Free Press.

Holm, J. (1982). *Women in the Military: The unfinished revolution*. Novata, CA: Presidio Press.

Institute of Medicine. (2010). *Operation Enduring Freedom and Operation Iraqi Freedom: Demographics and Impact*. Washington, DC: National Academies Press. doi:10.17226/12812

Institute of Medicine. (2013). *Returning home from Iraq and Afghanistan: Assessment of readjustment of veterans, service members and their families* (pp. 33–46). Washington, DC: National Academies Press.

Keib, R. (1982). Vietnam veteran fact sheet. *Stars and Stripes, The National Tribune*. Washington, DC: National Tribune Corp.

Kemp, J., & Bossarte, R. (2012). *Suicide Data Report*. Washington, DC: U.S. Department of Veteran Affairs.

Lang, K. (2016). *Facts you should know about Desert Storm*. Fort Meade, MD: Department of Defense News Media Activity.

Lee, J., Sanders, K. M. & Cox, M. (2014). Honoring those who have served. *Academic Medicine, 89*(9), 1198–1200. doi:10.1097/ACM.0000000000000367

Leipold, J. D. (2012). *Women veterans mark 60th anniversary of Korean War*. Arlington, VA: U.S. Army News Service, U.S. Army.

Lifton, R. (1973). *Home from the war*. New York, NY: Basic Books.

National Center for Veterans Analysis and Statistics. (2018). *Office of Policy and Planning, Statistics at a Glance*. Washington, DC: Department of Veteran Affairs.

Norman, E. M. (1988). Post traumatic stress disorder in military nurses who served in Vietnam during the war years 1963-1973. *Military Medicine, 153*, 238–242. doi:10.1093/milmed/153.5.238

Obama, B. (2010). *Remarks by the president honoring Veterans Day in Seoul, South Korea*. Retrieved from https://obamawhitehouse.archives.gov/the-press-offi ce/2010/11/10/ remarks-president-honoring-veterans-day-seoul-south-korea

Office of Mental Health (OMH) and Suicide Prevention. (2018). *Veteran Suicide Data Report 2005-2016*. Washington, DC: U.S. Department of Veteran Affairs.

Office of Public Affairs. (2018). *America's Wars*. Washington, DC: U.S. Department of Veteran Affairs.

Scott, C. (2012). *Veterans Affairs historical Budget Authority FY 1940-2012*. Washington, DC, Congressional Research Service.

Severo, R., & Milford, L. (1989). *Wages of War: When America's Soldiers Came Home: From Valley Forge to Vietnam. Forbidden Bookshelf* (Vol. 5). New Yor, NY: Open Road Publishing.

Shane, L. (2018, February 12). VA spending up again in Trump's fiscal 2019 budget plan. *Military Times*. Retrieved from https://www.militarytimes.com/veterans/2018/02/12/va-spending-up-again-in-trumps-fiscal-2019-budget-plan/

Schwartz, L. (1987). Women and the Vietnam experience. *Image: Journal of Nursing Scholarship, 19*. Winter 1987. doi:10.1111/j.1547-5069.1987.tb00001.x

Schwartz, L. (1998). Health problems of American women veterans of the Vietnam War. In *Human Exposure Epidemiology, Risk Assessment and Management: Halogenated Environmental Organic Pollutants* (Vol. 38, pp. 215–219). Stockholm, Sweden: Swedish Environmental Protection Agency.

Schwartz, L. (2008). *Testimony Congressional Hearing: Mental Health Treatment for Families: Supporting Those Who Support Our Veterans, House Veterans Affairs Committee 110th Congress 2nd Session*. Retrieved from https://archives-veterans.house.gov/witness-testimony/linda-spoonster-schwartz-rn-drph-faan

Starr, P. (1972). *The Discarded Army: Vietnam Veterans After Vietnam*. New York, NY: Charterhouse.

Stout, M. (2018). *Agent orange and the fight for justice for Vietnam veterans*. Silver Spring, MD: Vietnam Veterans of America Inc.

U.S. Department of Veteran Affairs, Office of Public Affairs. (2016). *Department of Veteran Affairs Organizational Snapshot*. Retrieved from https://fr.slideshare.net/granimal/department-of-veterans-affairs-15652856

U.S. Department of Veteran Affairs. (2017). *Federal benefits for veterans, dependents and survivors*. Washington, DC: US Government Printing Office.

U.S. Department of Veteran Affairs. (2018a). *Federal benefi ts for veterans, dependents and survivors*. Washington, DC: U.S. Government Printing Office.

U.S. Department of Veteran Affairs. (2018b). *VA benefi ts book. Office of public and intergovernmental affairs*. Washington, DC: U.S. Government Printing Office.

U.S. Department of Veteran Affairs. (2018c). *Veterans compensation benefits rate table effective 12/1/18*. Washington, DC: Veterans Benefi ts Administration

Veterans Administration. (1967). To care for him who shall have borne the battle. Washington, DC: U.S. Government Printing Office.

Veterans for Common Sense. (2016). *IOM Gulf War Report "Turns science on its head."* Retrieved from https://www.prnewswire.com/news-releases/iom-gulf-war-report-turns-science-on-its-head-researchers-say-568463821.html

Vietnam Veterans of America. (2017). *VVA self-help guide: Service connected disabled compensation for exposures to Agent Orange*. Silver Spring, MD: Agent Orange Committee, Vietnam Veterans of America.

Vogt, K. S. (2015). Origins of military medical care as an essential source of morale. *Military Medicine, 180*, 604–605. doi:10.7205/MILMED-D-14-00492

Interprofessional Collaboration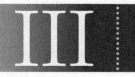

12 Achieving Health Equity: Exemplars in Engaging Global Communities

Margherita Procaccini Clark and
Franchesca A. Cifuentes-Andrade

CHAPTER OBJECTIVES

- ◉ Understand how Lansing Community College Career Ladder Nursing Program partnered with local organizations to impact the health of women and children in Uganda without the risk and cost of traveling abroad
- ◉ Gain a global understanding of the economic and environmental living conditions in the Kigezi region, rural Uganda
- ◉ Identify low-cost sustainable interventions implemented in the Kigezi region to help promote a culture of health and wellness among women, children, and families living in villages in rural Uganda

KEY CONCEPTS

Ambient learning	Service learning
Food insecurity	Servant leadership
Moment of obligation	Sustainability
Purpose-driven	Transformational leadership

KEY TERMS

Altruism	Transformative
Civic leadership	Nongovernmental organization (NGO)
Collaboration	Oral rehydration salts
Community-based organization (CBO)	Pedagogical
Inquiry	Purchasing power
Multidisciplinary	

■ Introduction
· ·

I think one's feelings waste themselves in words; they ought all to be distilled into
actions which bring results.

—Florence Nightingale

It was Florence Nightingale, the founder of modern nursing, who said we need to take actions that create results instead of wasting time talking about something without results. Nurse Nightingale inspires nurses across the world to provide service to others. The nursing profession is founded on service. In higher education, service learning is a pedagogical approach that combines community service and learning to benefit both the growth of the student and the community stakeholders involved. The Center for Teaching and Learning at University of Washington describes service learning as "learning that actively involves students in a wide range of experiences, which often benefit others and the community, while also advancing the goals of a given curriculum" ("Service Learning," n.d.). Service-learning projects incorporate structured preparation, training, and student reflection and allow students to learn beyond the traditional classroom. Amid supportive faculty and administrators, students who engage in service-learning projects are granted the opportunity to collaboratively implement purpose-driven initiatives at a local, regional, national, or even international level based on the partnerships cultivated by faculty and administrators. Service-learning projects deepen and democratize the learning process for all those involved (Longo & Saltmarsh, 2011); therefore, incorporating service learning as part of the nursing curriculum in the Career Ladder Nursing Program at Lansing Community College (LCC) in Lansing, Michigan, was a natural fit, given the foundational tenets of nursing.

The multidisciplinary team of faculty and staff at LCC's Career Ladder Nursing Program has developed a strong framework for civic leadership, which allows students to engage with various communities and professionals through transformative service-learning projects. This chapter elaborates on the outcomes of a significant collaboration between LCC's Nursing Program and Kigezi Women and Children Health Initiative (Kigezi Women), a small nongovernmental organization (NGO) operating in the community that is committed to empowering women and children in rural Uganda. Through investigative and research work as part of their service-learning projects, nursing students at LCC were able to put their knowledge and skills to use to support Kigezi Women address the nutritional, health and wellness, and literacy needs of women and children located across the globe.

▪ About Kigezi Women and Children Health Initiative

Since its inception in December 2016, Kigezi Women has served over 1,000 women and children across three villages in rural Uganda: Bwisa-Kakore, Nangara, and Kigarama. Kigezi Women is committed to empowering women and children through three key strategies: (a) improving literacy rates and access to skill-based trainings; (b) improving health conditions and access to adequate healthcare; and (c) increasing women's earnings, purchasing power, and household income. Kigezi Women was founded by Dr. Olivia Kamayangi, a native of Uganda and a practicing physician in the Midwest of the United States (Figure 12.1). With her husband, Gian Luca Gamberini, Dr. Kamayangi started Kigezi Women because she believes that the key to improving the quality of rural life lies in addressing the basic needs of the most vulnerable, women and children. Dr. Kamayangi elaborates on why health and education is at the core of Kigezi Women's work:

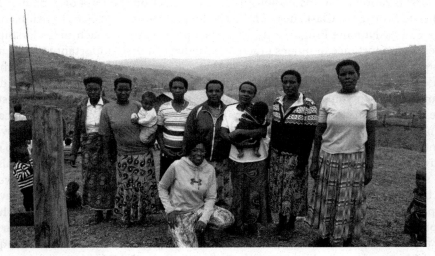

FIGURE 12.1 DR. KAMAYANGI WITH VILLAGE HEALTH LEADERS IN BWISA-KAKORE, UGANDA, DEC 2017.

Photo Credit: Gian Luca Gamberini.

Our objective is to provide women with bold livelihood options that enhance their dignity, economic status, and increase their decision-making power. Empowered and well-informed women will be in position to improve their children's livelihood, provide them with more appropriate nutrition options, teach them better hygiene practices, and guarantee the best health possible. We recognize the unbelievable efforts women in these rural communities make every day to provide for their children, and our main goal is to support them in their wish for the improved life of their children. We focus on children's health as the main instrument of building a better future for the whole community. (O. Kamayangi, personal communication, December 30, 2017)

Kigezi Women's initial work at the early stages of the organization's development was possible due to key collaborations with larger institutions like LCC and the Career Ladder Nursing Program. With LCC's support, Kigezi Women has been able to impact the lives of over 1,000 women and children across three villages through small interventions such as providing vital medicine, bolstering peer-to-peer networks, offering training, and providing access to clean energy via solar panels. To learn more about Kigezi Women and their work, visit the website (kigeziwomen.org).

■ Service Learning in Action

LEADERSHIP AND COLLABORATION

The collaboration between LCC's Career Ladder Nursing Program and Kigezi Women was the result of a nurse's inquiry, which brought devoted people together to connect on a common thread of hope, love, and teaching. This collaboration was possible because of the effort and courage of individuals intentionally reaching out to communities, organizations, and institutions to create impact on the lives of people in need. Margherita Procaccini Clark, dean of the Health and Human Services Division and the Career Ladder Nursing Program at LCC, has a particular approach to leadership and stresses the importance of nurses practicing inquiry: "It is so important to learn about a person's story or a community's story so that you can know how to make an impact. If you don't take the risk to ask questions and learn about situations that are different from your own you miss out on the ability to impact others through modest and simple interventions that may have a big impact" (M. Clark, personal communication, December 2018). Nursing faculty, administrators, and staff are dedicated to cultivating students and nurses who are servant and transformational leaders—leaders who show initiative, assume risks, take action and ownership, and seek to change individuals and social systems (Sousa & van Dierendonck, 2017)—and leaders who are effective and impactful. Developing civic knowledge and engagement at the local and global levels is a key part of LCC's essential learning outcomes adopted by the institution as a whole.

For over 20 years, LCC's nursing program has been participating in service learning. There are four levels in the Career Ladder Nursing Program. Each level has a requirement of 4 hours of service learning with a reflection narrative. Nursing students engage in a total of 16 hours or more of service-learning activities in the local community with a variety of community-based organizations (CBOs) serving the underserved. Cristo Rey Community Center (CRCC) and The Davies Project (TDP) are two main CBOs in the greater area of Lansing, Michigan, that provide opportunities for nursing students to engage with members of the community. Other local organizations with which the nursing program has partnered include Saint Vincent Children's Home, Ronald McDonald House, Lansing Rescue Mission, Willow Elementary Grade School, Sexton High School, and many more. These CBOs are ripe for opportunities to teach and share knowledge, engage students in civic responsibilities, and cultivate socially aware and conscience professionals. Through these diverse interactions, nursing students can develop a level of awareness and leadership that will inform their practice for years to come. For more information about these CBOs, see the section Resources at the end of this chapter.

Because of a chance encounter between Dean Clark and Dr. Kamayangi, one question and one conversation expanded into a long-term partnership that created opportunities for students, faculty, administrators, Lansing CBOs, and community members to engage in projects that contribute to the improvement of the health and wellness of an international community of women and children. These kinds of partnerships and collaborations offer nursing students the opportunity to gain an international experience without expense or risk of traveling abroad, which can be challenging for community college students and staff.

RECOMMENDATIONS AND INTERVENTIONS

Nursing education is founded on the tenets of the nursing process: assessment, diagnosis, planning, implementation, and evaluation (Nursing Process, n.d.). These tenets are the framework for all actions of inquiry and curiosity. Sixty-four LCC nursing students engaged in service-learning projects that focused on three main issues: (a) health risks faced by mothers with low literacy skills; (b) children under the age of 5 experiencing life-threatening dehydration as a result of diarrhea, vomiting, and fever; (c) young girls aged 10 to 12 with hygiene supplies to care for menstruation needs in order to continue attending school. Simple and sustainable interventions were developed, adopted, and implemented locally by Kigezi Women staff. LCC nursing students designed individual pamphlets that explained in English and in the native language, Rukiga, how to stop microbes, use the oral rehydration salts (ORS) and diverse nutrients, and create a microgarden (see Figures 12.2 and 12.3 for a sample pamphlet). Pamphlets were printed and laminated at LCC as an in-kind donation. These pamphlets were delivered to Kigezi Women staff in Uganda who utilized them as educational tools when providing health trainings to mothers (see Figures 12.4 and 12.5). Each family received the pamphlets to take home to help reinforce what they had learned in the health trainings. These pamphlets provide more opportunities for

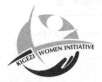

Stop Microbes, Wash Your Hands
Yerinde obukoko burikureeta endwara, naaba engaro

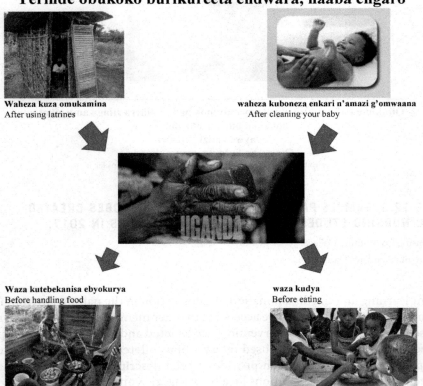

FIGURE 12.2 SAMPLE PAMPHLET ON STOPPING MICROBES CREATED BY LCC NURSING STUDENTS DISTRIBUTED TO FAMILIES IN 2017.

LCC, Lansing Community College.
Photo Credit: Gian Luca Gamberini.

EKIRIKURETA ENDWARA EZIMU EZITURIKUBASA KWERINDA
CAUSES OF PREVENTABLE DISEASES:

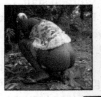 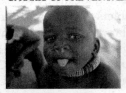 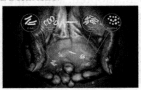

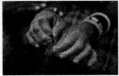 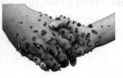

Kunaba engaro N'ESABUNDI nikiyamba OKWERINDA encungura, endwara zimwe
z'ekitigu nezomwiso
HAND WASHING WITH SOAP IS SHOWN TO PREVENT DISEASES SUCH AS:
Cholera, dysentery, typhoid, hepatitis A, upper respiratory infections

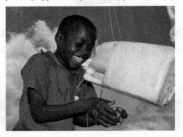

Oijukuke kufundikira ebyokurya kwenda ngu eshohera zitagwamu zikatamu
obukoko burikureta oburweire
Onywe amizi gatekire
Ogyezeho kutanya omumuhanda
Remember to always cover your food to prevent flies contaminating it
Drink boiled water
Avoid defecating in open air

FIGURE 12.3 SAMPLE PAMPHLET ON STOPPING MICROBES CREATED BY LCC NURSING STUDENTS DISTRIBUTED TO FAMILIES IN 2017.

LCC, Lansing Community College.
Photo Credit: Gian Luca Gamberini.

ambient learning and the dissemination of information in the natural environment by allowing these teaching tools to be accessible to other members of the family to review and also learn the applicable interventions as depicted and written on the pamphlets.

Recommendations and proposed interventions offered by LCC nursing students are depicted in Table 12.1, which provides a brief description of each issue and the approach to implementing solutions locally by Kigezi Women staff.

Issue: Acute Diarrheal Diseases and Dehydration

The World Health Organization (WHO) lists acute diarrheal diseases as the leading cause of death in infants and young children in developing countries around the world (WHO, 2017). The WHO was founded in 1948 and is a specialized agency of the United

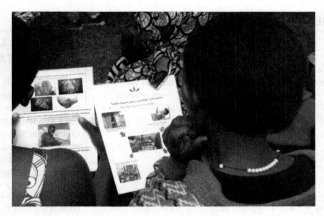

FIGURE 12.4 MOTHERS IN RURAL UGANDA RECEIVE PAMPHLET CREATED BY LCC NURSING STUDENTS WITH NUTRITIONAL INFORMATION IN 2017.

LCC, Lansing Community College.
Photo Credit: Gian Luca Gamberini.

Nations. The primary purpose of the WHO is to lead global health responses of its partners related to international health within the United Nations. The WHO partners with world experts working together with shared interests to improve the health of the world's citizens (WHO, n.d.). Dehydration is one of the several symptoms of acute diarrheal diseases along with high fever, vomiting, and severe diarrhea as reported by the WHO, which if untreated, can result in the demise of the infant or young child (WHO, 2017). A simple, cost-effective treatment is administering ORS at the earliest sign of dehydration (listlessness, dry skin, warm skin, watery stools, sunken eyeballs, and change in level of consciousness, increased thirst, dry mucous membranes, and

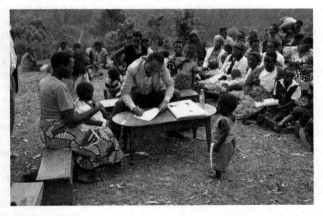

FIGURE 12.5 KIGEZI WOMEN STAFF PROVIDING TRAINING TO UGANDAN MOTHERS UTILIZING PAMPHLETS CREATED BY LCC NURSING STUDENTS AS EDUCATIONAL TOOLS.

LCC, Lansing Community College.
Photo Credit: Gian Luca Gamberini.

TABLE 12.1 ISSUES, RECOMMENDATIONS, AND INTERVENTIONS

ISSUES	RECOMMENDATIONS AND PROPOSED INTERVENTIONS	APPROACH AND IMPLEMENTATION
Acute diarrheal diseases and dehydration	Distribute ORS and bottled water to mothers. Inform mothers on how to mix and administer ORS to a sick child or a relative.	Nursing students, faculty, and administrators collaborated to create educational tools in the form of a laminated pamphlet that instructs mothers on how to properly mix and administer ORS packets when children are experiencing diarrhea and fever.
Food insecurity and access to high-protein nutritional foods	Provide access to plant-based protein seeds to enhance and diversify diet.	Health trainings instructed families on how to grow protein-rich, plant-based foods by setting up microgardens. Funding was provided to partner with Ugandan women to share the cost of purchasing one chicken or rabbit per household and increase access to protein. A few mothers piloted creating microgardens near their homes and Kigezi Women provided seeds to test out how families could have access to green leafy vegetables for daily use in meal preparation. Many women are subsistence farmers and must travel long distances to gather the food they grow on other plots.
Hand and personal hygiene	Promote the importance of hand-washing and personal hygiene and make connection to overall health. Provide washable, reusable menstruation pads with sanitary belts to young women and mothers.	Important hygiene practices were discussed in smaller community group meetings among women and through the use of educational plays developed by the women themselves to promote a culture of hygiene among families in the villages. Village Health Leaders (see Figure 12.1) used educational tools to continue promoting a culture of hand hygiene through the frequent use of tippy taps (water receptacles). Menstruation pads and sanitary belts were also provided to young girls and women by LCC nursing students. Menstruation pads were designed to be reusable and sewn by hand with volunteers at LCC.

LCC, Lansing Community College; ORS, oral rehydration salts.

later signs of deep tongue furrows). The ORS is a compounded mixture of glucose and electrolytes (sodium chloride, potassium, glucose, and citrate; WHO and United Nations Children's Fund [UNICEF], 2006). It was in the late 1960s that ORS treatment reduced adult patient deaths from 50% to zero and gained the title "A Miracle Cure." In the early 1970s, the ORS treatment expanded to include children (WHO, 2011).

The rural villages of the Kigezi region are overwhelmed by poverty, early death, malnutrition, poor hygiene, lack of protein-rich foods, and little to no running water or electricity, just to name a few of the daily challenges that families face. LCC nursing students and faculty, in partnership with Dr. Olivia Kamayangi, MD, a native of the Kigezi region of Uganda, created and prepared teaching materials for use during the ORS trainings with mothers. Dr. Kamayangi also provided translation from English to Rukiga, the local language (see Figures 12.2 and 12.3). With these teaching materials, Kigezi Women staff implemented workshops about dehydration and rehydration and the use of ORS with the women in the village of Bwisa-Kakore and Nangara. Five packets of ORS were distributed per child to each family, and through the health trainings, the women and mothers were empowered to be able to treat early signs of dehydration themselves and provide lifesaving interventions for their children as they sought proper medical care. Since the introduction of ORS packets, Dr. Kamayangi reports zero child deaths related to dehydration have been recorded in the village of Bwisa-Kakore and Nangara (O. Kamayangi, personal communication, September 2018).

Issue: Food Insecurity and Access to High-Protein Nutritional Food

The WHO, along with other international organizations, reported that the absolute number of undernourished people in the world is now estimated to have increased from around 804 million in 2016 to almost 821 million in 2017 (Food and Agriculture Organization of the United Nations [FAO], International Fund for Agricultural Development [IFAD], UNICEF, World Food Programme [WFP], & WHO, 2018). Approximately, one out of every nine people in the world is undernourished, and evidence shows that severe food insecurity may be increasing in almost all regions of Africa as well as in South America (FAO, IFAD, UNICEF, WFP, & WHO, 2018). The FAO, a specialized agency of the United Nations that leads international efforts to defeat hunger, reports that 60% of those undernourished around the globe are women and about 80% of the world's extreme poor live in rural areas, most of them dependent on agriculture (FAO, IFAD, UNICEF, WFP, &WHO, 2018). This is the reality for those living in rural Uganda. The women who are part of the Kigezi Women network are often subsistence farmers who till the land to provide for themselves and their families. Subsistence farmers often travel long distances to gather the food they grow on other plots, which do not belong to them. The food available for consumption lacks nutritional content, and families are not able to afford protein-rich foods. Malnutrition is a serious health and welfare problem affecting children under 5 years of age and is the leading factor that affects mortality and morbidity rates. According to the Uganda Demographic and Health Survey of 2011 by the Uganda Bureau of Statistics (UBOS), 4 in 10 Ugandan children under 5 years of age (33%) are stunted (short for their age), 6% are wasted (thin for their height), and 14% are underweight (low weight for age; UBOS and ICF International, 2012).

In Kigezi, a rural Ugandan geographic area, carbohydrates and vitamins are relatively easy to access but proteins are often lacking. Access to poultry meat would guarantee a stable supply of protein for women and children. Funding was provided by Kigezi

Women to partner with the village women to share the cost of purchasing one chicken or rabbit per household through the "One Egg-One Child Project." The goal of the One Egg-One Child Project is to identify other sources of protein for mothers to provide to their children to strengthen their immunity, and to increase growth and muscle strength. The mothers sought the help of the Kigezi Health Initiative to partner with them and purchase hens and roosters. The women initially proposed that they could save their money and pay for 80% of the cost, asking if the Kigezi Women as an organization could pay the other 20%. They estimated the funds would be ready in 22 months. However, the organization proposed to shorten the time frame by providing 80% of the funding, while the women provided 20%. The project was launched and implemented in 4 months in the villages of Bwisa-Kakore and Nangara, reaching 129 families and a total of 239 children in 2018. Kigezi Women intend to grow this project into a chicken-lending scheme with multiple participants to allow various families to grow their own eggs and chickens. However, some chickens did not survive because of lack of access to veterinary care. The women indicated that rabbits survive well and reproduce faster and have substituted rabbits for eggs to improve protein consumption.

Microgardening
The concept of microgardening is uncommon in rural Uganda. LCC students and Kigezi Women introduced microgardening to address the issue of access to land. Trainings offered by Kigezi Women staff using the pamphlets created by LCC nursing students instructed families on how to grow protein-rich, plant-based foods by setting up microgardens. A group of mothers opted to pilot creating microgardens near their homes and Kigezi Women provided seeds to test out how families could have access to green leafy vegetables for daily use for meal preparation. In rural Uganda, most women are subsistence farmers, living off the land, working in agriculture, and must travel long distances to gather the food they grow on other plots. The land the women till is located miles away from their homes and the food they produce is not readily available for use. The introduction of microgardening was an important intervention for gaining immediate access to plant-based foods, protecting their harvest, and ensuring a steady food supply all year long, irrespective of weather changes. To ensure food security, 129 mothers in the villages of Kakore and Nangara were provided carrot, spinach, and entura seeds (a local form of green vegetable) and trained on how to develop a microgarden. Follow-up distributions included the aforementioned seeds as well as beans and groundnuts.

Issue: Hand and Personal Hygiene
In Uganda, as in many sub-Saharan African countries, causes of death among children under 5 are respiratory infections and oral–fecal transmitted diseases like cholera, dysentery, typhoid, and hepatitis A. Hand soap washing according to the WHO and the UNICEF is an inexpensive measure to prevent life-threatening conditions. Through raising awareness of the importance of the use of soap and handwashing, especially among mothers of children under 5 years old, the women are on a path to cultivating a stronger culture of health and hygiene and eradicating preventable diseases across the villages of Bwisa-Kakore, Nangara, and Kigarama and beyond. In December 2017, the Kigezi Women's Initiative distributed soap, reusable sanitary pads, and held educational workshops with emphasis on the importance of hand hygiene and prevention of oral–fecal transmitted diseases. Latrines were outfitted with "tippy taps," a water receptacle that pours water out of a small spout, to increase frequency of handwashing

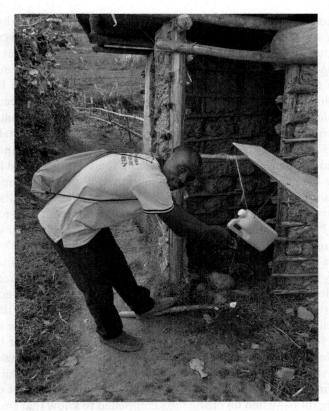

FIGURE 12.6 KIGEZI WOMEN STAFF MEMBER USING A TIPPY TAP TO WASH HANDS.

Photo Credit: Gian Luca Gamberini.

particularly after going to the latrine (see Figure 12.6). For women, especially young women attending school, experiencing their menstruation cycle can be challenging to go about daily life without the proper hygiene supplies. Women unable to conceal that they are experiencing their cycle face stigma and are even prohibited from attending school, affecting their ability to receive an education. Therefore, LCC nursing students made reusable menstruation pads and sanitary belts to provide to the young girls and women to wear while on their cycle. The menstruation pads were designed to be reusable and sewn by hand with volunteers at LCC. LCC staff and students convened volunteer organizations such as the Saint Jude's Catholic Church and the Women's Sewing Ministry along with LCC Divisional Staff to contribute and help out.

◼ Conclusion

Opportunities for service learning overseas are cost-prohibitive for many students in college and even more so for students in community colleges. At the LCC and the Career Ladder Nursing Program, students have the opportunity to participate in service-learning projects connected to organizations located abroad and engage in developing meaningful solutions that have the power of impacting the health and wellness of women and children in rural Uganda, East Africa. Providing service to others is inherent in the nursing profession; the faculty and administrators at LCC cultivate service-learning characteristics while teaching nursing students: giving, caring, and sharing. These faculty and administrators provide opportunities in local, regional, national, and global engagement in their students. Through service-learning projects, students are able to engage with real-world people and experiences that prepare them to become transformational leaders. Students learn that their time, talent, and treasure can have a life-changing impact through participating in immunization clinics, food drives, and projects abroad while completing their studies at the LCC. Students have tied fleece blankets; stuffed comfort pillows used to provide comfort support to chronically ill and disabled children; provided foot care to older adults and disabled; raised funds for local, national, and international charities; and gathered supplies for the LCC Food Pantry. Student nurses learn to give back early in their careers, which creates the framework for altruism and lifelong service to others.

Nursing leaders are cultivated through experiences and opportunities that surround everyday life; these leaders see opportunity and act on those encounters. Laura Galinsky described people who engage in social, environmental, and economic problems and are driven by a "moment of obligation"—a specific time in their lives when they felt compelled to act (Galinsky, 2013). The opportunity to serve the Kigezi Women and Children Health Initiative was the result of a chance encounter between Dean Clark and Dr. Kamayangi and Mr. Gamberini. Their commitment to making an impact and leadership resulted in the involvement of LCC's Career Ladder Nursing Program, acting, and giving of time, talent, and treasure. It takes the action of one person—a moment of obligation—when he or she feels compelled to know that small actions can make an enormous change. Nurses see and act. How will you seek opportunities to improve your community and beyond?

■ Critical Thinking Exercise

Service learning is an action-oriented approach to address an identified community need where students engage with local, regional, national, and/or global communities to improve their quality of life, solve a public health issue, or teach citizens a sustainable trade. This critical thinking exercise can be executed in any of the aforementioned locations; the intent is for the learner to identify a community, different from his or her own. If students are unable to travel abroad, they can seek organizations that provide refugee services in their area.

1. Conduct a survey (through focus groups with interpreters) of an identified diverse culture to ascertain needs related to:
   a. Food and nutrition safety
   b. Health and wellness
   c. Education
   d. Values
   e. Literacy
   f. Home living conditions

This part of the exercise incorporates observation, analysis, interpretation, and reflection.

2. List the top three to five needs and create teaching materials to address the needs highlighted in #1. Include the language of record for the community surveyed and the English translation. Be cognizant of using accurate pictures that denote the culture and using appropriate dress.

This part of the exercise incorporates evaluation, inference, explanation, problem-solving, and decision-making.

■ Discussion Questions

1. The use of ORS is a successful intervention for rehydration because of the combination of glucose and salt in an oral solution. Describe the physiology of glucose and salt absorption in the body.

2. Traveling overseas can be costly, which is a major barrier for students with limited resources to participate in global student-learning experiences. The cost of travel and immunizations can exceed $3,000. What are some innovative options for students to contribute to the work in Uganda or other developing countries without being geographically present?

3. Given the environmental and economic conditions in the Kigezi region of Uganda, what are the additional methods to provide sustainable opportunities to these women at low or no cost?

4. A moment of obligation is when a person is compelled to act at a specific time in his or her life. Think about your own *moment of obligation* that you may have personally experienced. Share your story, describe what you felt, explain why you felt compelled to act, and share what you did.

■ Resources

Association of American Colleges and Universities. (n.d.). *Global Learning VALUE Rubric*. Washington, DC: Author.

Cristo Rey Community Center (CRCC): Cares for the spiritual and social needs of individuals and families by offering services that encourage self-sufficiency and recognize the dignity of the human person. https://cristoreycommunity.org

García, A. N., & Longo, N. V. (2013). Going global: Re-framing service-learning in an interconnected world. *Journal of Higher Education Outreach and Engagement, 17*(2), 31–55.

Kigezi Women and Children Health Initiative: Committed to elevating the dignity of women in rural Uganda. http://kigeziwomen.org

The Davies Project (TDP): Provides community-based, nonmedical support for local families facing serious, long-term health challenges with a child. https://thedavies project.org

Lansing Rescue Mission: Works to meet physical and spiritual needs in Michigan's capital area. http://bearescuer.org

Ronald McDonald House of Mid-Michigan: Works to keep families close to the care their sick children need, providing comfort, support, and resources for families just steps from the hospital. https://rmhmm.org

Saint Vincent Catholic Charities' Children's Home: Cares for children and families, offering 30-day comprehensive clinical assessment or case planning, stabilization, and treatment for children aged 5 to 17. http://stvcc.org/services/childrens-home

World Food Day. (n.d.). Retrieved from http://www.fao.org/world-food-day/home/en/

■ References

Food and Agriculture Organization of the United Nations, International Fund for Agricultural Development, UNICEF, World Food Programme, & World Health Organization. (2018). *The state of food security and nutrition in the world 2018: Building climate resilience for food security and nutrition.* Rome, Italy: Food and Agriculture Organization of the United Nations.

Galinsky, L. (2013, April 15). Find your moment of obligation. *Harvard Business Review.* Retrieved from https://hbr.org/2013/04/find-your-moment-of-obligation

Longo, N. V., & Saltmarsh, J. (2011). New lines of inquiry in reframing international service learning into global service learning. In R. G. Bringle, J. A. Hatcher, & S. G. Jones (Eds.), *International service learning: Conceptual frameworks and research* (pp. 69–85). Sterling, VA: Stylus Publishing.

Nursing Process. (n.d.). *The 5 steps of the nursing process.* Retrieved from https://www.nursingprocess.org/Nursing-Process-Steps.html

Service learning. (n.d.). Retrieved from http://www.washington.edu/teaching/teaching-resources/engaging-students-in-learning/service-learning

Sousa, M., & van Dierendonck, D. J. (2017). Servant leadership and the effect of the interaction between humility, action, and hierarchical power on follower engagement. *Journal of Business Ethics, 141*(1), 13–25. doi:10.1007/s10551-015-2725-y

Uganda Bureau of Statistics and ICF International. (2012). *Uganda: Demographic and health survey 2011.* Kampala, Uganda and Calverton, MD: Authors.

World Health Organization. (n.d.). Retrieved from https://www.who.int/

World Health Organization. (2011). *Bugs, drugs & smoke: Stories from public health.* Geneva, Switzerland: WHO Press.

World Health Organization. (2017). *Diarrhoeal disease.* Retrieved from https://www.who.int/news-room/fact-sheets/detail/diarrhoeal-disease

World Health Organization and United Nations Children's Fund. (2006). *Oral rehydration salts: Production of the new ORS.* Geneva, Switzerland: Author.

13

A Health System's Interprofessional Approach to Impact Health Equity

Barbara Wadsworth, Chinwe Onyekere,
Karen Fitzpatrick Smith, Sandra Ross, Shonalie Roberts,
Sharon Larson, and Barry D. Mann

CHAPTER OBJECTIVES

- Demonstrate how a health system drove a focused effort on diversity, respect, and inclusion for all
- Explain a number of innovative interprofessional approaches to identifying disparities in care and addressing health equity
- Demonstrate a number of interprofessional programs that positively impacted patients, health professionals, and a health system

KEY CONCEPTS

Health equity	Strategic planning
Population health	Clinical environment workgroups
Student advocates	Interprofessional

KEY TERMS

Diversity	Collaboration
Respect	Health equity
Inclusion	Population health
Community	

■ Introduction

This chapter uses Main Line Health (MLH), a health system in suburban Philadelphia, as the backdrop to understanding interprofessional collaboration. As a medium size health facility, our organization wants to be "the *best* place to *give and receive* care" while serving our community through our mission, vision, and living our values. The most important values and core work include safety, quality, diversity, respect, inclusion, and health equity through identifying and decreasing disparities and affordability. These tenets drive us every day while balancing the challenges of ensuring that mission and margin are met. Through the strong, courageous leadership of our CEO, Jack Lynch, our organization is committed to and drives work focused on health equity, disparities, social determinants of health, and most importantly, creating an environment of inclusion for all. Throughout this chapter, there are numerous examples of how our health system is leading the way to create a culture of excellence for all.

Through collaborative work, partnerships, and interprofessional teams, our organization is able to positively impact our community. Described in this chapter is the organization's prioritization, commitment, and work related to the #123Equity Campaign, system-wide diversity education, the Pursuing Equity initiative of the Institute for Healthcare Improvement (IHI), an annual Healthcare Disparities Colloquium, a patient-centered Medical Student Advocate (MSA) program, a youth-centered Health Career Collaborative (HCC), as well as a Center for Population Health Research, and a hospital-owned wellness farm. We, the authors of this chapter, believe that these programs are easily replicable and could and should be implemented in other communities. These programs demonstrate that through interprofessional collaboration and partnership, small groups can have an immediate and a sustainable impact on their communities.

■ MLH Strategic Plan: Mission, Vision, and Values

While consumerism drives where patients seek care, medical science is expanding exponentially, new payment models demand cost efficiency, and the healthcare industry's economic foundation has shifted focus from volume to value. Progressive health systems across the country are prioritizing their commitment to the goals of eliminating harm, focusing on population health and tackling the challenges of disparities in care. The vision of MLH strives to emphasize these values, and by doing so, to become the partner of choice in achieving optimal health status for each member of our community.

The MLH Strategic Plan is the blueprint for achieving the goal of providing the safest and highest quality care to all who utilize our community health services. Using interprofessional collaboration with physicians, community partners, and our informed and integrated staff, we strive to meet patient needs across the broad continuum of health concerns.

One foundation of the MLH strategic plan is our community health needs assessment (CHNA), which MLH, like most other nonprofit healthcare organizations, must complete every 3 years. The CHNA identifies the critical health needs of the communities we serve, and the information, when appropriately analyzed, informs our system of significant opportunities to improve the health status and health equity of our constituents in the various zip codes in which they live.

In its most recent CHNA, MLH identified our communities' needs to (a) address chronic diseases (asthma, diabetes, and obesity) and health behaviors (smoking, diet); (b) increase access to mental health resources; (c) provide opportunities for older adult well-being; and, while considering all these, (d) provide more affordable healthcare and eliminate healthcare inequities. Focused on addressing the socioeconomic determinants of health in our most vulnerable populations, MLH has, therefore, targeted initiatives in the areas of obesity, diabetes, cardiovascular, stroke, cancer, lung disease, senior care, as well as ensuring a culture of diversity, respect, and inclusion (DRI) throughout our health system.

If the CHNA is seen as a fundamental tool in assessing needs, the Academy of Medicine's STEEEP (safe, timely, effective, efficient, equitable, and patient-centered) domains is seen as the fundamental process by which care is delivered and metric by which it is assessed. The STEEEP mantra is well recognized and ubiquitously referenced by all—from the executive team to the frontline staff. The STEEEP domains are the categories through which we share data and drive our physicians, providers, partners, and staff to deliver on the tenets of our strategic plan.

On the evidence-based foundation of the CHNA and the quality-focused process of STEEEP, our system leadership has developed, disseminated, and demanded an overlay of DRI. The specifics of the DRI movement are explicated later in this chapter. The CHNA data analysis, the STEEEP process, and the DRI culture may then be seen as a Venn diagram that represents and actualizes our mission, vision, and values.

The leadership makes the principles of DRI the center of the strategic plan to better serve the diverse patient population and achieve its commitment to its communities and patients. All leaders, managers, and supervisors have completed a 2-day learning experience on DRI demonstrating our commitment to this leadership.

The open, respectful, inclusive, and caring environment across the health system is what keeps our employees engaged. Our organization fosters an environment where employees, physicians, and volunteers work as an integrated healthcare team across our system and within our communities to provide a superior patient experience.

The MLH leadership system illustrates the MLH system's priorities and a high-level view of its operational workflow (Figure 13.1).

Embedded in this work are the frameworks for MLH Quality and Patient Safety and Performance Excellence 2020 (PE2020). The PE2020 framework serves as the uniting force—the nucleus—of all our efforts, connecting and informing performance improvement projects through system-wide standards and metrics. The operation committees measure progress toward goals through our STEEEP domains with regular organizational performance reviews, with the aim of delivering a STEEEP experience every time, everywhere, and for everyone across MLH. In FY2019, PE2020 was focused on four critical goals or pathways to excellence: eliminating harm; top decile performance; eliminating disparities in care; achieving affordability.

■ Interdisciplinary/Interprofessional Collaboration

MLH prides itself on the fact that system leadership teams represent collaborations of individuals from different professions working together in clinical environment workgroups (CEWs) to achieve best patient outcomes, which aligns our definition of the interprofessional team with the World Health Organization's (WHO's) expectations (WHO, 2010). CEWs are determined by clinical program focus (e.g., medicine, surgery, OB/GYN, emergency medicine/ICU). CEWs report to the Systems Clinical Operations (see Figure 13.2), which then reports to the Senior Executive Committee led by the system CEO. While the leadership structure is heavily matrixed with presidents, regional vice presidents (VPs), and system directors, most clinical teams have a physician and nurse leader, forming a dyadic leadership. Indeed this leadership dyad is modeled by an executive duo: a chief medical officer (CMO) and a chief nursing officer (CNO), who routinely lead dyadically.

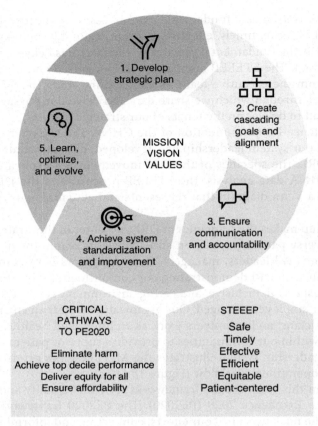

FIGURE 13.1 MAIN LINE HEALTH LEADERSHIP SYSTEM.

Source: From Main Line Health. (2016). *Community Health Needs Assessment.*

Further explanation and membership of the system and campus clinical operations, as well as the service lines and programs, are provided in the following.

SYSTEM CLINICAL OPERATIONS

System-level executive leadership provides operational oversight of system clinical operations, clinical program performance, and clinical infrastructure. Membership includes the CNO, CMO, VP for quality and patient safety, hospital presidents, system CEW leaders, and clinical infrastructure leaders. The latter include regional VPs of patient services, regional VPs of medical affairs (VPMA), and regional VPs of administration, as well as the chief medical information officer, and systems' chairs of emergency medicine, medicine, surgery, and OB/GYN.

CAMPUS CLINICAL OPERATIONS

Campus-level executive leadership provides operational oversight of campus clinical operations, clinical program performance, and clinical infrastructure. Membership

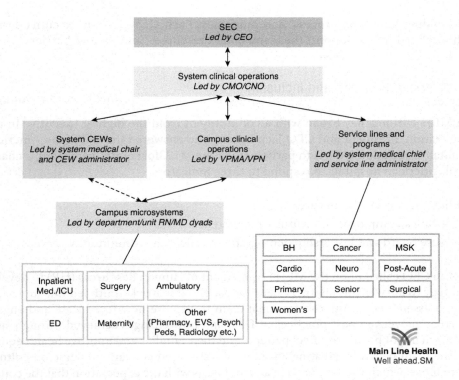

FIGURE 13.2 CLINICAL OPERATIONS: COMMITTEE REPORTING STRUCTURE.

BH, behavioral health; CEW, clinical environment workgroup; CMO, chief medical officer; CNO, chief nursing officer; EVS, Environmental Services; MSK, musculoskeletal; SEC, Senior Executive Committee; VP, vice president; VPMA, vice president of medical affairs.

Source: From Main Line Health. (2016). *Community Health Needs Assessment.*

includes the campus clinical leadership team of the regional VPMA, regional VPs of patient services, and administration/presidents working with campus clinical operation leaders and supporting contributors: patient safety specialists, case management, clinical informatics, infection prevention, and so on.

SERVICE LINES/CLINICAL PROGRAMS

Service lines/clinical programs and CEWs are commonly used organizational structures to manage the clinical environment. Service lines/clinical programs are structured around clinical conditions. The goals are to organize and design standardized care processes to treat patients across the continuum of healthcare and optimize efficiency and mitigate risk through communication and engagement. CEWs are an overlapping structure to service lines/clinical programs that manage the clinical environments that support clinical programs in their care delivery. They serve as the basis for our primary work systems.

All the clinical work is coordinated interprofessionally. Each team embraces the STEEEP domains, sets goals to accomplish the work, and maintains a dashboard of results. The clinical work is focused around standardization, evidence-based practice, and building structure, process, and outcomes. Each CEW has an executive leader with a defined role to support the team, obtain resources, and remove barriers.

▪ Diversity, Respect, and Inclusion

The MLH DRI journey began with a commitment from the highest executive in our organization, President and CEO Jack Lynch, who answered the call of the American Hospital Association (AHA) to participate in the "#123forEquity" campaign, a charge for all American hospitals to respond to three indicators:

1. Eliminate disparities in care.
2. Educate all employees on cultural competence.
3. Ensure board and leadership demographics reflect the communities served.

The CEO called upon the MLH Department of Human Resources (HR) to develop a strategy to answer this charge. Coauthor Karen Fitzpatrick Smith led this undertaking and assembled an interprofessional team to explore how to educate and engage 11,000 employees in best practices of DRI, and how changes achieved through such education might positively affect patients and their families and improve health equity.

The team began by creating an internal web-based education course on cultural competence, which was launched to all employees with the expectation that the course would be completed within 1 year. The course incorporated case studies and experiences that impacted our patients, families, and staff. This online course was a primer to more advanced, formal education and was required as part of the health system's leadership expectations.

The next step in this journey was to create an infrastructure of DRI. Consideration was given to designating a chief diversity officer (CDO). The contention of our senior vice president of Human Resources was that by assigning a single individual to the role of CDO, others in the organization, particularly the leadership, would fail to realize that accountability for DRI is the responsibility of all members of the organization. The decision was made that rather than employing a CDO, the focus would be to empower all leaders to understand, embrace, and lead with a focus on being inclusive of all, seeking out disparities, identifying opportunities for improvement, and addressing issues in their respective departments.

DRI was added as one of the core values at MLH (Figure 13.3) and a fundamental tenet of the system's strategic plan (Figure 13.4). Besides promoting these core values because "they are the right thing to do," MLH addressed and defined the true "business case": this work is fundamentally important for organizational wellness, the engagement of our employees, and the experience of our patients. The message of DRI, we concluded, needed to reach every employee.

A system-wide, interprofessional steering committee was created with specific workgroups focused on infrastructure (Information Technology [IT], Finance, & Communications), internal and external relationships (Talent Management, Business/Vendor Relationships, Education, Talent Management and Community) as well as a Disparities in Care workgroup (Figure 13.5). The Disparities in Care workgroup focuses its time on patient care, metrics, and evidence that identifies opportunities for

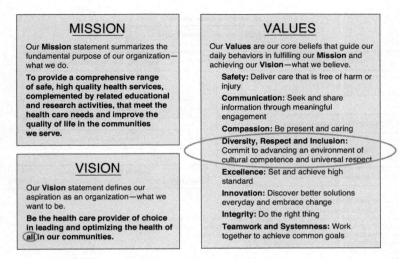

FIGURE 13.3 MLH MISSION, VISION, AND VALUES.

MLH, Main Line Health.

Source: From Main Line Health. (2016). *Community Health Needs Assessment.*

improvement in health equity. Additionally, each of the 11 MLH entities has a Diversity Council with specific charters regarding work, activities, education, and events that are shared with the entire health system.

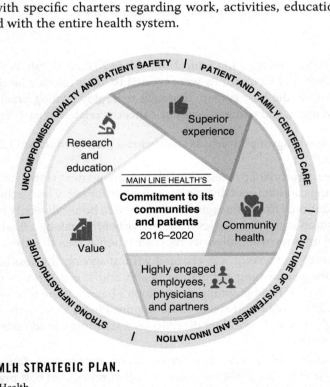

FIGURE 13.4 MLH STRATEGIC PLAN.

MLH, Main Line Health.

Source: From Main Line Health. (2016). *Community Health Needs Assessment.*

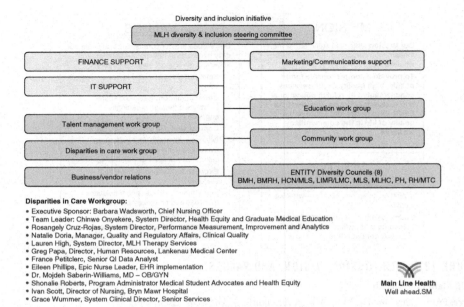

Diversity and inclusion initiative

MLH diversity & inclusion steering committee

FINANCE SUPPORT

IT SUPPORT

Talent management work group

Disparities in care work group

Business/vendor relations

Marketing/Communications support

Education work group

Community work group

ENTITY Diversity Councils (8)
BMH, BMRH, HCN/MLS, LIMR/LMC, MLS, MLHC, PH, RH/MTC

Disparities in Care Workgroup:
- Executive Sponsor: Barbara Wadsworth, Chief Nursing Officer
- Team Leader: Chinwe Onyekere, System Director, Health Equity and Graduate Medical Education
- Rosangely Cruz-Rojas, System Director, Performance Measurement, Improvement and Analytics
- Natalie Doria, Manager, Quality and Regulatory Affairs, Clinical Quality
- Lauren High, System Director, MLH Therapy Services
- Greg Papa, Director, Human Resources, Lankenau Medical Center
- France Petitclerc, Senior QI Data Analyst
- Eileen Phillips, Epic Nurse Leader, EHR implementation
- Dr. Mojdeh Saberin-Williams, MD – OB/GYN
- Shonalie Roberts, Program Administrator Medical Student Advocates and Health Equity
- Ivan Scott, Director of Nursing, Bryn Mawr Hospital
- Grace Wummer, System Clinical Director, Senior Services

Main Line Health
Well ahead.SM

FIGURE 13.5 MLH DIVERSITY, RESPECT, AND INCLUSION ORGANIZATIONAL INFRASTRUCTURE.

MLH, Main Line Health.

Source: From Main Line Health. (2016). *Community Health Needs Assessment.*

System workgroups including Education, Talent Management, Vendor Relations, Disparities in Care, and Community were created to focus on specific elements of the work and determine the best system approach to deploy leading practices, focus on process improvement, and address issues or concerns related to each group.

- The Education workgroup's role was to develop a plan to educate 11,000 employees in DRI.
- As part of the recruitment process, the Talent Management workgroup was charged with presenting candidates of diverse backgrounds for every leadership opportunity in the organization. Hiring managers are required to honor diversity in interviewing for every position at the director level and above before making a final selection. The team focused on improving minority representation across all jobs.
- The Community workgroup was charged with analyzing the results of the MLH CHNA (a survey informing population health and social services planning conducted every 3 years) and planning events/topics based on the results of the assessment (MLH, 2016). MLH entities became responsible for sharing monthly diversity messages with staff and including diversity as a standing agenda item for monthly leadership assemblies.
- The Disparities in Care group's mission was to obtain accurate data on patients to analyze disparities in care in the organization. MLH referenced best practices on how to collect patient's self-identified race, ethnicity, and language (REAL) information. This information was a critical first step in beginning to stratify data and identifying disparities in care (Health Research & Educational Trust, 2014). One key best practice

EXHIBIT 13.1 MAIN LINE HEALTH *WE ASK BECAUSE WE CARE* CAMPAIGN

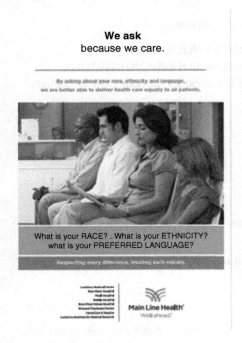

Initiatives

- **RELiable data initiative:** Created a system-wide, evidence-based approach to collect patien's race and ethnicity

- **320 Registrars trained:** Registrars trained in june2015 in evidence-based practices for collection of REL data

- **Invison updates:** Timestamp added. Alerts registrars if the questions have been asked.

- **Benchmark and targets:** Created benchmark and target goals for REL data across MLH that is tracked on the disparities in care workgroup report.

Source: From Main Line Health. (2016). *Community Health Needs Assessment.*

was to train all MLH registrars to ask questions about REAL rather than relying on assumptions. Once all of the registrars were trained, MLH implemented the Robert Wood Johnson Foundation's Aligning Forces for Quality national campaign, *We Ask Because We Care* (http://forces4quality.org/node/4185.html; see Exhibit 13.1).

- The Vendor Relations workgroup was charged with increasing the number of underrepresented minority vendors. This required MLH leaders to set expectations for increased engagement with minority vendors.

The program leader obtained a 1-year certification in Diversity Management in Healthcare. A consultant was hired to work with MLH to host employee focus groups to learn about the experiences of our staff and further understand the work environment. Special focus groups were assembled based on characteristics of staff including race/ethnicity, age, gender, sexual orientation, and position/level within the organization. The feedback from these groups identified unconscious biases and became the basis of diversity-related topics covered in a mandatory DRI education program that was facilitated as a 2-day learning experience for all leaders and a 1-day program for all other employees (see Box 13.1 for specifics).

LGBTQ Inclusive Care and Health Equity

In the context of our DRI initiative, it was both natural and mandatory to pursue the elimination of disparities among the LGBTQ community. In this arena, we first

BOX 13.1 MLH DRI Learning Experience

Creating an inclusive workplace: the DRI learning experience

- A 2-day (self-discovery) education program for MLH leaders
- A 1-day (self-discovery) education program for MLH individual contributors
- Designed internally through the MLH HR Education and Development department
- Topics include:
  - Race
  - Implicit bias
  - Generational differences
  - Power and privilege
  - LGBTQ/LGBTQIA in healthcare
  - Temperament differences

DRI, diversity, respect, and inclusion; HR, Department of Human Resources; MLH, Main Line Health.

Source: From Main Line Health. (2016). *Community Health Needs Assessment.*

worked to improve our electronic medical record (EMR) intake process to include LGBTQ-related patient data as described earlier.

System-wide, we adopted a new policy with regard to gender-neutral bathrooms. We had a choice—to either simply put up a sign with male/female identifiers or to add a statement about the importance of gender identity and expression. The MLH leadership team chose the latter in order to make a clear statement to our staff, patients, visitors, and community members about our commitment to equity in this arena. System policies were updated to incorporate inclusive language, including the language of our bereavement policy, which expanded the definition of "family." New policies were created to protect employees from being terminated based on their sexual orientation, gender identity, and gender expression. A curriculum was developed to train providers on inclusive care practices and the unique healthcare needs of the LGBTQ community.

Ultimately, our Bryn Mawr Family Practice residency program, through special training and experiential learning, became the first practice identified as LGBTQ Inclusive Care provider, a program that was officially launched in June 2018. While all of our practices provide superior care to patients, the physicians and staff in our "Inclusive Care" practices undergo additional training related to the specific needs of the LGBTQ community.

■ A Health Equity Strategy: The Framework of the IHI

After the adoption of the DRI platform mentioned earlier, MLH committed to a pursuit of health equity in all aspects of care. Partly due to its recognition for launching the DRI Initiative, MLH was selected, along with eight other health centers—diverse in size, geography, and patient populations served—to participate in the IHI's 2-year initiative, titled "Pursuing Equity." The Pursuing Equity initiative set out to break new

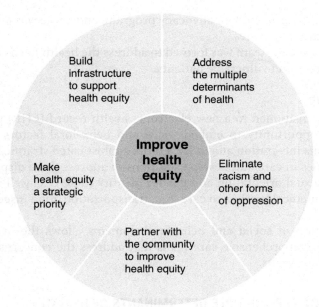

FIGURE 13.6 IHI PURSUING EQUITY FRAMEWORK.

IHI, Institute for Healthcare Improvement.

Source: Adapted from Wyatt, R., Laderman, M., Botwinick, L., Mate, K., & Whittington, J. (2016). *Achieving health equity: A guide for health care organizations* [IHI White Paper]. Cambridge, MA: Institute for Healthcare Improvement. Institute for Healthcare Improvement retains copyright. All rights reserved.

ground by explicitly addressing institutional racism and by identifying ways in which healthcare organizations can impact equity in areas such as employee wellness and social determinants of health, in addition to reducing clinical disparities at the point of care (IHI, 2017). The initiative aimed to reduce inequities in health and healthcare access, treatment, and outcomes by implementing comprehensive strategies to create and sustain equitable health systems.

Considering ourselves fortunate to participate in this wonderful initiative, we then adopted its five-pillar framework to further our work (Wyatt, 2016; see Figure 13.6).

The IHI pillars and our system responses are recorded in the following.

PILLAR 1: MAKE HEALTH EQUITY A STRATEGIC PRIORITY

Embed Core Values in the Strategic Plan

As discussed in the beginning of this chapter, through the lens of the DRI initiative (see the preceding text for details), health equity is now firmly embedded in the health system's strategic plan.

PILLAR 2: BUILD INFRASTRUCTURE THAT SUPPORTS EQUITY

Equity Appointees

A system director of "health equity" was appointed, community health services was transformed to community health and equity, a program administrator was appointed to our medical student advocacy program, and a role was created for a fellow in Health Care Disparities.

In addition, a special team was formed to address the health needs of the community's most complex and vulnerable patients.

Leveraging the EHR

In 2018, MLH transitioned to a new electronic health record (EHR) platform, Epic, and seized the opportunity to embed social and behavioral factors into the electronic record. This integration allows for a more sophisticated stratification of data to uncover disparities in care and develop solutions to address these disparities. We are now capturing sexual orientation and gender identity (SOGI) as well as information on patients' nonmedical barriers to care (e.g., transportation, food insecurity, income) within the EHR.

The integration of social and behavioral domains allows the interprofessional team to develop comprehensive care plans that address the concerns of vulnerable and high-risk populations.

PILLAR 3: IMPACT THE MULTIPLE DETERMINANTS OF HEALTH

The core ground work of equity is to understand the key underlying socioeconomic determinants of health that bring to bear inequitable outcomes. Many have colloquially expressed this by saying that one's *zip code* has a greater impact on one's life span and health quality than one's *genetic code* (Roeder, 2014). In our geographic area, the Lankenau Medical Center (LMC) serves one of the healthiest counties (Montgomery County, ranked fourth) and the unhealthiest county in Pennsylvania (Philadelphia County; County Health Rankings & Roadmaps, 2019), which presents big challenges to providing high-quality care to our patients.

In MLH's pursuit of equity, this fundamental understanding has led to several initiatives. By way of introduction, the establishment of our Healthcare Disparities Colloquium led to the creation of the MSA program, which then gave rise to the development of an Emergency Room High Utilizer Analysis. In sync with these developments, MLH created a Center for Population Health Research and leveraged the land surrounding the LMC campus to create the Delema G. Deaver Wellness Farm to promote a focus on healthy food access for our patients. These intertwining and interprofessional initiatives are described in the following.

The Annual Healthcare Disparities Colloquium

For the past 8 years, MLH has hosted an annual system-wide Health Care Disparities Colloquium intended to identify disparities in healthcare processes and practices as they might exist—unknown to us—within our system. *The interest in research into social determinants of health through the work of collaborative interprofessional teams of faculty, residents, and nurses has been significantly enhanced in our system since the opportunity to present such research projects has been afforded by the annual colloquium.* Since 2012, MLH physicians and interprofessional teams have presented more than 70 research studies focusing on a variety of important topics such as health literacy, transportation barriers to primary care, food access and nutritional health, unconscious bias, disparities in stroke rehabilitation, and the disparities in outcomes of breast cancer and mother/baby mortality in the African American population.

Medical Student Advocate Program

The uncovering of disparate outcomes revealed in the early Healthcare Disparities Colloquium stimulated the creation and development of the MLH MSA program, now in its sixth year. The MSA program uses volunteer medical students from Philadelphia College of Osteopathic Medicine to help identify nonmedical barriers to care and connect patients to established resources in order to address their needs. The MSA program provides future physicians with a unique educational opportunity that allows them to develop skills in establishing doctor–patient relationships, understand the psychosocial factors shaping health outcomes, and engage with other healthcare professionals (Onyekere, Ross, Namba, Ross, & Mann, 2016).

MSAs are embedded in patient-centered medical home (PCMH) teams at Lankenau Medical Associates (LMA), an internal medicine and subspecialty residency practice at the LMC, which serves many of our most vulnerable patients.

PCMH teams comprise nurses, social workers, nurse practitioners, health educators, physicians, and medical assistants. Via a social need survey screening tool (Exhibit 13.2), MSAs identify a range of nonmedical patient needs, including transportation, child care, food access, and utility assistance.

Patient surveys are reviewed at a PCMH team meeting dedicated specifically to addressing psychosocial needs. Subject to survey outcomes and patient willingness, patients are triaged to social workers, health educators, case managers, or an MSA for follow-up. This interprofessional team-based care incorporated into a weekly interprofessional forum provides for improved care coordination and population health management.

The value of interprofessional collaboration was demonstrated in the MSA comment, "Social work, nursing, and physicians come together and add their skill sets and their backgrounds to the patient. And that's where medicine is going." Through actively addressing real-life problems, students developed a deep appreciation of the scope of primary care in addition to a thorough understanding of the roles of other health professionals (Onyekere et al., 2016). The program has expanded to include five clinical sites, including MLH's Lankenau Medical Center Emergency Department (a level II trauma center) and Spectrum Health Services, a federally qualified health center in West Philadelphia. Since 2012, at MLH, a total of 102 MSAs have served 1,513 patients, identified 3,688 nonmedical needs, and provided 1,535 referrals to community resources for patients.

ED High Utilizer Study

Integrated with the efforts of the MSA, the LMC initiated a project to analyze the underlying nonmedical needs (e.g., transportation, utilities, food insecurity, housing) that might lead to the high frequency of ED visits by members of the vulnerable populations who have become known as "ED superutilizers." In this pilot project, an interprofessional team-based approach was used to identify and address the medical and psychosocial needs of patients who had been "treated and released" from the Lankenau Medical Center Emergency Department more than three times over a 15-month period. An interprofessional team was established including a nurse case manager, primary care physician, nurse practice manager, social worker, clinical psychologist, hospital administrator, MSA, ED nurse and nurse manager, and medical assistants (Interprofessional Education Collaborative, 2016). We referred to the team by an acronym—the **EDU** Committee (short for **EDUCATION: E.D.** High Utilizer **C**ommittee

EXHIBIT 13.2 MEDICAL STUDENT ADVOCATE PATIENT SOCIAL NEEDS SURVEY

Lankenau medical associates social needs survey

Provide the best phone number to reach you   ———————

May we leave a message at this telephone number? Yes or No

Indicate the best tiem to call: Days: **M Tu W Th F Sat Sun**

Time of day: **AM PM**

Please place sticker here

We want to care for all your needs, not just medical. This survey will help us to identify your concerns, If you check any of the items listed on this page, a member of our team will contact you.

Please circle whether the following statments are often true, sometimes true or never true for your household in *the last 12 months*.

1. **We worried whether our food would run out before we got money to buy more.**
   Often true   Sometimes true   Never true
2. **The food that we bought just didn't last and we didn't have money to get more.**
   Often true   Sometimes true   Never true

	Check if you would like help	Please explain
Affording your medications or diabetes testing supplies	▢	
Health insurance	▢	
Transportation	▢	
Home repairs/maintenance	▢	
Child care	▢	Number of children ages:
Paying rent	▢	
Paying for utilities (electic, gas, water)	▢	
Employment or career issues	▢	
Having too much time alone	▢	
Activities of daily living (e.g., cooking, dressing, bathing, eating)	▢	
Nutrition (e.g., following a special diet, eating healthy)	▢	
Quitting smoking	▢	
Loss of housing or eviction	▢	
Other problems (please describe)		

Your answers to this survey are confidential.

Source: From Main Line Health. (2016). *Community Health Needs Assessment.*

for **A**dvocacy, **T**argeted **I**ntervention, and **O**ngoing **N**urturing). The pilot program initially included six patients who had a combined total of 89 "treat and release" ED visits in 2015 and 83 in 2016. After identifying and addressing their barriers to care, those six patients' total "treat and release" visits were remarkably reduced from 89 to 6, and the decrease was maintained for an entire year.

The following is a summary of the specific histories of a few of the patients served by the program, which illustrate the benefit of a deeper dive into the background of an individual's socioeconomic determinants of health.

Patient 1

A 62-year-old male with uncontrolled psychiatric illness, uncontrolled chronic medical issues (including diabetes), and chronic abdominal pain, presented to the ED more than 25 times in 2015. He began seeing a primary care provider (PCP) in 2016, almost weekly, to help reduce his reliance on the ED. Once trust with the patient was gained, he mentioned he had no electricity or heat in his home. The EDU Committee intervened and with the coordinated efforts of the care team, heat and electricity were restored in the patient's home. In the past 3 years, the patient has had almost no ED visits.

Patient 2

A 43-year-old female with severe asthma presented to the ED more than 25 times in 2015 and 13 times in 2016. The EDU Committee (via an MSA) identified that the patient was not picking up her three inhalers from the pharmacy due to copays that she could not afford. The EDU Committee intervened and worked with pharmaceutical companies to waive her copays. Resolution of this easily remedied problem (once identified!) has ended visits related to her medication issues.

Patient 3

A 64-year-old male with complicated medical issues, including AIDS, heart failure, and gout consistently visited the ED more than once per month for exacerbations of his chronic medical illnesses. The EDU Committee discovered that the patient, who was prescribed 19 to 20 drugs, was not taking his medications because they were too complicated for the patient to understand and manage. The EDU Committee worked with a pharmacy to prepackage the patient's medications, clarify what should be taken when, and deliver them monthly. His PCP calls the pharmacy once a week to complete a medication reconciliation. Three months postintervention, the patient's CD4 count was improved and his ED visits became rare.

Patient 4

A 47-year-old male with gout and other chronic medical issues frequently presented to the ED (17 times in 2015), usually for gout flares. The EDU Committee discovered he was not making his outpatient appointments and learned he had transportation challenges to/from appointments. The committee (via social work) arranged medical transportation for the patient, virtually eliminating his use of the ED for his primary care.

The results of this pilot program demonstrate the importance of conducting a deeper dive, often into nonclinical needs of patients, in order to positively impact health outcomes and reduce recurrent ED visits. MLH is now partnering with its Medicaid-managed care payer to scale and explore ways to sustain this program.

PILLAR 4: ELIMINATE INSTITUTIONAL RACISM AND OTHER FORMS OF OPPRESSION

Everyone concedes that the fourth pillar of the IHI platform is formidable: to eliminate institutional racism is a long-held goal of centuries and not an easy task for a health system.

MLH did indeed implement a movement to effect improvement in unconscious bias and identifiable *personal racism*. This movement was described earlier in this chapter as the mandatory facilitator-led DRI Learning Experience, intended to increase employee understanding and awareness of cultural competency and the value it brings to colleagues and patients. As part of that mandatory training, a segment on power and privilege, delivered via a video and question/answer session, introduces the concept of institutional racism.

At our Healthcare Disparities Colloquium in 2017, institutional racism as a societal issue was introduced to the wide cross section of system attendees. Our explanation was based on elucidation of (a) the inequitable distribution of educational opportunities in our surrounding communities and (b) on the fact that around the country in academic centers, medical clinics for the underserved based on Medicaid insurances often serve as proxies for clinics of ethnic and/or racial minorities. Informal feedback indicated that the presentation was understood, illuminating, and enlightening.

PILLAR 5: PARTNER WITH COMMUNITY ORGANIZATIONS.

Recognizing that achieving equity cannot occur solely within the confines of its health system, MLH has been actively and successfully employing strategies to partner with community organizations. Herein are described as examples three key partnerships: (a) Greener Partners, (b) Together for West Philadelphia, and (c) the HCC and summer camps.

Greener Partners

Greener Partners, an organization working to create healthier communities through food, farms, and education, partners with MLH to develop and to maintain the Delema G. Deaver Wellness Farm at LMC (Greener Partners, n.d.).

We are fortunate that the LMC was built nearly 75 years ago on a golf course, the rolling hills of which allowed for the creation of the Delema G. Deaver Wellness Farm at the LMC. Through research at the MLH Center for Population Health (discussed in the following), we became aware that only 10% of adults in West Philadelphia eat adequate servings of fruits and vegetables daily. In this geographic region, approximately 34% are obese and about 27% have multiple chronic diseases. The vision of MLH is to use the Delema G. Deaver Wellness Farm to improve access to healthy foods for this population, reinforcing the link between nutrition and health, and to support PCPs in identifying and addressing food insecurity. The LMC collaborates with Greener Partners, whose farm experts have helped us plan and continue to support us to maintain a year-round organic, half-acre farm on our hospital campus that is now fully integrated into healthcare delivery. The goal is to harness the power of locally grown food to strengthen our community's health; see Figures 13.7 and 13.8.

For the past 4 years, the Deaver Farm has been harvesting over 30 different types of produce. The farm offers the opportunity to expose patients to the benefits of fresh fruits and vegetables at regular appointments with their PCP or with their OB/GYN provider. Pop-up "farmers' markets" (produce is offered at no cost to patients but presented in a farm stand format) and nutrition demonstrations (Figure 13.9) provide opportunities for patients to receive free produce and nutrition education (Bate, 2018).

Education generally includes a recipe provision and meal preparation demonstrations. By holding these activities in a primary care setting, MLH meets the patients where they are—without adding the additional burden of travel. It also offers an avenue for providers to open a discussion around healthy eating and nutrition. The farm offers the opportunity to address the food insecurity and chronic disease management

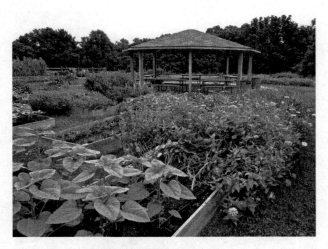

FIGURE 13.7 MLH DELEMA G. DEAVER WELLNESS FARM.

MLH, Main Line Health.

Source: From Main Line Health. (2016). *Community Health Needs Assessment.*

needs of MLH's most vulnerable patients and supports population health initiatives in demonstrating how hospitals can play a vital and important role in creating a culture of health (Bate, 2019).

Together for West Philadelphia

The LMC is located at the intersection of two designated communities, the "Main Line" suburbs of Philadelphia associated with wealth and West Philadelphia, which over recent decades has come to be seen as an under-resourced community (see Figure 13.10). The Main Line is situated in Montgomery County, which usually carries a designation as one of the healthiest among the 67 counties of Pennsylvania, whereas West Philadelphia is a component of Philadelphia County, now regarded as the 67th of 67 counties in health ranking (see Exhibit 13.3).

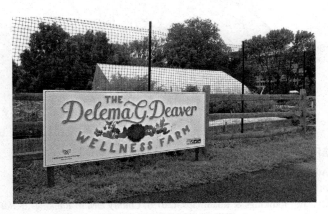

FIGURE 13.8 MLH DELEMA G. DEAVER WELLNESS FARM.

MLH, Main Line Health.

Source: From Main Line Health. (2016). *Community Health Needs Assessment.*

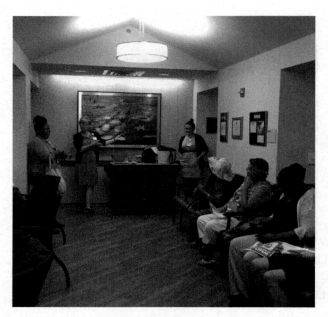

FIGURE 13.9 POP-UP FOOD DEMONSTRATION CLASS IN LANKENAU MEDICAL ASSOCIATES.

Source: From Main Line Health. (2016). *Community Health Needs Assessment.*

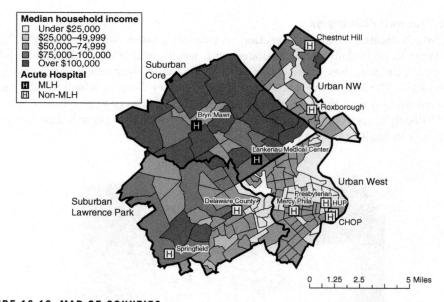

FIGURE 13.10 MAP OF COUNTIES.

*Five-Year Inflation-Adjusted Income to 2010.

Note: Census tracts with small sample sizes are non-shaded.

Source: From County Health Rankings & Roadmaps. (2019). *County Health Rankings & Roadmaps: Building a Culture of Health, County by County.* Retrieved from https://www.countyhealthrankings.org/reports/state -reports/2019-pennsylvania-report

EXHIBIT 13.3 ZIP CODE MAP

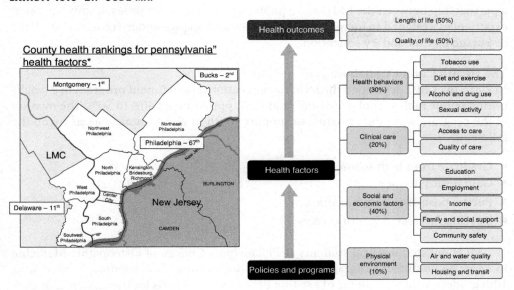

Source: From Map: Robert Wood Johnson Foundation, University of Wisconsin Population Health Institute; Ranking Scale: Reprinted with permission from University of Wisconsin Population Health Institute, County Health Rankings & Roadmaps. (2019). *County Health Rankings & Roadmaps: Building a Culture of Health, County by County.* Retrieved from https://www.countyhealthrankings.org/reports/state-reports/2019-pennsylvania-report; and Main Line Health. (2016). *Community Health Needs Assessment.*

Stimulated by the IHI Pillar 5 and supported by IHI leadership, the MLH IHI team reached out to academic and community partners in and surrounding West Philadelphia to "break silos" and to seek collaboration—based on an assumption that through collaboration, the impact of advocacy could be maximized. Together for West Philadelphia—a collaborative (and now, a 501c3 organization) within West Philadelphia among more than 20 community, public, and private sector stakeholders—was born to foster shared projects in order to maximize impact in the areas of health, education, food access, and opportunity. The board of 28 volunteers has operationalized the organization's work into six subcommittees, substantially corresponding to the socioeconomic determinants of health: (a) health equity, (b) education, (c) food justice, (d) employment, (e) housing, and (f) senior well-being. The fledgling organization is privileged to have the encouragement and support of our U.S. Congressional representative whose constituents live in the five zip codes that constitute Together for West Philadelphia's focus area.

Health Career Collaborative and Summer Camp

As known from research in the socioeconomic determinants of health, it is clear that one's level of education is a key determinant of predictable life span and health quality. Accordingly, MLH began to explore how to make a meaningful contribution in addressing inequities in education—even when the primary mission of the health system is healthcare, not early education. The discussion herein, therefore, focuses on MLH's efforts to introduce underserved and at-risk students to the broad spectrum of health careers by leveraging our relationships with local high schools and colleges. In this summary report, two ongoing efforts are described: (a) the HCC, which began as a partnership between the LMC and a public high school; (b) a series of summer camp experiences designed to increase health literacy and inspire under-resourced students to pursue postsecondary education.

The Health Career Collaborative

In 2007, the LMC developed the HCC, an educational enrichment program in a neighboring public high school whose dropout rate approximated 40% to 50%. The mission of the program was (and remains) to support youth in disadvantaged areas to: do the following:

- Graduate from high school
- Gain health literacy
- Pursue postsecondary education
- Develop interest in health careers

MLH enlisted medical students at Philadelphia College of Osteopathic Medicine to serve as volunteer program mentors and instructors. The mentors worked with 10th graders, using the theme of exciting ED cases as the basis for discussion of important social issues and health topics impacting the community. After demonstrating success, three additional medical school–high school alliances were formed in the Philadelphia area (Sidney Kimmel Medical College at Jefferson University, Drexel College of Medicine, and Lewis Katz School of Medicine at Temple University), and the four groups began working as a coalition under the direction of MLH's chief academic officer and a cohort of experts in education.

With financial support from the Aetna Foundation, 11th and 12th grade curricula were established (see Figure 13.11), and in 2014, the program was successfully replicated in Atlanta, demonstrating that the HCC could be implemented wherever there are students in need of engagement and enthusiastic mentors ready to engage them.

As a primary goal of the program was to introduce the broad spectrum of health careers to the underserved classroom, medical students found themselves partnering with nursing students and students from the allied health professions in a collegial effort to expose high school students to the processes and rewards of their own professional studies.

This interprofessional collaboration at the mentor level was expanded to include members of the various local chapters of the National Association of Health Services Executives (NAHSE), whose members represent a wide range of administrative careers in healthcare. This partnership allowed MLH to broaden exposure to the wide scope of careers in healthcare, provide additional networking and educational opportunities to motivate high school students, and enhance the interprofessional dialogue of student mentors.

In 2018, the HCC was adopted by the American College of Surgeons as a domestic offering of community volunteerism in its initiative called "Operation Giving Back," and the program has spread rapidly ever since. The program is now in 13 cities and includes partnerships between 22 medical schools and 26 high schools (Gefter et al., 2018). The HCC's easily reproducible curriculum, as well as instructional videos and materials, is accessible through the program's website (www.healthcareercollaborative.com). From this website, student mentors can review lessons, print materials, and

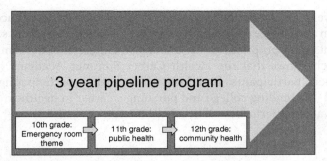

FIGURE 13.11 3-YEAR CURRICULUM OVERVIEW FOR THE AMERICAN COLLEGE OF SURGEONS HEALTH CAREER COLLABORATIVE.

Source: Used with permission from Dr. Barry D. Mann.

watch instructional videos designed to explain best program practices. The creation of web-accessible, easily reproducible curricula is intended to minimize preparation time required by volunteers and increase the potential for participation. Each site's implementation is assessed and supported by the HCC national program director who meets with faculty and medical students virtually on a regular basis.

The HCC has reached over 2,500 high school students. Postparticipation surveys (2014–2018) demonstrated that the program is well liked by students, appreciated by their teachers as a focus of student engagement, and feasible to replicate. Tenth-grade students reported the HCC helped them learn about different healthcare career options, plan for how to reach career goals, and understand how healthcare workers care for patients. Eleventh-grade participants noted the program made them aware of the importance of public health and taught them about medical conditions, self-care, and safety. A high percentage of students—86% of 10th graders and 71% of 11th graders—reported they are considering healthcare careers. Teachers noted that participants learned broadly applicable skills and that the program stimulated interest in health-related careers and created optimism about furthering education.

Health Career Summer Academy

Relationships with the high school students in the HCC resulted in the realization that there is a lack of educational opportunities for youth in under-resourced areas in the summer. It has been shown that students without satisfactory intellectual stimulation during the summer experience a phenomenon often referred to as "summer slide," which results in loss of academic gains from the prior school year. An awareness of these facts and our system achievements with the HCC program propelled us to engage academic partners in our surrounding community to jointly sponsor a series of Health Career Summer Academy camps. The primary goal of the camps is to broaden the perspectives of impressionable students by reinforcing the importance of education and demonstrating how they can apply science and health concepts to a variety of attainable careers in healthcare.

The Health Career Summer Academy began as a 1-week pilot program for middle school students of the Chester Upland School District on the campus of West Chester University and was a major success. The program has since been replicated at Rosemont College, Arcadia University, Saint Joseph's University, University of the Sciences, and Friends' Central High School. The college or school supplies the grounds and counselors (college student role models) and establishes a plan for recruiting campers, focusing on students who live in an environment in which barriers to educational success exist. The health institution and college collaborate to develop a 1-week curriculum suitable for student engagement and appropriate for the training and interests of the camp counselors.

Our research shows that the Health Career Summer Academy has a positive impact on student participants. Based on self-reporting, participating students are more interested in attending college and pursuing a career in healthcare in the future and more motivated to perform well in school (Gefter et al., 2018).

■ Conclusion

As we conclude our description of MLH's implementation of the five IHI pillars of health equity, it is appropriate that we recognize herein the insight and commitment of the LMC hospital president, Phillip D. Robinson. Phil's ideas and development of the Delema G. Deaver farm, his insights into community partnering, his embrace of health equity, and his unwavering support to those under his inspirational leadership have truly forged the way for the innovations we have detailed earlier.

Over the past decade, the MLH system has implemented initiatives that have directly impacted those we serve including our various communities of patients, employees, physicians, and partners. We have leveraged interprofessional relationships to broaden the educational horizons of our leaders, staff, and employees, and we have used interprofessional collaboration to further health equity and to narrow the chasm of inequality. With renewed optimism we suspect that other health systems are similarly capable of channeling interprofessional collaboration for success in the quest for health equity. As health organizations continue to focus on identifying and eliminating health disparities, learning from the evidence-based literature, and challenging their interprofessional teams to apply best practices, we will find ourselves moving together on a journey of improving health equity for all.

■ Critical Thinking Exercise

Respond to each of these scenarios as though you (a nurse) were a member of an interprofessional team consisting of a physician, case manager, clinical psychologist, and social worker.

Case Study A: Jessica, a 24-year-old single mother, who just delivered her second child, is your patient in a family medicine practice. Her elder child is 4 years old. Jessica is interested in returning to school to obtain an associate's degree, which could have a direct impact on the health of herself and her family. Considering your role as a member of an interprofessional team, how could you support her in this endeavor? How would you integrate the patient history and care plan that you have developed to inform how the interprofessional team works with Jessica to meet this important goal?

How would you address this problem in a clinical setting? How would you include the physical assessment and patient history into the care plan? Each student should participate in the discussion of how to best support Jessica. Then map out the plan to assist her in meeting her end goal. Should goals or milestones be included in the plan, both short term and long term? Would the team recommend monthly meetings to assess the plan and identify barriers to Jessica's success?

Case Study B: Mrs. Johnson is a 68-year-old obese diabetic with chronic congestive heart failure who has had two recent hospital admissions precipitated by fluid overload and probably lack of adherence to her diuretic regimen. Though Mrs. Johnson states she wants to lose weight and control her salt intake, she and her husband report stopping at the local McDonald's daily. When questioned about her excessive visits to McDonald's, she states that she has no access to fresh food. How can your team members, from diverse disciplines, minimize the chances of her readmission to the hospital?

Case Study C: You are asked to speak with Jason, an 87-year-old man with multiple chronic conditions who reports to you that he has not obtained his medications in over a month. How would you engage your interprofessional team to support Jason in addressing this issue?

■ Discussion Questions

1. Discuss why health equity should be a strategic priority for a health organization.
2. Discuss the advantages of taking an interprofessional approach to healthcare delivery versus working as a single provider.
3. Describe how interprofessional teams can advance health equity initiatives to improve population health.
4. Discuss how your practice of nursing can support interprofessional teamwork to address disparities of care.

■ Resources

Institute of Medicine. (2014). *Capturing social and behavioral domains and measures in electronic health records: Phase 2.* Washinton, DC: National Academies Press.

■ References

Bate, D. (2018, November 29). *Take two aspirin and a bunch of Swiss chard: Hospital farm aids to promote patient wellness.* Retrieved from https://whyy.org/articles/take-two-aspirin-and-a-bunch-of-swiss-chard-hospital-farm-aims-to-promote-patient-wellness

Bate, D. (2019, July 10). *Pennsylvania hospital grows a farm to encourage patient wellness.* Retrieved from https://www.wbur.org/hereandnow/2019/07/10/pennsylvania-hospital-farm

County Health Rankings & Roadmaps. (2019). *County Health Rankings & Roadmaps: Building a Culture of Health, County by County.* Retrieved from https://www.countyhealthrankings.org/reports/state-reports/2019-pennsylvania-report

Gefter, L., Spahr, J., Gruber, J., Ross, S., Watson, L., & Mann, B. (2018). Addressing health disparities with school-based outreach: The Health Career Academy Program. *Journal of Racial and Ethnic Health Disparities, 5*(4), 700–711. doi:10.1007/s40616-017-0414-5

Greener Partners. (n.d.). Get to know all *about us.* Retrieved from https://greenerpartners.org/about-us-2

Health Research & Educational Trust. (2014). *A framework for stratifying race, ethnicity and language data.* Chicago, IL: Author. Retrieved from http://www.hpoe.org/Reports-HPOE/REAL-data-FINAL.pdf

Institute for Healthcare Improvement. (2017, April). *Initiatives: Pursuing equity.* Retrieved from http://www.ihi.org/Engage/Initiatives/Pursuing-Equity/Pages/default.aspx

Institute of Medicine. (2014). *Capturing social and behavioral domains and measures in electronic health records: Phase 2.* Washington, DC: The National Academies Press.

Interprofessional Education Collaborative. (2016). *Core competencies for interprofessional collaborative practice: 2016 update.* Washington, DC: Author. Retrieved from https://hsc.unm.edu/ipe/resources/ipec-2016-core-competencies.pdf

Main Line Health. (2016). *Community Health Needs Assessment.* Retrieved from https://www.mainlinehealth.org/about/community-health-needs-assessment/archive

Onyekere, C., Ross, S., Namba, A., Ross, J., & Mann, B. D. (2016). Medical student volunteerism addresses patients' social needs. *Ochsner Journal, 16*(1), 45–49. Retrieved from https://www.ncbi.nlm.nih.gov/pmc/articles/PMC4795500

Roeder, A. (2014, August 4). *Zip code better predictor of health than genetic code.* Retrieved from https://www.hsph.harvard.edu/news/features/zip-code-better-predictor-of-health-than-genetic-code

World Health Organization. (2010). *Framework for action on interprofessional education & collaborative practice.* Geneva, Switzerland: Author.

Wyatt, R, Laderman, M., Botwinick, L., Mate, K., & Whittington, J. (2016). *Achieving health equity: A guide for health care organizations* [IHI White Paper]. Cambridge, MA: Institute for Healthcare Improvement.

14 The Critical Discussion of Race and Racism Toward Achieving Equity in Health Policy

Mia Keeys

CHAPTER OBJECTIVES

- ⊙ To describe pivotal Congressional policies, judicial rulings, and social events that have significantly altered the health of U.S. communities of color; of gender, religious, sexual identity, and language minorities; as well as differently abled bodied persons.

- ⊙ To evaluate the economic and workforce costs associated with avoidable, yet ongoing health inequities as a consequence of federal policies.

- ⊙ To explore the new frontier of health inequities in augmented intelligence, precision medicine, and advanced technological use in healthcare decision-making.

■ Introduction

Disparities in health are not only alarming but also taxing on individual health outcomes, the American public, and are a cost burden to the nation's entire healthcare system.

Disparate health outcomes are also long-standing and determine the ways in which health policies are presently designed. This chapter presents a robust conversation on the historical and present ways in which race and its operationalization—racism—play out in health systems and heighten inequities. The chapter unpacks how race and racism have been embedded into our social and health institutions and are guiding national policies, namely policies that ultimately determine the differential states of wellness of people living in the United States.

■ SECTION I: Social Darkness and Disruption: The Birth of a Raced Nation

RACE AS SOCIAL DARKNESS

What *Is* Race?

More specifically, what does it mean to *be raced*? More than an affixed skin color attributed to genetics, race is one of our nation's most hardy social processes of "othering," which plays out within sociocultural situations, within our oldest social institutions, and is entrenched within the policies and practices that govern those social bodies. As a prelude to a more robust conversation on the historical ways in which race and its operationalization, racism, have been instituted into our country and are guiding national policies—especially policies that ultimately determine the equitable wellness of people living in the United States—we must revisit a time before our country was born.

Throughout this chapter, I specifically aim to demonstrate that while the physical idea of race may vary among social contexts, racial formation (Omi & Winant, 1994) is an invariant feature and residual of a violent colonial legacy, which contributes to the persistence of present-day disparate health outcomes among postcolonial communities across the world. Yet race is uniquely expressed in the U.S. context. Herein, I also analyze how community-wide experiences of violence impact the health of peoples who—as a result of persistent poor health—have *become raced*, have become "othered," in terms of a subpar lived experience or cultural legacy of trauma, but also of resistance, an effect I will hereafter refer to as "Social Darkness." Social Darkness is the result of a series of mechanisms that structures of colonialism and imperialism have used to arbitrarily yet considerably stratify populations and inculcate biased social institutions. For example, religion, gender, miscegenation, notions of manifest destiny, apartheid, Jim Crow segregation, and race have all been used, in their verb tenses, by colonial powers to elevate one sector of a community, while simultaneously caste-*ing*, other-*ing*, or darken-*ing* other peoples of the same community. Social Darkness is a result of, and also a social tool, that has historically marred and marginalized populations. It is known by a community's endured legacy of violence rooted in vestiges of peculiar institutions, including colonialism, slavery, apartheid, and postcolonialism, illuminating an historical path on which communities are marked by generations of colonial and imperialistic power aggressions—and are thus darkened by rites of social stratification. Even as the United States has instituted polices in recognition and toward the preservation of some of its most vulnerable citizens, vast health disparities persist among certain communities. Indeed, the words of Dr. Harriet Washington ring true into the present day: "the overarching presence of two Americas, one healthy and White and the other filled with sick, disaffected people of color, has haunted our discussions" (2006, p. 12). The vestiges of colonial violence remain pronounced and darken the lives of those whom policy redresses are purported to protect. In this way, where one finds the most ill communities, one has located the phenomenon of Social Darkness. The idea of race is largely recognized in these places of visibly heterogeneous racial makeup. By expanding race as a health disparity experience, rather than merely a physical attribute, health political decision makers have the opportunity to propose health measures that may transform racially patterned public health travesties in places where racial health disparities are not formally recognized nor addressed. The United States comprises over 325 million people (U.S. Census Bureau, 2018) with more than 435 Congressional districts across vastly different geographies and terrains. But, deeper than this, just how do we differ, what are the myriad geneses of our differences, and why is acknowledging these differences a crucial part of our current social existence and our nation's success? I address these and other critical concerns throughout this chapter.

The beginning of this chapter focuses predominantly on the manifestation of Social Darkness, consequent of the violent victimizing of First Peoples in the Western Hemisphere to present-day peoples of color, each of whom has endured centuries of colonial violence under the auspices of differential sociopolitical policies. While one can elect to evaluate the outcomes of these policies on the communities, we exclusively focus on the effects of these policies as evidenced by the persistence of disparate racial health statuses. This chapter yields insight into factors that expand mainstream understanding of how race, and more insidiously, racism, operates in contemporary society, and the deleterious health effects of ignoring the impact of racial history on federal policy design. Finally, the chapter ends with a brief discussion of policy areas that, if addressed with a fuller understanding of the operationalization of race—racism—would go far to address national racial health disparities.

RACE AS DISRUPTION

Differences, or disparities, oftentimes are born out of phenomenological disruptions. Disruptions are sudden and shocking in their subsequent societal impact, like the tremor of an earthquake or the spill of a massive oil tanker into open waters. Otherwise, disruptions can be gradual, yet no less socially consequential, like climate change, the construction of a market complex in a gentrifying neighborhood, or the spread of avian flu. Disruptions interrupt the planned or expected routines of life, rearranging social networks and thwarting the trajectory of sociohistorical events. We often retrospectively assign negative or positive valence to these unanticipated social events, which may be evaluated from familial, community, state, national, international, and systematic perspectives.

Whether theorized as an innovation or a deviation, disruptions serve "both as a chronicle of the past (this has happened) and as a model for the future (it will keep happening)" (Lepore, 2014, p. 7). Thus, a disruption is always rooted in history, and it moves in a nonlinear course toward the future. The nuclear nature of disruption is exponentiation. It always changes the course of a people, their expression of their cultural practices, and often their life chances, in one massive way or another, for generations upon generations.

In a modern American social context, what remnants of past disruptions linger in full, exaggerated force today? One example might be the creation and imprint of race, which has metastasized in form to permeate all social institutions in the United States, including our premier executive, judicial, and legislative bodies. One could think of the process of race-ing, of Social Darkening, as disruption and as a causal mechanism implicating the health, resources, religious rites, and economic situation of a community—whether the processes are deleterious or beneficial. Once a society has become othered along the lines of race, "racialization develops a life of its own" (Bonilla-Silva, 1997, p. 475).

There is no biological distinction between human beings along racial lines. Perhaps there is no other work that thoroughly breaks through the falsehood of biological determinism than Stephen J. Gould in his book, *The Mismeasure of Man*, the purpose of which is to "demonstrate both the scientific weaknesses and political contexts of determinist arguments" (Gould, 1980, p. 53). *Biological determinism* contends, "differences between human groups . . . arise from inherited, inborn distinctions and that society, in this sense, is an accurate reflection of biology" (Gould, 1980, p. 52). Biological determinism considers the current overall social status of a population as a proxy for where they should and ought to be in society. In essence, science was applied to justify the ascription of social worth to groups by ostensibly locating their inherent intelligence as a single quantity, nonbiased measure (Washington, 2006). Being that the science of craniometry is based on the belief that intelligence is located in the head (Gould, 1980), scientists of old, such as Samuel Morton, would use biological justifications to bolster essentially racially prejudiced social agendas. This use of the scientific argument to justify differential treatment and social reward is the foundation of "reification" and "racial ranking," what Gould argues are the two major fallacies of biological determinism (Gould, 1980). Gould exposes the fallacy of biological determinism as well as the deep cultural damage that the proponents of the theory perpetuated. For instance, Gould uses the natural scientist Samuel Morton's seminal work, the *Crania Americana,* to expose the prejudicial science behind Morton's craniometric arguments of racial ranking. Morton's main argument was that Native Americans and Blacks ranked lower on the scale of intelligence, as "proven" by smaller brain capacity and thus stunted intellectual development. To refute his claims, thereby defending his own position that Morton erred enormously, Gould points out several discrepancies in Morton's methodology. Foremost, as Gould notes, Morton's sample over-represents Native persons who are corporeally smaller—and thus have smaller heads—than not only other Native groups but also those of European descent, the effect of which skewed the mean of Native American skulls to the left. According to Gould, Morton also failed to consistently admit skulls from Caucasian persons who were also of smaller stature, and thus head size, in his sample, as the effect would have skewed the group mean similar to that of Native persons. Moreover, Gould uncovers that Morton did not explain confounding effects of sex, in addition to body size, on the size of a skull. Each of these methodological errors—or omissions—is not in the least insignificant, as Morton's "a priori conviction about racial ranking [was] so powerful that it directed his tabulations along pre-established lines" (Gould, 1980, p. 101). Gould's critique and deeper analysis does not end with 19th century scientists; he takes task with more recent work, as well. Toward the end of his tome, Gould expounds on the idea of Murray and Herrnstein's *The Bell Curve* (1994) as nothing short of the social philosophical expression of biological determinism, which has had—and continues to have—dire sociopolitical impact. He goes on to concisely state, "prior prejudice, not copious numerical documentation, dictates conclusions" (Gould, 1980, p. 112) with respect to beliefs about entire communities.

In spite of well-evidenced conclusions that races are not significantly biologically different at the onset, in the U.S. context, the phenotypically contended notion of race is one that is largely uncontested since "skin color or parentage often makes one's publicly constructed race inescapable" (Haney-Lopez, 1996, p. 41), and the historical deconstruction of the race as a social advent an improbable or infrequent scholastic venture. As demonstrated earlier, in the not too distant past, the idea of "biological race" was the dominant definition under which natural and social scientists operated. That is, "there exist natural, physical divisions among humans that are hereditary, reflected in morphology, and roughly but correctly captured by terms like Black, White, and Asian" (Haney-Lopez, 1996, p. 6). Currently, while disciplinary schisms prevail with respect to the most accurate definition, many social scientists agree that race is an entity inextricably rooted at the historical intersections of European social, political, and economic domination, the active contestation, and yet the eventual subjugation, of original peoples. Sociologist Eduardo Bonilla-Silva contends as much, saying, "historically, the classification of a people in racial terms has been a highly political act associated with practices such as conquest and colonization, enslavement, peonage, indentured servitude" (Bonilla-Silva, 1997, p. 471). As Howard Winant, another sociologist, notes, the meaning of race has shifted over social contexts, from the imperialistic, colonial sense, to biologically based justifications, to the modern ideation of it being a social construction with political consequences. Humans—conquerors, imperialists, disruptors—are the architects of race, rather than abstract forces of society (Haney-Lopez, 1996). Man reifies race by designing racial formation systems in what Omi and Winant deem as, "the socio-historical processes by which racial categories are created, inhabited, transformed, and destroyed" (2002; p. 124) in societies structured in dominance and subjugation, governed by laws that serve as "a system of control or coercion" (Haney-Lopez, 1996, p. 81).

With these main points in mind, uncovering the specific historical forces as the onsets of race as social disruption cannot be fully addressed without historical narrative. Thus, let us take a moment to interrogate the disruptive, nascent formation of race operationalized in the Western Hemisphere as early as 15th-century European colonialism. This narrative cannot be fully explained in a linear fashion as numerous factors collided to impact the construction of Social Darkening, of race-ing during this period. "Construction" here refers to "complex social processes wherein race initially emerged as a socially disruptive process of subjugating an entire community" (Haney-Lopez, 1996).

Moreover, just as there was the onset of mass social *disruption* in the form of subjugation, there was a social *disruptor*, an antagonist (or protagonist, depending on your orientation), Christopher Columbus, who is arguably primarily responsible for the birth of race in the Americas, and thus, throughout the world. Relying on the historical narrative form of various populations as a unit of analysis—Native Americans, peoples of African descent in the Americas, and even previously "non-White" European Americans—one can initially broach these questions through a sociohistorical interrogation of Christopher Columbus's trans-Atlantic journey, the enormity of which is rarely considered in social scientific or policy narrative spaces as the dominating onset of Western subjugation along racial lines. While not intended to be exhaustive, this analysis of the Columbus–Native domination–subjugation matrix offers a firm foundation for an important conversation, and a nascent depiction of subjugation that bred and then reproduced Social Darkening, which birthed race and, eventually, racial inequities expressed as health disparities between Whites and Socially Darkened communities throughout the United States.

CHRISTOPHER COLUMBUS, THE PATRIARCH OF RACE

Christopher Columbus did not intend to come across a Caribbean isle, to mistakenly deem the indigenous Arawak people of the said isle as "los indios" (meaning, "dark people"), nor was he ever under the impression that his discovery was a breakthrough of any great magnitude (Axtell, 1988). Irrespective of his mistakes, misperceptions, and disappointments, the consequences of his "New World" discovery are embedded within the revered framework of America's social institutions. Celebratory commissions—federal holidays, esteemed statues, or highly valued artworks depicting a noble-standing Columbus with Native peoples, genuflecting and gracious, in the name of his legacy—are national strongholds attesting to the multicenturial endurance of his feats. John Vanderlyn's painting, "Landing of Columbus at the Island of Guanahani," on the ceiling of the Capitol Rotunda in the District of Columbia is one such work. One would also be remiss if overlooking the large marble statue of Columbus outside the east wing of the Capitol building. The adjectival form of his name—Columbian—has been used as a proxy connoting support of the gallant and civic ideals, which the United States espouses (Schlereth, 1992). Even impressionable young children in America come to know the name of Columbus. Childhood rhymes sang in elementary classrooms pay homage to the Genoese commoner who, after several advances, finally convinced King Ferdinand and Queen Isabella of Spain to sponsor his quest to the East through the

West in the late summer of 1492 (Schlereth, 1992). Earlier that year, the Spanish army defeated the Muslim Moors at Granada, albeit sustaining heavy casualties and loss of resources. Thus, it became imperative that monarchs find other ways to restore the diminished coffers of the Spanish kingdom. Columbus's appeal to venture across the sea in search of savory spices and, especially gold, connoted a lucrative business deal; after two previous rejections, their majesties acquiesced to granting their sponsorship of Columbus's intrepid voyage.

By extension, they also agreed to the economic, religious, physical, ecological, cultural disruption and absolute devastation of an entire population.

On August 3, 1492, Columbus steered a three-ship fleet across the Atlantic Ocean (Heat-Moon, 2002). As captain of the first ship, the *Santa Maria*, he led the way toward what he thought was an innovative, yet straightforward western sea route to the Indies, as the *Nina* and the *Pinta* followed sail. While his sense of geography was dubious and his subsequent proclamations of having reached the Indies were not manifest, Columbus was no nautical novice. For several years prior to this journey, Columbus was a seafaring slave trader on African coasts under the auspices of the Portuguese crown (Tinker & Freeland, 2008). At a time when cartographers were truly beginning to accept the round-world hypothesis, the "Admiral of the Ocean Sea" (Axtell, 1988) would eventually traverse the Atlantic Ocean to the landmass of Hispaniola (today Haiti and the Dominican Republic) for a total of four voyages in the name of the Spanish monarchy between 1492 and 1506. After approximately 2 months at sea, and directly before his first landing, Columbus claimed to have spotted land at daybreak. Archived accounts from his *Diario de a Bordo*—the ship's outboard log—would later confirm Columbus's initial thoughts regarding the beneficial prospects of his landing (Heat-Moon, 2002). Undoubtedly, economics motivated his venture. "I was very attentive and worked hard to know if there was any gold," Columbus claimed (as cited in Todorov, 1999, p. 8). His high prayers echoed his golden hopes, and his avarice he justified with religious and political dogma: "Our Lord in his goodness guide me that I may find this gold . . . so that their Highnesses might be pleased and might thus judge this situation on the basis of a number of large stones filled with gold" (as cited in Todorov, 1999).

Understanding the success of the social disruptor, Columbus, is a factor dependent on thoroughly understanding Columbus, the man, pious and ambitious or, ambitious through his piety, beyond his avarice. In fact, his last expression before sailing from Europe was an act of absolution of his sins prior to embarking on his journey across the ocean. On those shores of embankment, Columbus readied himself for a jihad, a quest that necessitated conquering whatever—and whomever—lay before him in the name of religion and royalty. This was the first frontier of social disruption and subjugation.

While many accounts, including some of Columbus's own aforementioned, attest to his rapacious appetite for gold and personal riches as the main impetus behind such a large undertaking, it was his conviction and belief in a God-granted inheritance, and an allegiance and obligation to the Spanish crown, which winded his sails into unchartered territory. Here, spiritual as well as material conquests were one in the same justification to Columbus, a disposition Least and Heat-Moon explain well:

> Columbus was in no way averse to financial compensation for his long efforts, but that was not the primary goal pushing him. For him, his compelling geographical concept, one in his mind underwritten by a deity, was the force that would drive the three ships on toward opening new riches to Europe. (as cited in Todorov, 1999, p. 40)

Overpowering Native peoples to advance his visions of golden grandeur came down to one word: colonialism.

Colonialism necessitated subjugation—a subjugation that needed to be rationalized by an uncontested sacrament, such as religion, and then operationalized by a stratifying social system, such as labor. Columbus had this to say about subjugating Natives: "How easy it would be to convert these people—and to make them work for us" (Morrison, 1942, p. 67); "they are fit to be ruled" (Todorov, 1999, p. 46), he would continue. The social disruptor would then implement a system of award and punishment to ensure the success of his mission. Naming the land San Salvador, or "Holy Savior," the Admiral harshly punished those Natives unwilling to convert to Christianity, granting converts with life, but not necessarily unbridled freedoms. Thus sprung forth a subjugated Native populace stratified by social labels "Christian" or "heathen"; keep in mind that neither distinction could be easily delineated on sight, as religious belief was not necessarily marked in this society by, say, a nun's modesty head covering or a monk's humble robes. This subjugation system was based on ethereal, internal conditions, like the status of one's soul, rather than on an irrefutable external mark, like one's skin complexion. It was bound to be refined by something more tangible, something that could more easily be manipulated as an othering mechanism. By naming the subjugated "los indios"—the "dark people"—Columbus cast the racialized net across the community, invented the racial category, "Indian," and fastened racial social meaning to the identity of a newly subjugated, newly Darkened, newly racialized peoples (Bonilla-Silva, 1997), simultaneously protecting his as well as "the interests of powerful actors in the social system" (Bonilla-Silva, 1997, p. 473).

Race is a volatile and dynamic construct. "The meaning of race is defined and contested throughout society, in both collective action and personal practice. In the process, racial categories themselves are formed, transformed, destroyed, and reformed," claim Omi and Winant (1994, p. 61). The abrupt rate at which racial systems developed, and thereby the racialization of a people—who were not previously considered a race—demonstrates the malleability of the social construct. The transformation of Native peoples to a race manifested as a result of interlocking social interruptions. This process of race by subjugation occurred in the context of religious, economic, physical, and cultural domination, generating religious, economic, physical, and cultural elites among the Europeans and subjects among Native people. Within these contexts, Columbus would govern the "dark people" (here we can already ascertain the burgeoning racial undertones of a subjugated class) with a voracious crusader's mission and an unremitting arm. Consequently,

> Myriad disparate Native American cultures were collapsed into a single monotonous racial 'Indian' by the Anglo emphasis on morphological difference as a trope for social and power inequalities. (Haney-Lopez, 1996, p. 54)

Now, in the words of Haney-Lopez, "a race, once created, does not take on a life of its own independent from the surge of social forces" (1996, p. 38). Force is exactly what Columbus would use to uphold this racialized social structure in San Salvador. To support his end, on his second trans-Atlantic voyage from Europe to Hispaniola, Columbus returned with a cavalry greater than 1,000 men and vicious dogs. Columbus once wrote that, "against the Indians, one dog is the equal of ten men" and proclaimed that his desire "was to pass by no single island without taking possession of it" (as cited in

Bigelow & Peterson, 1998, p. 101). Tooled with these instruments of force—religious and racial stratification and dogs—he then established the oldest Spanish settlement on the isle, Isabella, in 1494. In the following year, Columbus enforced a law of tribute—known as the *encomienda*—whereby Spanish soldiers subjected Native men and women, aged 14 years and older, to mine gold and surrender their ore to the Spanish governorship. In his book on the subject, Lesley Byrd Simpson (1929) contends that the *encomienda* legally legitimated the subjugation of the Native peoples at the behest of the European colonizers. "The Spaniards could not have lived without the forced labor of the Indians," Simpson continues (1929, pp. 8–9). Forced religious conversion operated right alongside forced labor under the *encomienda*. In addition to the consequences associated with the offense of maintaining an unchristian lifestyle, those who did not acquiesce to this tribute, or procure sufficient amounts of gold, were also subject to severe punishment, including the chopping off of their hands. Notable Spanish historian, Bartolome de Las Casas, a clergyman who resided on the island with Columbus and his party, recounted his observations of such heinous acts:

> Others, and all those that they desired to let live, they would cut off both their hands but leave them hanging by the skin, and they would say to them: "Go, and take these letters," which was to say, carry the news to the people who have hidden themselves in the mountains and the wilderness. (2003)

In fact, so moved and bothered by the odious treatment that the Native peoples endured at the hands of the colonial power enforcers, Las Casas would eventually advocate for a foreign labor base to emigrate to Hispaniola as relief to the Arawaks. His advocacy within the social context of European economic development in the Americas, it would turn out, would also eventually implicate the institutionalization of chattel slavery in the Americas (Franklin & Moss, 2001).

Let us digress a bit.

In the beginning of the land to become known as the Americas was the community. What followed—a socially disruptive ideology subjugation based on religiosity, race-ing, and labor wherein the said community became Socially Darkened—swept through the community, like a blinding storm. Yet, prior to the arrival and occupation of the European colonizers, the Native peoples in the Americas

> Cultivated corn, tubers, cassava, and peppers; they fished and caught crabs; they spun and wove cotton, made decorated pottery, and fashioned ornaments of shell and bone. Their frame houses had palm-thatch roofs, and they were expert in moving large dugout canoes over the open sea . . . most significantly, once they understood the Spanish plans, they were not willing to become servants and certainly not slaves. (Heat-Moon, 2002, pp. 35–36)

Not only were the Native peoples rich in resources—as demonstrated earlier—but also sophisticated and sustained in their own technologies, namely having to do with irrigation of their crops.

> The economy was based on a form of *conuco* agriculture. Fields were arranged in mounds called *conucos* three feet high, and at times nine feet in circumference in order to improve drainage, slow the process of erosion, and allow the storage of manure tubers in the ground. (Tinker & Freeland, 2008, p. 47)

Yet the disruptive onset of the *encomienda* changed the flow of this natural abundance. The Europeans were largely unschooled in complex agricultural practices (Tinker & Freeland, 2008). Consequently, ecological devastation through the deforestation of Native forests and the European insistence of overplanting cash crops, including sugar cane and cotton, led to topsoil erosion of the once very fertile lands; this destruction lasts into the present day, exacerbated by climate change and natural disasters (McClintock, 2003). Destruction of the land led the way to declines in health of the Native peoples, who, after losing their primary source of subsistence, became much more susceptible to European defeat through disease. Specifically,

> By 1519, the island had experienced the worst and most devastating wave yet of epidemic disease (smallpox), and the Crown had begun authorizing the importation of massive numbers of enslaved Indians to supplement the island's dwindling active labor supply. (Guitar, 1997, p. 9)

This is the first instance of significant differential health outcomes among the residents of Hispaniola, wherein the greatest disease burden befell that Socially Darkened population.

Individual incident of suffering is one phenomenon to behold; it is a wholly different marvel when subjugation becomes systematic. *Encomienda* was the systematized structure that solidified a relationship based on labor and social hierarchy. By superimposing a socioeconomic system based on domination by one group and subjugation of another, a racial order was the accompanying discord.

Even more egregious, the disruptive onset of European subjugation of Native peoples in the Americas was overwhelming and multifaceted, approaching nothing short of genocide. There is evidence that as early as 1496, Native population numbers were so terribly decimated through deaths associated with European-forced laboring conditions that the colonizing regime was forced to find replacement workers in the gold mines and crop fields. In the specific case of the Native American peoples overtaken by the rogues of Columbus, physical, cultural, territorial, economic, and social annihilation were undeniable effects of the late 15th century disruptive encounters between European powers and Native American victims. Historians Sherburne Cook and Woodrow Borah (1971) maintain that Native population numbers hovered between 7 and 8 million prior to the arrival of Columbus. By the mid-16th century, however, the Native population under Spanish subjugation was all but depleted. Dobyns estimated the population of American Natives to have declined at depopulation rates of 1/20 or 1/25 (at exponential declines) before having reached nadir, the lowest point just before repopulation, or no recovery whatsoever. Dobyns asserts, "the idea that social scientists hold of size of the aboriginal population of the Americas directly affects their interpretations of New World civilizations and cultures" (1966, p. 395).

In addition to religious, economic, labor, and ecological warfare, the smallpox epidemic demonstrates that "the European conquest of the American Indians was initially a medical conquest, one that paved the way for the more well-known and glorified military conquests and colonization" (Thornton, 1987, p. 47). Thus, "by eliminating earlier populations of American Indians, the Old World diseases prepared the way for European military conquest and full colonization" (p. 62).

Native laborers did not succumb passively, however. Many would seek solace from the oppressive conditions of their labor by escaping into their shrouded lands (Karras

& McNeill, 1992)—which were still largely unknown spaces to the terrain-ignorant European—through collective and organized revolts against the European or even through self-sacrifice and suicide. Scholars contend that "the *encomienda* [emphasis added], at least in the first fifty years of its existence, was looked upon by its beneficiaries as a subterfuge for slavery" (Simpson, 1929, p. xiii). However, due to the rapidity of Native deaths by disease and as a result of many actively desisting from laborious conditions, the Spanish soon found that Natives were not "good" slaves. In turning to the African continent for reprieve, "racialized social orders emerged after the imperialist expansion of Europe to the New World and Africa" (Bonilla-Silva, 1997, p. 473).

European disruption was a veritable decimation of the economics, religious rites, physical well-being, ecology, culture, and health of 15th-century Native life in the Americas. It profited European nations along these same lines by making way for a more staid, persistently lucrative system of subjugation well after Columbus was dead and gone; yet his legacy lingered in the sociopolitical practices of later European conquests. In their classic tome, historians John Hope Franklin and Alfred A. Moss Jr. noted,

> No where was Indian slavery profitable. Even it if had been, it would have been insufficient for the robust agricultural life that the European colonies were fostering in the seventeenth century. (2001, p. 38)

With Native population numbers almost nil approaching the 16th century, European colonizers turned to the African continent to replenish their labor base in gold mines, on plantations, and on ranches, making way for an inexhaustible labor network between European colonizing nations and the exploited lands and peoples of the Americas and of Africa. And so, the way of Native-based subjugation for labor began to shift toward African-based chattel slavery. This combination of disruptions exacerbated conditions in which subjugation based on something more tangible than religion—skin color— could then flourish. By the early 16th century, the word "naboria"—not "Negro," "nigger," or "Black"—was the term synonymous with "slave"; it gained traction with reference to the Native laborers to the Spanish crown in the New World. In 1512, the well-endowed *encomenderos* (European plantation owners) of Hispaniola commandeered hundreds of naborias during this time. Just 7 years later, 4,000 "bozales," or African slaves, captured at the behest of the Spanish crown, arrived to work on the sugarcane plantations alongside the naborias, beginning the onset of the large-scale and systematic overlapping enslavement of the Native Indians and Africans enslaved in the Americas, which became "the first commercial license for the bulk importation of *bozales*, slaves direct from Africa, to the Indies" (Guitar, 1997, p. 13). Thus,

> Spanish . . . conquerors enslaved Indians as well as Africans in Central and South America during the sixteenth century, but by the seventeenth century almost all slaves in the Americas were of African origin . . . in 1500 Africans and persons of African descent were a clear minority of the world's slave population, but that by 1700, Africans and persons of African descent had become the majority of the world's slave population. (Karras & McNeill, 1992, pp. 46–47)

In these ways, the *encomienda* was the seed of religious and labor-based subjugation in the Americas between Europeans and Native peoples, paving the way for the centuries-long, institutionalized subjugation of Africans and African-descendant peoples in the Americas. Yet, *encomienda* differed in some ways from the protocols by which chattel slavery would eventually come to be characterized. For instance, Native laborers were not legal property of the Spanish, and their terms of contractual agreement were drawn to specify the expected labor, in exchange for "one-and-a-half gold pesos annually," or the equivalent of what could earn laborers one linen outfit per year. Native laborers also worked during a specified season, called the "*demora*," which arguably lasted from between 5 and 9 months, returning to their home villages following the seasonal end of their tributary contract.

Social disruption theory would posit Columbus's failure-cum-success in terms of profitably enterprising a market approach to labor that had not before been broached with such voracity and violence. From epidemiological and demographic perspectives, in terms of years of life lost due to Columbus's impact on the Native American population in the early days of Hispaniola, by the end of his rule, "seven and a half million human beings were subjected to murder, torture, oppression, slavery, and cultural dislocation" (Tinker & Freeland, 2008, p. 36).

The Governor Columbus of Isabella ruled with a gold-plated fist for 8 years before the Spanish crown extradited him to Spain, arrested him for misconduct, and stripped him of his titles and wealth. In spite of the monarchy's efforts to quell the actions of their sponsored Columbus, the social disruption of race by subjugation had already been irrevocably set, and had ballooned beyond Columbus, making more accessible the way for colonizers other than the Spanish to then follow suit for centuries to come. Here we re-emphasize a sociohistorical view of the race concept as "races are peoples *created* [emphasis added] by history" and "groups [are] subsequently defined by the social significance of their morphology and ancestry" (Haney-Lopez, 1996, p. 38). A Marxist perspective argues that "circumstances directly encountered, given and transmitted from the past" (Marx, 1852, p. 103) always form social contexts in which social forces develop. Once these social contexts are accorded racial meaning, it follows that social identities are formed along racial lines as well. Thus, the social significance related to particular sociocultural histories, as well as phenotypic embodiments, frames race.

The legality of chattel slavery on the basis of race of the Atlantic New World would not dissipate until well into the 19th century. The 14th and 15th Amendment to the American Constitution abolished slavery in the United States (Blackmon, 2008); countries including Cuba and Brazil lagged and relinquished their systems respectively in 1886 and 1888 (Karras & McNeill, 1992). In the years following the fall of slavery as a formal institution in the United States, and the period of Reconstruction set in, many Blacks moved from their previous owners' plantations in the South, spreading out across the South, North, and the West. Having never occupied larger cities, Blacks moved to urban areas in droves.

> In 1890, 12 percent of the 7.5 million African Americans lived in cities, although only 4 percent had been urban in 1860. Many spent most of their time in White households as domestic servants. (Washington, 2006, p. 153)

Sites across the regions of the United States, under the auspices of the Freedman's Bureau, began erecting schools and public health clinics to serve the social and health needs of recently freed Blacks. However,

> When the freeman's camps dissolved, no public health support replaced them. Poverty and desperation trapped southern Blacks into an insidiously indirect new form of slavery—sharecropping. The exploitative, abusive medical care of slave owners

was replaced by no medical care at all for most poor Blacks, and disease and death ran rampant through Black populations. (Washington, 2006, p. 152)

It is no surprise then that, "in 1900, the life expectancy at birth in the United States was 47.6 years for Whites and 33.0 years for non-Whites, who were mainly Blacks" (Williams, Lavizzo-Mourey, & Warren, 1994, p. 26). Arguably, race-ing via subjugation is a European colonial and political instrument with persistent, modern implications for the health of our nation. Only policies that are rooted in the full understanding of this dark history can remedy disparities and usher in an equitable future for all of America.

■ SECTION II: Race, Policy, and Health Equity: Then

RACE IN THE POLICY SPACE: PART I

In terms of policy, just what *is* race? Why should policy designers be concerned as to whether the process is cognizant of the import of race or racism?

In the United States, race is generally understood to be a discrete physical and cultural phenomenon, wherein phenotype is perceived as a reliable proxy for one's social classification. Politically, racial categorization determines, to a large extent, distribution of resources by population. For instance, regarding the idea of Whiteness, physician and sociologist Jonathan Metzl argues, "I do not mean White as a biological classification or a skin color but as a political and economic system" (Metzl, 2019, p. 16) wherein Whiteness is so valued that it is not unheard of for persons who are White to cling to their racialization and to be willing to die for one's racial social positioning than yield concessions for the sake of equity, which would benefit everyone, including—especially poor—Whites (Metzl, 2019).

In 1977, the Office of Management and Budget (OMB) implemented Directive 15, which determined five racial groups, under which all persons accounted for in the United States would be delineated. Then, all federal data would be categorized accordingly:

- American Indians/Alaska Natives (AIAN)
- Asian/Pacific Islander (API)
- Hispanic
- White
- Black

Moreover, up until 1989, the race of one's mother determined the race of her child, with the exception of Pacific Islanders (a child was Pacific Islander if either parent was) and Whites (a child was White if both parents were). This "one-drop" rule invariably determined race. But, as social policies changed, so too did race become variable, albeit not well defined, and certainly not determined by any objective, scientific means. As racial determinations change, policies follow. Yet, as we have already witnessed with respect to the European conquest of First Peoples in the Americas, policies have been drawn in order to delineate races and sociopolitical outcomes along racial lines too. The latter is a trend that we now explore from the 19th century through to the 21st century.

RACIALIZED POLICIES IN THE 19TH AND 20TH CENTURIES

Prior to 1830, the indigenous population numbered approximately 125,000 in the Native lands of present-day Georgia, Tennessee, Alabama, North Carolina, and Florida (Ehle, 1988). All of this changed once the nation's new president laid down the law of the land. The Indian Removal Act of 1830 was a treatise enforced by Major General turned President Andrew Jackson. It forced indigenous peoples residing in the southeastern area of present-day United States to relocate to lands west of the Mississippi River. This forced relocation was explicitly intended to make room for White settlers and to advance President Jackson's mission to expand the burgeoning country's territory westward. Over the course of about 8 years, between 1831 and 1839, Seminole, Cherokee, Choctaw, Creek, and Chickasaw Indians marched from their homes in what today equates to half the land in the state of Alabama, and almost a quarter of the state of Georgia, into uncharted territory. Before the close of the 19th century, there were a total of nearly 70 such removal treaties, which the Jackson administration enforced on 100,000 indigenous of the nation. It is estimated that a quarter of those indigenous peoples died during what has become known as "The Trail of Tears" of 1838. This period of time also marked the advent of Indian Reservations.

In the decades following the Trail of Tears, health trends of indigenous peoples continued to decline. Lack of access to traditional lands and the foods that naturally grew in the soils they cultivated exacerbated their vulnerabilities to disease, malnutrition, and other traumas, with not just individual and tribal-wide consequences, but more persistently, generational disruptions to cultural practices that more likely preserved their health.

It is no exaggeration that the policies and practices of the past matter today with respect to the health of Native peoples. A recent Indian Health Service (IHS; 2019) report shows American Indians and Alaska Natives die at higher rates than other Americans from alcohol-induced deaths (564% higher), chronic liver disease and cirrhosis (356% higher), diabetes mellitus (217% higher), unintentional injuries (146% higher), assault/homicide (111% higher), and intentional self-harm/suicide (68% higher).

The federally sanctioned IHS continues to document and strives to undo this lowered health status that darkens indigenous peoples' quality of life.

In 1862, a little more than 30 years following the Indian Removal Act, President Abraham Lincoln signed into law the first of five iterations of the Homestead Act. The original law dictated that settlers be granted with 160 acres of land, provided they could pay the filing fee (of about $18), live on the land for 5 years, and commit to building and maintaining their home on the land. In law, land allotments were to be made available to any and all persons who fell under the categories of "head of family" or "21 years of age or older," including single women, immigrants, and the previously enslaved.

In effect, however, discrimination ran rampant across the land distribution process. Previously enslaved Blacks experienced peak barriers to gaining access to the benefits of the law:

> This social and economic transformation never occurred. The Southern Homestead Act failed to make newly freed blacks into a landowning class . . . What is more important, blacks had to face the extra burden of racial prejudice and

> discrimination along with the charging of illegal fees, expressly discriminatory court challenges and court decisions, and land speculators. (Oliver & Shapiro, 2006, pp. 14–15)

Compared to the approximately 1.6 million White applicants who benefited from Homestead policies, only about 4,000 to 5,000 Blacks gained land through the Homestead Act enacted in the 19th century. The Homestead Act remained in effect for well over a century (Merritt, 2017).

Then and now, property rights matter with respect to health and wellness. Both the Indian Removal Act and the Homestead Act demonstrate the significant connection between access to resources and maintenance of sustainable health practices. Sustainable access to water and soil, from which to grow traditional foods and other resources, determines families' livelihoods. Moreover, lack of ownership means generational, transferable wealth is decimated and cycles of poverty are perpetuated. Then and now, where one lives is less a reflection of exercising democratic choice and more a mirroring of the ways in which broader, insidious social processes—such as residential segregation and similar inequality social structures—impact the choice of individuals and families over time. Wellness of a community and wellness of individuals are tandem functions.

Individual behaviors do play a considerably significant role in wellness, but the choices one can make toward this point are inevitably determined by one's "place" in society—"place" here being physical, as in an address in a particular neighborhood subjected to conditions that vary across blocks, and "place" as in socioeconomic status (SES) as well.

The 1865 to 1877 Period of Reconstruction following the Civil War and the abolition of slavery (1865) came with progress. Black men were legally granted the right to vote.

Contemporaneously, a vast portion of the young Black community underwent a "great migration" from southern cotton fields to the industrial cities of the north (Wilkerson, 2010). No longer accepting remnants of the peculiar institution of slavery or of the slim pickings of sharecropping, they negotiated a new way of life. This period can just as easily characterize the early 20th century as can a crisis of identity and hardship. Access to academic venues by which to make sense of the new was often not an option. Without widescale access to formal education and perhaps without the patronage of a White beneficiary, there initially existed scant valid scientific speak of the rampant poverty or the deep discrimination facing Blacks.

The years 1934 and 1935 were critical years for federal policy affecting the wellness of Americans. President Franklin Delano Roosevelt's New Deal program was an investment in public works programs to quell unemployment and to increase the purchasing power of the nation's disenfranchised following the Great Depression years. The 1934 National Housing Act established the Federal Housing Administration (FHA), which was implemented to regulate lending and underwrite processes for home mortgages. While the intention of the FHA was to galvanize homeownership among all American residents, the legacy of the FHA rings similar to the housing and land-related restrictions imposed on Blacks in the previous century's Homestead Act. More overtly than the impact of the Homestead Act, the FHA mortgage home loan eligibility process was delineated along racial lines. Blacks faced significant barriers to securing these coveted housing loans. "Indeed, of the over 120 billion dollars in federal home-owner subsidies that were disbursed between 1934 and 1962, only 2% went to families of color" (Belcher, 2016, p. 92). In his June 2014 article, "The Case for Reparations," contemporary writer Ta-Nehisi Coates (2014) cites the "compounding moral debts" associated with housing discrimination. This *redlining* resulted in social and moral unraveling geographically bound. Oliver and Shapiro vividly describe the cycle of degradation:

> City services begin to decline, contributing to blight. As the community declines, it becomes the center for antisocial activities: drug dealing, hanging out, and robbery and violence . . . Racialized state policy contributed to this pattern, and the pattern continues unabated today. (2006, p. 43)

Not until 1968—almost 35 years later—was the Fair Housing Act made law, which was meant to undo the suppression of the Federal Housing Administration (FHA). Yet the damage had cut deeply into the social fibers of the nation.

While the FHA operated as a mechanism to depress one form of wealth building through homeownership, another New Deal milestone offered promise and security into older age. The Social Security Act (SSA) of 1935 is arguably one of the most revolutionary economic measures implemented in our nation's history. Also under the Roosevelt administration, the SSA's structure based on taxes withheld from able-bodied workers to support the nation's older adults (over the age of 65 years), the invalid, pregnant mothers, and the most vulnerable children, also provided an economic safety net for retired workers. However, as outlined in section 210 of the SSA, these benefits applied to all workers in the United States except for agricultural workers and domestic servants, who, at this time, accounted for almost half of all workers contributing to the American economy.

Ostensibly, this exclusion was a tax structural decision, not overt racial class exclusion. However, the impact on Black and Brown people, who occupied the majority of these low-paid agricultural and domestic positions, is unmistakable (Belcher, 2016). The New Deal also established the Aid to Families with Dependent Children (AFDC) as a direct cash aid source to especially single-parent families with small children. The historical impact of labor unions on the American families' ability to build toward the American Dream also cannot be understated. The Wagner Act of 1935 allowed for unions to leverage collective bargaining and to negotiate better working conditions. Yet, it too excluded people on the basis of race and did so for decades after its implementation (Belcher, 2016).

Thereafter, the wealth nexus divide between people of color and Whites spread like disease. The establishment of corporate and industrial developments catapulted a White middle class and truncated the emergence of an equal Black middle class. By the mid-20th century, our nation's wealth divide and the impact of national policies on the realities of American peoples had become stark. In the words of Oliver and Shapiro, "Policies have created differential opportunities for blacks and whites to develop disposable income and to generate wealth" (2006, p. 41).

In the era following the Roosevelt years of policy, as the nation entered into elongated periods of defense and diplomacy—World War II (1939–1945) and the Vietnam War (1955–1975)—the health of the nation did seem promising for the average American: smallpox had become a communicable disease of the past; polio and influenza deaths in children declined by more than half, given the widespread availability of vaccines; prenatal care service utilization was up and infant mortality rates were down; heart disease–related mortalities had decreased on average; smoking rates were consistently decreasing among adults and youth; and elderly deaths from preventable diseases had slowed. Many of these progressions could be attributed to an uptick in health education and public health prevention programs of the 1970s (National Center for Health Statistics, 1982).

However, while the nation celebrated the vestiges of its hearty defense abroad, race wars blazed across the American home front, and the health of Blacks suffered for it.

Homicide rates among Black males and females aged 15 to 24 years of age were five and four times higher than homicide rates of White males and females of the same age group. The country as a whole experienced decreases in communicable and chronic disease conditions, yet there were staggering heart disease rates among Black men and women between the ages of 25 years and 44 years. By this time, Jim Crow segregationist laws and practices had ruled the United States for the better part of the 20th century, barring non-Whites from critical health spaces, including hospitals. The damage had taken its toll, creating cultural practices of exclusion and expectations based on Blacks' general mistrust of the medical system and disparate access to quality healthcare services. George Bernard Shaw could not have been more clairvoyant when, in 1909, referring to the state of healthcare in the early 20th century, he admonished, "the tragedy of illness at present is that it delivers you helplessly into the hands of a profession which you deeply mistrust" (Shaw, 1906). While he was speaking of the state of his own nation in the United Kingdom, this sentiment can veritably be applied to the levels of mistrust that many Blacks experienced with respect to the U.S. healthcare system throughout the 20th century (Washington, 2006). The significance of distrust of medical establishments cannot be overlooked with respect to their contributions to ongoing health disparities. Long histories of medical abuse of Blacks at the hands of White physicians and scientists make this reticence understandable, yet also deeply unfortunate. One who does not trust care providers or hospitals—or suffers from what Harriet Washington terms as "iatrophobia"—will most certainly avoid presenting for care, often to his or her peril, which is unfortunately more likely to be earlier in life compared to Whites.

The rise of social movements in answer to the growing wealth and health disparities set the nation ablaze in the 1960s. The strategic advocacy (sometimes fatal), sacrifices, and outspokenness of civil rights leaders, including Bayard Rustin, Malcolm X, Dorothy I. Height, Ella Baker, and current Member of Congress, Representative John Lewis (D- GA), for example, carried the nation into its Civil Rights period. Milestone legislation in the Civil Rights Act (1964) and the Voting Rights Act (1965) embodied the shift of the nation in terms of instituting policies that would optimistically turn the tides of centuries-long inequities along racial lines. The former act authorized federal enforcement of desegregation in public spaces, whereas the latter prohibited any form of discrimination against persons historically blocked from exercising their 15th Amendment right to vote.

In 1965, then President Johnson also signed into law measures that would become perhaps the most significant health policies of the 20th century: Medicare and Medicaid. The former, as a federal trust fund program, is the healthcare system's flagship entitlement program. Medicare provides health coverage for people aged 65 and older, to people under 65 years with certain disabilities, and to anyone with end-stage renal disease (ESRD). To date, it covers 57 million Americans (48 million seniors; 9 million disabled persons). Through Medicare, beneficiaries can access most health services including inpatient and outpatient care, preventive health services, and prescription drugs (Kaiser Family Foundation, 2019). Medicaid differs in that it is an assistance partnership program between federal and state jurisdictions. Its initial intent was to provide low-income people with cash assistance, and it has evolved into a federal health insurance program providing access to high-quality, but low-cost healthcare (Kaiser Family Foundation, 2019) for eligible consumers. Both programs are operated by the Centers for Medicare and Medicaid Services (CMS) under the U.S. Department of Health and Human Services (HHS).

The impact of Medicaid and Medicare was not confined to the healthcare delivery space; the legislation would critically shift social norms, reverberating throughout the country's social institutions, and this was not at all lost upon proponents and dissenters of the milestone. "Social programs such as Medicare and Medicaid carry particularly racial histories" (Metzl, 2019, p. 13). For example, when Medicaid and Medicare were implemented in 1965, especially Whites in the U.S. South experienced consternation because the law required hospitals to desegregate as a condition to receiving federal funding (Metzl, 2019). Much more was bound to change during this critical stage of America's history. In the years following the Civil Rights period and the implementation of Medicare and Medicaid, "black health status improved dramatically for a decade" (Byrd & Clayton, 2001, p. 215). Specifically, the policy implications of the 1960s cannot be overstated:

> The 1964 Civil Rights Act, hospital desegregation rulings in the federal courts, passage of Medicare and Medicaid, the Voting Rights Bill, and the health center movement created a Civil Rights Era in health care for African Americans. (Byrd & Clayton, 2001, p. 215)

Finally, by the 1970s, the federal government presented legislation "in response to the failing health status of Native Americans" (Fusselman, 2012, p. 392). The Indian Health Care Improvement Act (IHCIA) of 1976 appropriated annual funds for the nationwide care system, the IHS, through 2000, after which IHS funds had to be reappropriated (Fusselman, 2012). Fortunately, with the implementation of the Patient Protection and Affordable Care Act (ACA), "the IHCIA is reauthorized 'permanently and indefinitely' with funds appropriated through fiscal year 2010 and every fiscal year thereafter until all federal funds are expended" (Fusselman, 2012, p. 393). While the health of Native Americans has improved since the egregious days of Columbus, and of Jackson, there remains a significant and vast disparity between them and White Americans. Further along in this chapter, we will have a more robust review of the significance of the ACA on the Native American population.

Legislation in the late 20th century began to consider the unique challenges of differently able-bodied persons in America. The Americans with Disabilities Act (ADA) of 1990, for all intents and purposes, very much set a legislative precedent to the formal establishment and recognition of federally classified protected classes not only on the basis of ability status but also on race/ethnicity, religion, national origin, sex, and age. Based on the ADA, it is illegal to bar anyone who falls within one, or at the intersection of several, of these protected classes. Without this law, swaths of the American population would be locked out of opportunity to live vibrantly.

As I cited earlier in this chapter, "in 1900, the life expectancy at birth in the United States was 47.6 years for whites and 33.0 years for nonwhites, who were mainly blacks" (Williams et al., 1994, p. 26). Among other notable social improvements in the 20th century, the implementation of laws on health and wealth building, education and opportunity literally elongated the life of all, but still had not closed the mortality gap between Whites and Blacks, a phenomenon which I roughly outline in Figure 14.1.

> By 1990, the comparable numbers were 76.1 years for whites and 69.1 years for blacks. Thus, during this century, substantial progress has been made in improving the health status of both blacks and whites, but blacks continue to bear a higher burden of death, disease, and disability. (Williams et al., 1994)

As the 21st century loomed, new administrations implemented key welfare legislation, such as the 1996 Personal Responsibility and Work Opportunity Act, otherwise known as the Welfare Reform Act, namely in answer to the burgeoning number of single-mother households and dwindling national employment rate. The overall intent of welfare reform was to discourage out-of-wedlock childbirths, increase work opportunities for heads of households—especially single mothers—and by effect, encourage the formation of nuclear families. Here, we can take a moment to reflect on a more intersectional and problematic implication of race, gender, and SES in welfare policies. As a construct, gender differentially impacts one's opportunities and access to opportunities, which in turn affects one's well-being. The way gender and race together play out in federal policies is generally from a lens of personal responsibility, which we will evaluate more, shortly, in this chapter.

The mechanism of SES also explains differences in health outcomes over the life course (Gorman & Read, 2006). I am especially thinking here of the "strong Black woman" theory offered by Tamara Beauboeuf-Lafontant (2009). High loads of chronic

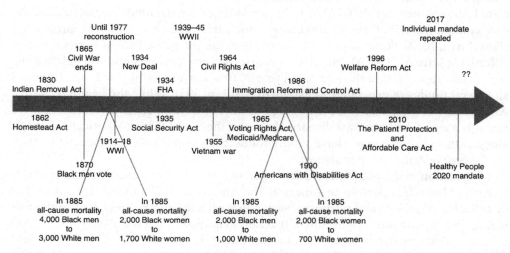

FIGURE 14.1 HEALTH POLICY MILESTONES AND MAJOR EVENTS IN THE UNITED STATES, 1830–PRESENT.

FHA, Federal Housing Administration; WWII, World War II.

stress in connection with depression and poor coping mechanisms due to lack of access to healthy coping mechanisms linked to SES essentially describe this theory. In terms of the value judgments inherent in the medical care decision process, a major assumption is that everyone deserves access to the highest/best levels of care. But this does not align with another major economic assumption that resources need to be equitably distributed across society to ensure this happens. Essentially, this is a welfare of society argument.

RACE VERSUS RESPONSIBILITY

Perhaps out of optimism, or in a haste to distance oneself from the sins of one's forefathers, many assert that race is inconsequential because everyone has an equal chance and responsibility to achieve greatness. This concept of personal responsibility saturates American culture. It is the philosophical mantle upon which American policy has for so long rested, pervading our social institutions and even dividing communities. It is the ideology that frames the formula of achieving the American Dream. It is, but is not exclusively, a signal of America's foundational conservatism. Even President Obama, in his 2009 inauguration speech, harkened to this very idea by calling for "a new era of responsibility" (NPR, 2009), alluding to a correctness of doing things in one's life in order to achieve the highest levels of success. To this day, the resounding tenor of American life is still "help yourself, save yourself, or be at fault." In this way, personal responsibility is the more socially desirable proxy for assigning culpability for one's conditions—social, economic, and health included. However, does personal responsibility apply the same to all people, regardless of their circumstances? No, it does not. This is the entire intent of this chapter, to demonstrate that throughout history,

> The history of race in America also helps explain why these topics cut to the heart of present-day debates about what it means to provide resources, protections, and opportunities for everyone in a diverse society versus providing resources and opportunities for a select few. (Metzl, 2019, p. 14)

While individual behavior does make a significant difference in one's personal trajectory, the health of individuals and that of communities is ultimately a factor of that community's relationship to sociological-determining factors, including policy.

Still others insist on subscribing to a color-blind theory that American society is "postracial," and that there are no present-day consequences of race and, more particularly, of racism. Social scholars like Barbara Trepagnier have studied this social naiveté at length, and can disabuse us of the notion that our nation is beyond race, that racism is no longer an issue. We must interrogate race and racism continuously, and in all social spaces, which differs from how individual people think about race and racism.

Interrogation at both levels is required in order to move beyond race (if ever that is actually possible, although I do not think it is as there will always be a mechanism of social divide that Socially Darkens communities in relation to another community). In her book, *Silent Racism: How Well-Meaning White People Perpetuate the Racial Divide*, Trepagnier explores how well-meaning White people make sense of and contribute to racism against individuals who are Black in the United States. She begins by illustrating the divergence of White and Black thoughts on racism. According to the author, Whites think of racism in terms of a dichotomy between "racist" and "not racist." The former assumes that racism is an act or statement that is virulent and hateful, more akin to the overt racism of the pre–Civil Rights era, and is thereby a rare occurrence today. The latter category tries to ignore racial differences and does not—or cannot—recognize as racist any act or statement that is not blatantly harmful to a person of color. Furthermore, this category excludes recognition of institutional racism. Both of these groups differ from the way the author describes the ability of persons who are Black to recognize racism. Blacks "see racism as permeating the institutions of society, producing racial inequality in employment, education, housing, and justice" (Trepagnier, 2006, p. 4). That persons who are White think in binary terms of racism and persons who are Black think in cyclical terms of racism is a discrepancy that perpetuates, subtlety, a collective paralysis and inability to undermine racial inequality. Now, let us look more closely at how this discrepancy may play out in clinical settings.

The operationalization of racism in the health space is often implicit, tacit, or hard to qualify. But the impact can be fatal. Implicit bias may have its influence on Black women's wellness. For instance, Black women are more likely to die after being diagnosed with breast cancer. This could be from delayed treatment and delayed treatment-seeking behavior if they had not formerly felt welcomed or empowered by their primary care provider (PCP). "Perceived discrimination has also been associated with lower levels of healthcare seeking and adherence behaviors" (Williams & Mohammed, 2009). Other scholars have identified similar findings that the impact of racism on the body is biologically harmful. Research has cited the associations between chronic experiences of racism and "higher risk of illness and obesity among African American women . . . sleep disturbances" and "greater rates of hypertension among adult African Americans" (Metzl, 2019, p. 15).

Whether or not one acknowledges his or her attitudes toward race, without doubt, health outcomes and economics are racially patterned and demonstrate great inequities. Simply put, "the racial system of America fails everyone" (Metzl, 2019, p. 20). Race implicates who holds power and resources, and it historically has been the rationalization for establishing social standards and norms, which has inevitably lent to the steadfastness of disparities in health across centuries (Byrd & Clayton, 2001). Poverty, economic and political marginalization, and health disparities all are current violent striations eroding at the bedrock of life quality for Socially Darkened communities in the United States. Such conditions that are by-products of a socially stratified nation impacted by historically embedded processes of domination—like slavery, colonialism, and postcolonialism—proceed to reproduce race. The world over, these symbolic effects place disparate harm on marginalized groups. But, particularly in the United States, "medical experts of every persuasion agree that African Americans share the most deplorable health profile in the nation by far, one that resembles that of Third World countries." (Washington, 2006, p. 20). This racialized experience is recognizable by an historical legacy of disenfranchisement, high rates of mortality, and lower life expectancy compared to White counterparts.

At this point, we have established that race is also a reliable proxy for economic patterns and health outcomes in the United States. Raced peoples face persistent and well-documented health outcomes and healthcare access disparities. This phenomenon prompted HHS, at the time under the direction of Secretary Kathleen Sebelius, to report that, disproportionately, raced peoples and low-income communities "experience reduced access to healthy lifestyle options and suffer higher rates of morbidity and mortality as compared to their higher-income counterparts" (2009, p. 9). Both biological factors and social factors, such as poverty, low SES, and lack of access to care, contribute to health disparities that exist along racial and ethnic lines.

Compared to their White American counterparts, for example, African Americans experience higher rates of premature death due to heart disease and stroke (Centers for Disease Control and Prevention [CDC], 2017). Nonelderly Black men (39%) and women (58%) experience significantly greater levels of obesity than do nonelderly White men (35%) and women (33%; see CDC, 2017). While Blacks account for 13% of the U.S. population, they make up more than 40% of new HIV incidences; the impact is especially grievous among Black men who sleep with men (MSM), who account for 73% of new HIV cases among Blacks in the United States (CDC, 2018a). Compared to White mothers and mothers-to-be, Black women are dying at three to four times higher rates during pregnancy, while giving birth, or during the postpartum period (CDC, 2018b). The list so goes on across other health metrics, with the exception of suicide rates.

Other vulnerable communities of color, such as those who are limited English proficient (LEP), face both racial and linguistic barriers to health services. Linguistic minorities experience more severe health outcomes consequent of medical errors and receive diminished quality of care compared to English-speaking patients (Ramirez, Engel, & Tang, 2008). These disparities are not only alarming but also costly to individual health outcomes, the American public, and are a burden to the nation's entire healthcare system. Namely, disparate health outcomes are associated with increases of inpatient and outpatient healthcare utilization, overuse of medications, and the number of specialty care requests, all of which exacerbate health system consumption and drive system costs.

The influence of race on health equity policy has implications spanning from the interpersonal, interorganizational, as well as national levels. Thus, race in policy and political arenas (viz., legislative and judicial branches of government) is about the decision-making process taking into full consideration that race, while not biological, has permeated our skin and races communities with respect to their wellness and opportunity outcomes. It takes enactment of comprehensive laws to both remedy the ills of our past and to usher in a healthier, more equitable future. We have evaluated what policy has done to population health outcomes across raced peoples. Moving forward, what is policy currently doing and what can policy do differently to assist Socially Darkened people toward becoming their healthiest selves?

The answer is this: *Legislation can veritably change people's lives.*

■ SECTION III: Race, Policy, and Health Equity: Now and Moving Forward
···

RACE IN THE POLICY SPACE: PART II

Enacted on the heels of the 2008 national recession, and during the high energy surrounding the election of the nation's first African American President, Barack Obama, the 2010 Patient Protection and Affordable Care Act (the ACA) was a veritable game changer with respect to closing racial gaps in healthcare access. ACA is likely the most thoroughly Congressionally debated legislation of our time. On the House of Representatives side alone, the bill went through 79 bipartisan hearings and markups over a 2-year period, and the Senate spent 25 consecutive days in session on health reform alone amounting to what was the second longest consecutive session in history.

At the outset, the primary goal of the ACA was to increase access to quality, affordable healthcare and to provide preventive care. Among racial and ethnic minorities, the largest gains existed among those with the largest uninsured rates, ultimately also contributing closures to economic as well as health access and health outcome disparities. Before the ACA, 30% of Hispanics and 30% of American Indians were uninsured. Black uninsured rates were at almost 20% (Kaiser Family Foundation, 2019). Since the ACA's inception, the health and healthcare access of minority populations has shifted in a nature akin to the impact of the Civil Rights Era milestone health legislation. Once its key elements—the individual mandate and full coverage of essential health benefits—were implemented in 2014, the nation witnessed an unprecedented exponentiation of historically medically underserved populations gaining access to healthcare providers. By 2017, the uninsured rate of Hispanics had significantly decreased to 19% and 22% for American Indians and to 11% for Blacks.

It is no debate that healthcare and system costs have been and are on the rise. Medical expenditures continue to increase at a faster rate than that of national inflation, and consume a significant portion of the national gross domestic product (GDP), and that of goods and services produced in the United States. These increases do not necessarily reflect the increase in population either but instead reflect the rise in health services, prices, and quality. Yet, in terms of the ACA's effect on the national economy, health-related costs have grown at their slowest rates in 50 years. According to the Congressional Budget Office, the ACA will generate total savings of more than $3 trillion over the next two decades. The uninsured rate for children has fallen by nearly half since 2008. For young adults, the uninsured rate has dropped by more than half since 2010 in large part to the ACA's crux tenet, the expansion of Medicaid to low-income persons residing in states that elected into the expansion. Moreover, Medicaid expansion is disproportionately important to rural patients. The ACA reduced the uninsured rate in rural counties throughout America by 8%. In states that have opted to expand Medicaid through the ACA, the uninsured rate has dropped by more than half, while in states that have not elected to expand Medicaid, the uninsured rate has dropped only a quarter. The absence of Medicaid expansion has made a critical impact on the health of Whites as well. For example, "When averaged across the population, Tennessee's refusal to expand Medicaid cost *every single* White resident of the state *14.1 days of life*" (Metzl, 2019, p. 13). Perhaps for the first time since the early 20th century, the impact of access to care is converging between Socially Darkened populations, most especially between Blacks and poor Whites.

Going into the 2016 presidential election, central issues captivated the Republican Party: repealing the ACA was a major mantle on which the party stood. At the time this chapter was written, the Trump Administration had instituted laws that erode the present health system and, consequently, the gains achieved under the ACA. Namely, under President Donald Trump, the individual mandate tenet of the ACA has been repealed, and we now begin to see a shift away from application to health insurance within the ACA marketplace. While it is not a perfect health policy, repeal of the ACA is not acceptable, or even feasible by economic, comprehensive insurance coverage, or health system means. In the absence of a comprehensive healthcare coverage plan like the ACA, the healthcare system will ultimately revert to pre-ACA individual marketplace conditions wherein sicker people were systematically excluded or marginalized via exorbitant premiums.

However, the ACA cannot be the culmination of health reform. While it has been a tremendous policy in remedy to the impact of barriers by race and SES to quality healthcare access, future health policies must bolster where it was weak and innovate in spaces where it does not have significant impact.

HEALTH INNOVATION, BIG DATA, AND INFORMATION TECHNOLOGY

Future health polices cannot be prescriptive; they must be forward thinking and innovative. In order to achieve health equity, policies must center on how they would positively impact communities in America with histories of political upheaval and social blight. The design of health policies must include a deep dive into the consumers'/beneficiaries' pasts. In this case, the consumer is the community. Some social scientists argue that "equitable access to quality healthcare, along with culturally appropriate public health initiatives and community support, is key to ameliorating the human ravages produced by the second-class health status of African American families" (Oliver & Shapiro, 2006, p. 241). I do not disagree, but the issue is more complicated than this. In truth, "more investment in healthcare does not automatically result in better health outcomes" (Metzl, 2019, p. 18). Even if we were to equalize access to healthcare, disparities in health status would still exist (LaVeist, Gaskin, & Richard, 2011) because the mechanism of other-ing communities still exists. Education is also not a "fix" to disparities; disparities persist irrespective of educational levels. In addition to continuous investments in the healthcare space, health policies must continuously bend toward equity.

If federal policies are not proactive, or if legislators do not pay close enough attention, then the next frontier of inequity in health and medicine will be unlike anything designers of mid-19th century health policy milestones would have ever imagined: the intersection of health and technology. As the cost of healthcare delivery continues to burgeon, and the health needs of the American people become more complex, traditional modes of care on their own—especially in historically medically underserved areas (MUAs)—(will) no longer suffice. The scope of medical care is moving firmly in the direction of telehealth and telemedicine. The healthcare reform debate is, in large part, an offshoot consequence of the unique, albeit costly, needs of MUAs' health settings and the growing advocacy for less costly and innovative remote-based medicine. Inequities in medical innovation and precision medicine will inevitably catch the nation's providers and legislators off guard if our policies are not designed with innovative foresight. There is great necessity of health policies to mirror new developments in health determinants, with less reliance on aggregate data that otherwise mask the nuances of mortality across racial lines and create a statistical false sense of health security. As physician and former member of Congress, Dr. Donna Christensen admonishes, "Health disparities are the civil rights issue of the 21st Century" (Washington, 2006, p. 3). Without foresight, we will again grapple with what W. E. B. DuBois (1903) declared in the early 20th century: the problem of the color line, particularly with respect to health outcomes.

Future policies should evaluate how to diversify and sustain a healthcare workforce in medically underserved populations as the health field integrates more heavily with technology, medical innovation, and big data. To date, "studies continue to demonstrate that, far from sharing in the bounty of American medical technology, African Americans are often bereft of high-technology care, even for life-threatening conditions such as heart disease" (Washington, 2006, p. 21). As our world becomes increasingly more digitally driven, the integration of big data will indeed determine the trajectory of health systems, hospitals, and services placed within communities, potentially revolutionizing norms of care delivery. In this way, the democratization of health information, including virtual community conversations around health, and the sharing of de-identified health information must become mainstream and interoperable across health systems to protect patients and amplify medical adherence, as well as protect providers from liable cases, only enhancing rather than inhibiting, their stewardship of care. Privacy and security of data is imperative in order to achieve human-centered design of health systems.

The role of data toward meeting the needs of communities must consider key questions:

- What do you do with the data?
- What are the bioethical concerns of data?
- How does one deal efficiently with "deluge of data" or "data tsunamis"?
- How does one ensure that there is proper representation in the data and that the data metrics themselves are not biased?

Most of the health disparities that exist are a result of living in a society that produces and reproduces disparities. As we evaluate what equity looks like with respect to health policy, there are a number of other policy subjects that deserve elevation in this space. While not all are straightforward health policies, such as policies at the intersection of health and technology, all can be transformative for the health of raced peoples in America, irrespective of one's race, immigration status, SES, ability, sexual orientation, English proficiency, and so on, potentially pushing the nation toward health equity.

PRESCRIPTION DRUGS: ACCESS, COST, AND TRANSPARENCY

One would be remiss if not to acknowledge that differential access to lifesaving medical innovations and medicines exacerbates quality care differences between populations. The role of federal policies in either abating or exacerbating high drug costs cannot be overlooked. The federal government partially pays for most new drug development, at least in the beginning stages of research (Spiro, Calsyn, & Huelskoetter, 2015). The Bipartisan Budget Act (BBA) of 2018 and its goal to reduce drug prices by requiring pharmaceutical companies to offer discounts on expensive drugs, predominantly for seniors who are Medicare Part D recipients, alludes to promising results. Released in May 2018, President Trump's proposed "Drug Pricing Blueprint" could help to reduce out-of-pocket costs for seniors receiving Part D benefits and ease the prescription drug cost burden for patients. However, if implemented, lifesaving drugs that treat protected classes—drugs including antidepressants, antipsychotics, anticonvulsants, immunosuppressants, antiretrovirals, and antineoplastics—could also be at stake. (The final rule upholds that drugs in these classes must continue to remain in formularies [CMS, 2018].)

The other side of the pharmaceutical drug and equity conversation has to do with racial representation in clinical trials. Clinical trials are not just about medical interventions.

Often, trials explore the best ways to prevent diseases in certain populations. Clinical trials need greater diversity, behavioral interventions, and knowledge about innovative treatments because limited information, education, access, and delays in treatment often mean life or death. For example, among African American women who suffer from the highest rates of the deadliest forms of breast cancer, trials are needed to generate a more granular understanding of why certain prevention strategies are unpalatable, underused, or difficult for certain communities to adopt as health habits, and their unique social challenges which make it hard for them to perceive of and pursue certain preventive options. Future policies must explicitly explore this dearth.

ALL POLICY IS HEALTH POLICY

Health policy is not just policy that is designed to address clinical concerns of health, healthcare financing, or healthcare delivery. In fact, equitable health policies may not explicitly fall within the category of health at all. Nor is it just about the science of health. As illustrated, the intersections between health and wealth are undeniable. The socioeconomic determinants of health—namely income, but also education, environmental elements, healthcare access, politics, and the like—contribute to, or detract from, the wellness of individuals. In addition to economic policies, transportation, zoning laws, and many more tangential fields all impact the public's health. Virtually any federal policy may have an impact on the health of populations in terms of messaging to and educating the public; distributing or redistributing resources; as well as regulating clinical and nonclinical realm practices. Equitable health policies are redistributive policies and policies based on closing economic gaps between Whites and Socially Darkened populations.

Given that the "unequal distribution of health-damaging experiences is not in any sense a 'natural' phenomenon but is the result of a toxic combination of poor social policies and programmes, unfair economic arrangements, and bad policies" (Commission on Social Determinants of Health, 2008, p. 1), future federal policies need not fall directly in the realm of the clinical world. But they must be well-informed of the historical elements that brought our nation to its present health divide across racial lines.

> Investing in communal health care solutions, workers' rights, better roads and bridges, research into climate change and opiate addiction, common-sense gun laws, or expanded social safety nets benefit everyone, not just the immigrant and minority. (Metzl, 2019, p. 19)

In order to effectively address the health disparities, which arise from the impact of social policies, we must first understand those policies and disparities. One of the best ways to prevent premature death of populations is by "increasing the purchasing power of the most affected groups" (Sen, 1992, p. 43), especially through the generation of a more culturally diverse health workforce and occupational opportunities.

Workforce policy is health policy that has the potential to bolster equity. Yet many people who would opt into careers in the health workforce often avoid doing so due to the great financial burdens associated with the training. Strengthening the National Health Service Corp and other loan repayment programs designed to increase the health workforce in rural, medically underserved areas and through IHS provider sites, for instance, would go a long way to address this issue. Such a move would not only enhance the health of populations we have discussed but would also help to distribute our physicians, nurses, mental health professionals, dentists, and other clinical providers in the areas with the most need. Additionally, modernizing the medical service reimbursement systems of Medicare and Medicaid is imperative if the nation is to preempt an exponential chasm of health outcome inequity.

■ Conclusion

This chapter is not meant to be exhaustive nor is it a treatise on all things related to race, health equity, and policy in the United States. Its sole intent is to generate critical thought and evaluation on the role of race—and the consequent role of being raced—historically and presently, and how that role has catapulted, in effect, inequitable health outcomes in our nation. While I maintain that there is no biological differentiation between races, sociopolitical factors have historically changed the biology of certain communities. Indeed,

> A closer look at the troubling numbers reveals that Blacks are dying not of exotic, incurable, poorly understood illnesses nor of genetic diseases that target only them, but rather from common ailments that are more often prevented and treated among Whites than among Blacks. (Washington, 2006, p. 3)

This is why our U.S. policies must both remedy past ills and remodel for the future. Very seldom will one find historical, sociological, epidemiological, demographic, and civil liberties or political arguments for health equity in one source. But this intersecting discussion is what is necessary to illuminate a hard truth: the critical study of race in policy design cannot be overlooked. Lawmakers must give primacy to this historical impact of race in America when making policies that impact those raced in America, for "the much bewildered racial health gap is not a gap, but a chasm wider and deeper than a mass grave" (Washington, 2006, p. 20). Without deep consideration of this point, we ought to select our own shovels and get digging.

■ Resources

Arendt, H. (1969). A special supplement: Reflections on violence. *The New York Review of Books*. Retrieved from http://www.nybooks.com/50/Arendt

Best, R. K. (2012). Disease politics and medical research funding: Three ways advocacy shapes policy. *American Sociological Review, 77,* 780–803. doi:10.1177/0003122412458509

Bonilla-Silva, E. (1999). The essential social fact of race. *American Sociological Review, 64,* 899–906. doi:10.2307/2657410

Bonilla-Silva, E., & Dietrich, D. R. (2008). The Latin Americanization of Racial Stratification in the U.S. In R. E. Hall (Ed.), *Racism in the 21st century: An empirical analysis of skin color* (pp. 151–170). New York, NY: Springer.

Bourdieu, P. (2001). *Masculine domination.* Redwood City, CA: Stanford University Press.

Bourdieu, P., & Wacquant, L. (1992). *An invitation to reflexive sociology*. Chicago, IL: The University of Chicago Press.

Butler, K. D. (2001). Defining diaspora, refining a discourse. *Diaspora: A Journal of Transnational Studies, 10*, 189–219. doi:10.1353/dsp.2011.0014

DuBois, W. E. B. (2009). *The gift of Black folk: The Negroes in the making of America*. Garden City Park, NY: Square One Publishers.

Edwards, B. H. (2001). The uses of diaspora. *Social Text, 19*, 45–73. Retrieved from https://muse.jhu.edu/article/31891

Fanon, F. (1952). *Black skin, white mask*. New York, NY: Grove Press.

Feagin, J., & Elias, S. (2013). Rethinking racial formation theory: A systemic racism critique. *Ethnic and Racial Studies, 36*, 931–960. doi:10.1080/01419870.2012.669839

Fields, K. E., & Fields, B. J. (2012). *Racecraft: The soul of inequality in American life*. Brooklyn, NY: Verso.

Gilroy, P. (1993). *The Black Atlantic: Modernity and double consciousness*. London, England: Verso.

Gilroy, P. (1994). Black cultural politics: An interview with Paul Gilroy by Timmy Lott. *Found Object, 4*, 46–81.

Gruesser, J. C. (2007). *Confluences: Postcolonialism, African American literary studies, and the Black Atlantic*. Athens: The University of Georgia Press.

Legal-Dictionary. (n.d.). Retrieved from http://www.legaldictionary.com

Malthus, T. R. (1798). *A summary view of the principle of population. An Essay on the Principle of Population* (1st ed.). London: J. Johnson, in St. Paul's Church-yard.

Massey, D. S., & Denton, N. A. (1993). *American Apartheid: Segregation and the making of the underclass*. Cambridge, MA: Harvard University Press.

Mbembe, A. (2001). *On the postcolony*. Berkeley: University of California Press.

Mbembe, A. (2003). Necropolitics. *Public Culture, 15*, 11–40. doi:10.1215/08992363-15-1-11

McKeown, T. (1979). *The role of medicine: Dream, mirage, or nemesis?* Oxford, England: Basil Blackwell.

Meriam, L. (1928). *The problem of Indian administration: Report of a survey made at the request of Honorable Hubert Work, Sec. of the Interior*. Brookings Institute. Washington, DC: Department of the Interior.

Minkler, M. (1999). Personal responsibility for health? A review of the arguments and the evidence at century's end. *Health Education and Behavior, 26*, 121–140. doi:10.1177/109019819902600110

Moten, F. (2013). Blackness and nothingness (mysticism in the flesh). *The South Atlantic Quarterly, 112*, 737–780. doi:10.1215/00382876-2345261

Murray, C., & Herrnstein, R. (1994). *The bell curve*. New York, NY: Free Press.

Sexton, J. (2011). The social life of social death: On Afro-Pessimism and Black Optimism. *InTensions*, 5. Retrieved from http://www.yorku.ca/intent/issue5/articles/jaredsexton.php

Shepperson, G. (1993). African diaspora: Concept and context. In J. E. Harris (Ed.), *The Global dimensions of the African diaspora* (pp. 41–50). Washington, DC: Howard University Press.

Smith, L. T. (2012). *Decolonizing methodologies: Research and indigenous peoples* (2nd ed.). London, England: Zed Books.

Ture, K., & Hamilton, C. V. (1967). *Black power: The politics of liberation*. New York, NY: Random House.

Vacher, L-C. (1979). A nineteenth century assessment of causes of European mortality decline. *Population and Development Review, 5*, 163–170. doi:10.2307/1972322

Walcott, R. (2004). Beyond the 'Nation-Thing': Black studies, cultural studies, and diaspora discourse (Or The Post-Black Studies Movement). In C. B. Davis (Ed.), *Decolonizing the academy: African diaspora studies* (pp. 107–124). Trenton, NJ: Africa World Press.

Wilderson, F. B. (2010). *Red, white, and black: Cinema and the structure of U.S. antagonisms*. Durham, NC: Duke University Press.

Williams, D. (2015). Racial bias in health care and health: Challenges and opportunities. *Journal of the American Medical Association, 314,* 555–556. doi:10.1001/jama.2015.9260

Wilson, W. J. (2012). *The truly disadvantaged: The inner city, the underclass, and public policy* (2nd ed.). Chicago, IL: The University of Chicago Press.

Zinn, H. (2003). *A people's history of the United States*. New York, NY. HarperCollins.

References

Artiga, S., Orgera, K., & Damico, A. (2019). *Changes in health coverage by race and ethnicity since implementation of the ACA, 2013–2017*. Retrieved from https://www.kff.org/disparities-policy/issue-brief/changes-in-health-coverage-by-race-and-ethnicity-since-implementation-of-the-aca-2013-2017

Axtell, J. (1988). *After Columbus: Essays in the ethnohistory of colonial North America*. Oxford, England: Oxford University Press.

Beauboeuf-Lafontant, T. (2009). *Behind the mask of the strong Black woman: Voice and the embodiment of a costly performance*. Philadelphia, PA: Temple University Press.

Belcher, C. (2016). *A Black man in the White House*. Healdsburg, CA: Water Street Press.

Bigelow, B., & Peterson, B. (1998). *Rethinking Columbus: The next 500 years*. Milwaukee, WI: Rethinking Schools.

Blackmon, D. A. (2008). *Slavery by another name: The re-enslavement of Black Americans from the Civil War to World War II*. New York, NY: Doubleday.

Bonilla-Silva, E. (1997). Rethinking racism: Toward a structural interpretation. *American Sociological Review, 62,* 465–480. doi:10.2307/2657316

Byrd, M. W., & Clayton, L. A. (2001). Race, medicine, and health care in the United States: A historical survey. *Journal of the National Medical Association, 93*(3, Suppl.), 11S–34S. Retrieved from https://www.ncbi.nlm.nih.gov/pmc/articles/PMC2593958

Centers for Disease Control and Prevention. (2017). *Prevalence of obesity among adults and youth: United States, 2015–2016*. Retrieved from https://www.cdc.gov/nchs/data/databriefs/db288.pdf

Centers for Disease Control and Prevention. (2018a). *Diagnoses of HIV infection in the United States and dependent areas, 2017* [HIV Surveillance Report Vol. 29. Retrieved from https://www.cdc.gov/hiv/pdf/library/reports/surveillance/cdc-hiv-surveillance-report-2017-vol-29.pdf

Centers for Disease Control and Prevention. (2018b). *Pregnancy Mortality Surveillance System*. Retrieved from https://www.cdc.gov/reproductivehealth/maternal-mortality/pregnancy-mortality-surveillance-system.htm

Centers for Medicare and Medicaid Services. (2018). *Contract Year (CY) 2020 Medicare Advantage and Part D Drug Pricing Proposed Rule (CMS 4180-P)*. Retrieved from https://www.cms.gov/newsroom/fact-sheets/contract-year-cy-2020-medicare-advantage-and-part-d-drug-pricing-proposed-rule-cms-4180-p

Coates, T-N. (2014). The case for reparations. *The Atlantic*. Retrieved from https://www.theatlantic.com/magazine/archive/2014/06/the-case-for-reparations/361631

Commission on Social Determinants of Health. (2008). *Closing the gap in a generation: Health equity through action on the social determinants of health*. Geneva, Switzerland: World Health Organization. Retrieved from https://www.who.int/social_determinants/final_report/csdh_finalreport_2008.pdf

Cook, S. F., & Borah, W. (1971). *Essays in population history, Vol. One, Mexico and the Caribbean*. Berkeley: University of California.

de Las Casas, B. (2003). *An account, much abbreviated, of the destruction of the Indies, with related texts (1620)*. Indianapolis, IN: Hackett Publishing.

Dobyns, H. F. (1966). An appraisal of techniques with a new hemispheric estimate. *Current Anthropology, 7*, 395–416. doi:10.1086/200749

DuBois, W. E. B. (1903). *The souls of Black folk*. Chicago, IL: A.C. McClurg & Co.

Ehle, J. (1988). *Trail of tears: The rise and fall of the Cherokee nation*. New York, NY: Anchor Books.

Franklin, J. H., & Moss, Jr, A. A. (2001). *From slavery to freedom*. New York, NY: Alfred A. Knopf.

Fusselman, K. E. (2012). Native American Health Care: Is the Indian Health Care Reauthorization and Improvement Act of 2009 enough to address persistent health problems within the Native American Community?" *Washington and Lee Journal of Civil Rights and Social Justice, 18*, 389–422. Retrieved from http://scholarlycommons.law .wlu.edu/cgi/viewcontent.cgi?article=1322&context=crsj

Gorman, B. K., & Read, J. G. (2006). Gender disparities in adult health: An examination of three measures of morbidity. *Journal of Health and Social Behavior, 47*, 95–110. doi:10.1177/002214650604700201

Gould, S. J. (1980). *The mismeasure of man*. New York, NY: W.W. Norton & Company.

Guitar, L. (1997). *No more negotiation: Slavery and the destabilization of colonial Hispaniola's* encomienda *system*. Université Antilles Guyane, Groupe de recherche AIP-CARDH. Retrieved from http://cai.sg.inter.edu/revista-ciscla/volume29/guitar.pdf

Haney-Lopez, I. (1996). *White by law: The legal construction of race*. New York: New York University Press.

Heat-Moon, W. L. (2002). *Columbus in the Americas*. Hoboken, NJ: John Wiley & Sons, Inc.

Indian Health Service. (2019). *Indian health disparities*. Retrieved from https://www.ihs. gov/sites/newsroom/themes/responsive2017/display_objects/documents/factsheets/ Disparities.pdf

Kaiser Family Foundation. (2019). *Overview of Medicare*. Retrieved from https://www .kff.org/medicare/issue-brief/an-overview-of-medicare

Karras, A. L., & McNeill, J. R. (1992). *Atlantic American societies: From Columbus through abolition 1492–1888*. London, England: Routledge.

LaVeist, T., Gaskin, D., & Richard, P. (2011). Estimating the economic burden of health inequalities in the United States. *International Journal of Health Services, 41*, 231–238. doi:10.2190/HS.41.2.c

Lepore, J. (2014). The disruption machine. *The New Yorker*. Retrieved from https://www .newyorker.com/magazine/2014/06/23/the-disruption-machine

Marx, K. (1852). *The Eighteenth Brumaire of Louis Bonaparte*. Retrieved from https:// www.marxists.org/archive/marx/works/download/pdf/18th-Brumaire.pdf

McClintock, N. (2003). *Agroforestry and sustainable resource conservation in Haiti: A case study*. Retrieved from https://projects.ncsu.edu/project/cnrint/Agro/PDFfiles/ HaitiCaseStudy041903.pdf

Merritt, K. L. (2017). *Masterless men: Poor Whites, slavery, and capitalism in the deep south*. Cambridge, UK: Cambridge University Press.

Metzl, J. (2019). *Dying of whiteness: How the politics of racial resentment is killing America's heartland*. New York, NY: Basic Books.

Morrison, S. E. (1942). *Admiral of the ocean sea*. Canada: Little, Brown & Company.

National Center for Health Statistics. (1982). *Health, United States, 1982* [DHHS Pub. No. (PHS) 83-1232]. Washington, DC: U.S. Government Printing Office. Retrieved from https://www.cdc.gov/nchs/data/hus/hus82acc.pdf

National Public Radio. (2009). *New president, new era of responsibility.* Retrieved from https://www.npr.org/templates/transcript/transcript.php?storyId=99634389

Oliver, M., & Shapiro, T. (2006). *Black wealth/White wealth: A new perspective on racial inequality.* New York, NY: Routledge.

Omi, M., & Winant, H. (1994). *Racial formation in the United States: From the 1960s to the 1990s (Critical Social Thought).* Abingdon, Oxford: Routledge.

Ramirez, D., Engel, K., & Tang, T. (2008). Language interpreter utilization in the emergency department setting: A clinical review. *Journal of Health Care for the Poor and Underserved, 19,* 352–362. doi:10.1353/hpu.0.0019

Rudowitz, R., Garfield, R., & Hinton, E. (2019). *10 things to know about Medicaid: Setting the facts straight.* Retrieved from https://www.kff.org/medicaid/issue-brief/10-things-to-know-about-medicaid-setting-the-facts-straight

Schlereth, T. J. (1992). Columbia, Columbus, and Columbianism. *The Journal of American History, 79,* 937–968. doi:10.2307/2080794

Sebelius, K. (2009). *HHS Action Plan to Reduce Racial and Ethnic Health Disparities: A Nation Free of Disparities in Health and Healthcare.* Retrieved from https://www.minorityhealth.hhs.gov/npa/files/Plans/HHS/HHS_Plan_complete.pdf

Sen, A. (1992). *Inequalities reexamined.* Cambridge, MA: Harvard University Press.

Shaw, G. B. (1906). *A doctor's dilemma.* London, UK: The Royal Court Theatre.

Simpson, L. B. (1929). *The encomienda in New Spain: The beginning of Spanish Mexico.* Los Angeles: University of California Press.

Spiro, T., Calsyn, M., & Huelskoetter, T. (2015). *Enough is enough: The time has come to address sky high drug prices.* Retrieved from https://www.americanprogress.org/issues/healthcare/reports/2015/09/18/121153/enough-is-enough

Thornton, R. (1987). *American Indian holocaust and survival: A population history since 1492.* Norman: University of Oklahoma Press.

Tinker, T., & Freeland, M. (2008). Thief, slave trader, murderer: Christopher Columbus and Caribbean Population Decline. *Wicazo Sa Review, 23,* 25–50. Minneapolis: University of Minnesota Press.

Todorov, T. (1999). *The conquest of America: The question of the other.* Norman: University of Oklahoma Press.

Trepagnier, B. (2006). *Silent racism: How well-meaning White people perpetuate the racial divide.* Boulder, CO: Paradigm Publishers.

Washington, H. (2006). *Medical apartheid: The dark history of medical experimentation on Black Americans from colonial times to the present.* New York, NY: Doubleday.

Wilkerson, I. (2010). *The warmth of other suns.* New York, NY: Random House.

Williams, D., Lavizzo-Mourey, R., & Warren, R. A. (1994). The concept of race and health status in America. *Public Health Reports, 109,* 26–41. Retrieved from https://www.ncbi.nlm.nih.gov/pmc/articles/PMC1402239

Williams, D., & Mohammed, S. A. (2009). Discrimination and racial disparities in health: Evidence and needed research. *Journal of Behavioral Medicine, 32,* 20–47. doi:10.1007/s10865-008-9185-0

U.S. Census Bureau. (2018). *Annual estimates of the resident population: April 1, 2010 to July 1, 2018: 2018 population estimates.* Retrieved from https://factfinder.census.gov/faces/tableservices/jsf/pages/productview.xhtml?pid=PEP_2018_PEPANNRES&src=pt

Pathways to Achieving Health Equity: Exemplars of Community and Intersectoral Partnerships

Raj C. Shah and Heather Miller

CHAPTER OBJECTIVES

- ⊙ Describe why community-engaged, intersectoral partnerships are considered important in achieving health equity
- ⊙ Examine models for pathways in which community-engaged, intersectoral partnerships can achieve health equity
- ⊙ Provide exemplars of how nursing has utilized components of community-engaged, intersectoral partnership models to foster health equity

KEY CONCEPTS

Health	Intersectoral partnerships
Health equity	Health in All Policies

KEY TERMS

Models	Leadership
Nursing	Collaboration
Mission	Additive results
Financial resources	Synergistic results
Partner resources	Antagonistic results

■ Introduction

WHY IS HEALTH EQUITY IMPORTANT?

"Health" is defined not just as the absence of disease or infirmity, but rather as "a state of complete physical, mental, and social well-being" (World Health Organization [WHO], n.d., para. 1). "Health equity" is commonly defined as the "attainment of the highest level of health for all people" (Office of Disease Prevention and Health Promotion [ODPHP], n.d.-a). However, why is health equity an important, multidimensional concept? As articulated by Nobel Prize economist Amartya Sen,

> Any conception of social justice that accepts the need for a fair distribution as well as efficient formation of human capabilities cannot ignore the role of health in human life

and the opportunities that persons, respectively, have to achieve good health – free from escapable illness, avoidable afflictions and premature mortality. Equity in the achievement and distribution of health gets, thus, incorporated and embedded in a larger understanding of justice. (2002, p. 660)

Social determinants are the conditions in which we live, work, and grow (Solar & Irwin, 2010). One schematic of determinants of health is shown in Figure 15.1, where the area of each concept box represents the potential magnitude of its potential impact and the number of embedded boxes represents how many potential pathways are required for the concept to influence health. The social determinants of health (ODPHP, n.d.-b) concept posits that social environment plays a significant role in determining an individual's overall health and well-being; however, the pathway to health is more complex. Social environments are shaped through choices made about how resources are shared among people in a society. The process of making and enforcing decisions is known as the structural determinants. Written and unwritten rules form the gradients of distribution of money, power, and resources (Osypuk, Joshi, Geronimo, & Acevedo-Garcia, 2014). Today, an inequitable distribution of resources exists among diverse and vulnerable populations (Braveman et al., 2011).

This inequitable distribution of resources has led to higher rates of morbidity and mortality in vulnerable groups and is termed health disparities (Deatrick et al., 2009; Dobal, Wesley, Gulstone, Archer, & Elias, 2017; ODPHP, n.d.-a). When health disparities are avoidable and unjust (Healthy People 2020, 2019; Wilkinson & Marmot, 2005), they are called health inequities. Addressing these avoidable inequities is a key method to achieving health equity (ODPHP, n.d.-a).

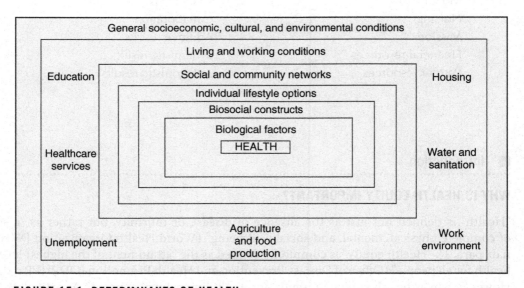

FIGURE 15.1 DETERMINANTS OF HEALTH.

Source: Data from Dahlgren, G., & Whitehead, M. (1991). *Policies and strategies to promote social equity in health.* Stockholm, Sweden: Institute for Futures Studies.

WHY ARE INTERSECTORAL PARTNERSHIPS CONSIDERED IMPORTANT FOR ACHIEVING HEALTH EQUITY?

Public sectors outside the health system continue to influence the health of populations and contribute to health inequities. Sectors include, but are not limited to, education, employment, housing, transportation, policy makers, and business (ODPHP, n.d.-b). These inequities require the health sector to engage in intersectoral partnerships to address the many interrelated factors that determine health.

"Intersectoral action" is defined as actions affecting health outcomes "undertaken by sectors outside the health sector, possibly, but not necessarily, in collaboration with the health sector" (Public Health Agency of Canada & WHO, 2008 p. 2,). The purpose of intersectoral action on health is to engage all viable stakeholders in the process of improving health and health equity, by considering multiple characteristics, such as politics, culture, and economics (Weinstein, Geller, Negussie, & Baciu, 2017).

As a pathway to achieving health equity, partnering with sectors outside the health system aids in a "Health in All Policies" (HiAP) approach. HiAP is an approach that can target root causes for health disparities and affect optimum health outcomes. HiAP is an integrative and collaborative strategy that recognizes health equity as multifaceted, and partners with multiple public sectors to consider the implications of policy-making processes to improve the health of all communities (Rudolph, Caplan, Ben-Moshe, & Dillon, 2013; WHO, 2013).

WHY IS NURSING RELEVANT IN ACHIEVING HEALTH EQUITY THROUGH INTERSECTORAL PARTNERSHIPS?

The profession of nursing in rooted in science, compassion, and advocacy. Nurses play a unique role in healthcare systems. The nursing profession accepts responsibility for improving healthcare delivery systems by treating persons with illnesses holistically and by influencing policy change. In 2011, the Institute of Medicine report, *The Future of Nursing: Leading Change, Advancing Health*, identified the fundamental role of nurses and their impact on transforming healthcare systems in order to improve the lives of their patients. Specifically, this report addressed the part nurses play in setting forth pivotal objectives in the 2010 Affordable Care Act (Altman, Stith Butler, & Shern, 2016). As stated in the report, "nurses should be full partners, with physicians and other health care professionals, in redesigning health care in the United States" (p. 189). Nurses possess the firsthand knowledge and training required to assess the needs of diverse populations and to develop collaborative partnerships in order to achieve health and wellness goals.

Being at the forefront of healthcare systems, nurses are best suited to lead health equity initiatives by establishing intersectoral partnerships. The American Association of Colleges of Nursing has specified the curriculum guidelines of nursing education to include a nurse's role in interprofessional education, cultural competency, and population health (Mezibov, 2000). These competencies are necessary for recognizing the needs that persist in diverse communities and for obtaining the knowledge to transform health through collaborative approaches. As advocates and educators, nurses provide insight on how health policy affects health equity.

WHAT ARE THE OBJECTIVES OF THIS CHAPTER?

This chapter builds on the themes of health, health equity, and intersectoral partnerships as they pertain to nursing professionals. First, the concept of intersectoral partnerships is described along with theoretical frameworks to describe how intersectoral partnerships work. A more in-depth analysis of one of the most studied models, the Bergen Model of Collaborative Functioning, is provided. In order to show the components of the Bergen Model in action, real-world exemplars are provided. Last, the importance of understanding and implementing intersectoral collaboration for nursing health professionals is examined.

◼ Intersectoral Partnership

WHAT IS THE DEFINITION OF INTERSECTORAL PARTNERSHIP?

One of the difficulties in understanding the concept of intersectoral partnership is that multiple terms have been used in the literature historically and contemporaneously to refer to the same concept. In this chapter, as in a recent review (Corbin, Jones, & Barry, 2018), "partnership" is utilized to encompass an arrangement where organizations and/or people join together to promote health. The partnership often is qualified as "collaborative" or "intersectoral," which are sometimes used interchangeably, but are different. A collaborative partnership could include persons or groups of a similar background, while an intersectoral partnership represents a recognized relationship between parts of different sectors of society that has been formed to take action on an issue to achieve health outcomes in a way that may be more effective, efficient, or sustainable than might be achieved by the health sector acting alone. As described by Roussos and Fawcett (2000), the broad aim of intersectoral partnership for community health is to improve population-level health. Intersectoral partnerships have been viewed as a public health practice to address the social determinants of health in order to reduce health inequities. Forming partnerships with governmental and nongovernmental sectors can lead to the formation of healthy policies and programs that target health equity (Newman, Baum, Javanparast, O'Rourke, & Carlon, 2015; Ndumbe-Eyoh & Moffatt, 2013).

> *An intersectoral partnership represents a recognized relationship between parts of different sectors of society that has been formed to take action on an issue to achieve health outcomes in a way that may be more effective, efficient, or sustainable than might be achieved by the health sector acting alone.*

WHAT ARE THE THEORETICAL MODELS FOR UNDERSTANDING INTERSECTORAL PARTNERSHIP?

In 2016, the Institute for Healthcare Improvement (IHI) published *Achieving Health Equity: A Guide for Health Care Organizations* (Wyatt, Laderman, Botwinick, Mate, & Whittington, 2016). This guide does not focus on describing health equity as an issue, but rather, focuses on identifying frameworks for achieving health equity within healthcare organizations. Some of these recommendations include, but are not limited to, ensuring health equity is a strategic priority, disseminating specific strategies to address the multiple determinants of health on which healthcare organizations can have a direct impact, decreasing institutional racism within the organization, and developing partnerships with community organizations to improve health and equity (Wyatt et al., 2016).

Three assumptions underlying the rationale for choosing intersectoral partnerships as a solution are (a) the goal cannot be reached by a single individual or group, (b) diversity of individuals and groups leads to more impactful solutions, and (c) shared interests among the participants make consensus on a solution or set of solutions possible (Roussos & Fawcett, 2000). Most work on understanding intersectoral partnerships has been based on analysis of particular cases with a range of variables suggested to explain why things worked based on the context of the case (Kegler & Swan, 2011). While such models may work for the particular case, they do not always enable the development and application of universal theoretical frameworks that can be tested in understanding multiple intersectoral partnerships. Theoretical models are important for a deeper understanding of intersectoral collaboration and for organizing empirical research (Kegler & Swan, 2011).

Currently, no universally agreed-upon theory of intersectoral collaboration exists; however, multiple frameworks have been proposed (Corbin et al., 2018). Table 15.1 describes the attributes of a select group of frameworks for intersectoral partnership that are based on theory with some empirical testing. While all the models depict how intersectoral partnership can lead to outcomes, they differ in the concepts and relationships of key inputs, activities, and outputs.

Of the frameworks described, the Bergen Model of Collaborative Functioning (Corbin & Mittelmark, 2008) has been the most evaluated (Corbin et al., 2018). The Bergen Model has been utilized by researchers to frame collaborative working arrangements, to guide practice, and to be an evaluation tool. A unique feature of the model is its focus on the impact of positive and negative interactions on the collaborative process. As depicted in Figure 15.2, the Bergen Model organizes collaborative function through a series of bidirectional, iterative interactions between inputs, collaborative processes, and outputs. The cyclical rather than linear process documents how complexity can be generated in intersectoral partnerships. The inputs include (a) a mission/purpose, (b) partnership resources, and (c) financial resources, which lead to the recruitment of additional inputs. As the inputs enter the collaborative realm, they can interact positively or negatively with the defined collaborative elements of leadership, communication, and structure/roles. The interactions influence the activities of planning for maintenance of the intersectoral partnership and the products that are generated through the collaborative effort.

The novel feature of the Bergen Model is that it incorporates a broader set of potential outcomes. The Bergen Model recognizes that the model could just result in additive effects (i.e., the sum of the effects of each sector in the collaboration) or could even result in antagonistic effects, where the collaborative generates less than what could have been done if the sectors continued to work without intersectoral collaboration. Finally, the desired outcome would be synergistic effects, where the collaborative work multiplies the impact of what would have occurred if each sector worked on its own. The outputs then feed back into the inputs and collaborative work as another level of interactions that add to the dynamic nature of the system. The dynamics and complexity make it sometimes very difficult to predict the outcomes of a particular intersectoral partnership to address a particular issue in a particular context; however, this property reflects better what happens in the real world.

TABLE 15.1 COMPARISON OF SELECT THEORETICAL MODELS FOR INTERSECTORAL PARTNERSHIPS

CHARACTERISTIC	MODEL			
TITLE	PARTNERSHIP SYNERGY	COMMUNITY COALITION ACTION THEORY (GROUP LEVEL MODEL)	BERGEN MODEL OF COLLABORATIVE FUNCTIONING	HEALTHY ALLIANCES
Reference	Lasker, Weiss, and Miller, (2001)	Butterfoss et al. (1996)	Corbin and Mittelmark (2008)	Koelen, Vaandrager, and Wagemakers (2012)
Key output(s)	Effectiveness	Committee satisfaction	Additive results	Health/Social outcomes
		Quality of work product	Synergy	
			Antagonistic results	
Key input(s)	None identified	Leadership roles	Mission	Lead agency
		Staff–committee relations	Partner resources	Coalition membership
		Organizational climate	Financial resources	Leadership and staffing
		Decision-making influence		Structures
		Community linkages		Processes
Key activity(ies)	Functioning	Participating	Maintaining	Synergizing
	Synergizing		Planning	Engaging
			Producing	Pooling resources
Interplay between input(s), activity(ies), and output(s)	Unidirectional and only horizontal	Unidirectional from inputs to activities but bidirectional between processes and outcomes	Bidirectional with inputs, activities, and outputs.	Unidirectional from inputs to activities to outputs; bidirectional within inputs and within activities

WHAT ARE REAL-WORLD EXAMPLES OF NURSING INVOLVEMENT IN INTERSECTORAL PARTNERSHIPS?

Nursing care extends beyond what is traditionally perceived in hospitals. The nursing profession is ubiquitous as nursing presence is found at many levels of community-based settings. Community health nurses deliver care in many environments such as schools, businesses, community organizations, and home-care agencies. Nurses

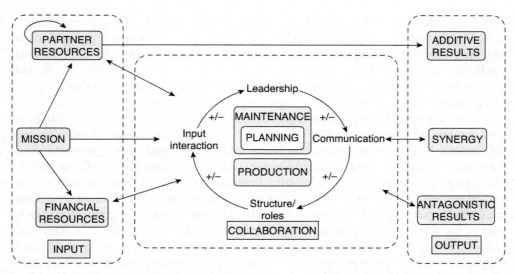

FIGURE 15.2 THE COMPONENTS OF THE BERGEN MODEL OF COLLABORATIVE FUNCTIONING.

Source: Data from Corbin, J. H., & Mittelmark, M. B. (2008). Partnership lessons from the Global Programme for Health Promotion Effectiveness: A case study. *Health Promotion International, 23*(4), 365–371. doi:10.1093/heapro/dan029

recognize that implementing a healthy lifestyle where one lives, works, and plays is crucial for preventive care initiatives. Nurses meet individuals where they are and integrate health strategies into their settings to achieve a more realistic means of improving health. In this section, national and local exemplars are provided with an emphasis on projects that included nursing participation.

National Intersectoral Collaboration

An illustration of this strategy was revealed through the partnership between the Robert Wood Johnson Foundation (RWJF), AARP, and AARP's foundation to form the Future of Nursing: Campaign for Action (https://campaignforaction.org). The purpose of this initiative is to transform health, healthcare, and build a healthier America through nursing advancement and leadership by addressing seven major issues: (a) improving access to care, (b) fostering interprofessional collaboration, (c) promoting nursing leadership, (d) transforming nursing education, (e) increasing diversity in nursing, (f) collecting workforce data, and (g) building healthier communities. As mentioned previously, this initiative works toward goals recommended by the Institute of Medicine (2011) report, *The Future of Nursing: Leading Change, Advancing Health.* Campaign for Action works on a community level to form intersectoral partnerships with local organizations in hopes of achieving health equity.

Another illustration focused on targeting population outcomes with nursing leadership is the Housing First movement work in Canada. The Housing First movement developed in New York City in the 1990s and was based on the principle that immediate provision of housing to homeless persons with mental health conditions followed by wraparound support services would be more effective than the traditional "treatment first, then housing" model (Tsemberis, Gulcur, & Nakae, 2004). In

2008, the federal government of Canada allocated 110 million Canadian dollars to the Mental Health Commission of Canada (MHCC) to undertake a research demonstration project to examine if the Housing First approach could work in Canada. Paula Goering, RN, PhD, an affiliate scientist at the Centre for Addiction and Mental Health and a professor at the University of Toronto Department of Psychiatry, was a coprincipal investigator for the design, implementation, and dissemination of the At Home/Chez Soi project (Goering et al., 2011). In order to conduct the randomized, controlled pragmatic field trial, the project team built relationships with over 200 mental health service providers along with 260 landlords and property management companies in five cities and more than 1,200 housing units (Geller, 2014). Then, engagement with criminal justice organizations, street-based homeless support providers, and hospital systems was needed to identify 2,148 homeless or housing unstable participants with mental health needs who were willing to consent to be part of the demonstration project. In the project, 1,158 individuals were eventually randomized to the usual care mechanism with information provided about local supports or the intervention arm of the study, where persons would be immediately placed in housing by paying for some of the rent with the remainder being paid to the landlords by the MHCC. Then, based on the severity rating of their mental health condition, wraparound support services through case managers at a staff-to-participant ratio of 1:16 were provided as intensive case management or as assertive community treatment with a staff-to-participant ratio of 1:10 with a psychiatrist, nurse, and peer specialist team. Over 2 years, 62% of participants in the Housing First intervention arm remained housed for the entire period while only 31% in the treatment-as-usual group did (Stergiopoulos et al., 2015). The intervention group also had less use of EDs and police detentions during the period with an average savings to the system of over 21,000 Canadian dollars per person with high needs and almost 5,000 Canadian dollars per person for moderate needs. Even though the study period ended in 2013, the housing and support activities provided by the intersectoral partnerships in all five test cities continued at most of the partners (Nelson et al., 2017). The model is being expanded for implementation in other places within and outside of Canada.

Local Intersectoral Collaboration

Academic medical institutions have been implementing faculty practice initiatives into their College of Nursing training programs. Implementing nursing faculty into local community settings empowers clinicians to form collaborative partnerships with community organizations to provide quality, evidence-based care to diverse communities and vulnerable populations, while educating student nurses on the significance of health implementation on a community level. In order to connect theory to practice, the exemplars that are provided highlight the key process steps and outcomes described in the Bergen Model. While recognizing that many other exemplars exist, these exemplars were selected to highlight multiple engagements with varied outcomes even a single entity can experience.

Rush College of Nursing Office of Faculty Practice, an extension of Rush University Medical Center (Chicago, Illinois), continues to care for underserved populations to advance the practice of health equity. The Office of Faculty Practice has formed partnerships with over 30 community organizations to provide excellent nursing services to those who need it most. By collaborating with sectors outside the health system,

Rush faculty practice clinicians have been able to target populations who commonly lack access to quality evidence-based health services. A person's living environment is a determinant of health, and homelessness contributes to poor health outcomes. Therefore, Rush Nursing Faculty Practice has identified housing as an important sector with which to partner in achieving health equity. Rush Nursing Faculty Practice has partnered with organizations such as North Side Housing and Support Services (see Exemplar 15.1). At North Side Housing, a Rush nurse provides health education, resources, and direct nursing care services for individuals who have or are currently experiencing homelessness. In addition to health services, North Side Housing connects the homeless populations with case managers who assist in providing comprehensive services. A Day Support Service Center has been initiated to connect those struggling to sectors that are crucial for one's health and economic stability; this includes housing, employment, and food services. Collaboration between sectors contributes to the goal of improving the lives of homeless persons by addressing the interrelated factors that determine health outcomes.

As described in Exemplar 15.2, the Rush Nursing Faculty Practice has also partnered with Flying Food Group, an airline catering company. The partnership integrated a nurse-managed clinic into the Flying Food Group corporation to provide urgent and primary care services to those working in their production kitchen. After performing a needs assessment and determining the workers were primarily low-income, faced cultural barriers, and had multiple chronic illnesses, Faculty Practice nurse practitioners began providing care that allowed for easy access to healthcare services. The "in-work" clinic benefited workers by contributing to continuity of care without having to jeopardize income by taking time off work. Employment means more than just financial stability; it is also crucial in maintaining proper health. The RWJF (2013) discusses the link between employment and health, and the challenges that persist beyond the loss of income. Unemployed Americans face many negative health effects including stress-related illnesses such as stroke, heart attack, heart disease, and depression. Additionally, many people are employed but are classified as the "working poor." This population also faces challenges in gaining access to proper health services. Similar to Rush Faculty Practice and Flying Food Group, the RWJF recognizes the benefits health promotion strategies have on both employees and business owners. Improving health

---

EXEMPLAR 15.1 North Side Housing and Supportive Services: Aligned Mission

Rush College of Nursing Office of Faculty Practice has partnered with North Side Housing and Supportive Services to provide comprehensive quality care to those experiencing homelessness. By comparing the collaborative partnership to the Bergen Model of Collaborative Functioning, it provides an analytical framework for examining the factors that contribute to effective, sustainable, and successful partnerships. The Office of Faculty Practice was able to identify factors that led the effective partnership. An *aligned mission* to serve vulnerable populations in a community-based setting played a key role in forming the partnership. Faculty Practice and North Side Housing missions were to provide and improve health for the homeless population by rendering comprehensive supportive services including integrating nursing education and clinical practice into care.

EXEMPLAR 15.2 Flying Food Group: Financial and Partner Resources

Rush College of Nursing Office of Faculty Practice have partnered with Flying Food Group to provide health services for individuals working for their company. By comparing the partnership to the Bergen Model of Collaborative Functioning, it provides information on components of the effective partnership. Flying Food Group's contribution to *financial resources* sustained funding for an environment, equipment, and staffing to deliver urgent and primary care health services. The Office of Faculty Practice provided *partner resources* that included excellent quality and evidence-based nursing services to meet health needs of the company.

---

and safety not only contributes to the well-being of employees but saves the business money. The RWJF (2013) found workplace health programs reduce sick leave, health plan costs, worker compensation, and disability costs by about 25%.

In Exemplar 15.3, the Rush Office of Faculty Practice identified similar elements that have led to synergistic outcomes (increased health outcomes) such as partner and financial resources, building trust, and frequent and meaningful communication in work between a state government department and a community-based mental health services provider. While there are many factors that influence positive collaborations, elements also can lead to failure of partnerships (see Exemplar 15.4 for interactions between healthcare delivery providers and school systems). Some of these elements included: (a) missions becoming misaligned, (b) poor communication, and (c) lack of structure. Many times this can lead to antagonistic results and result in a loss of time, money, and resources. Although antagonistic results are seen as negative, some partnerships may see this outcome to be a learning experience. Determining what factors contributed to the antagonistic outcomes can help in the design and operation of future intersectoral partnerships.

EXEMPLAR 15.3. Trilogy Behavioral Healthcare: Synergistic Results

In 2012, the U.S. Supreme Court ruled that individuals with mental illness have the moral right to live and thrive in the community with supportive services. This formed the Colbert Consent decree that allowed individuals living in institutions for mental disease (IMDs) to leave long-term nursing facilities and live a more independent lifestyle with the support of community-based health workers. The State of Illinois Department of Healthcare and Family Services formed a partnership with Trilogy Behavioral Health Care to carry out the Colbert class member program. Through the Bergen Model of Collaborative Functioning, *synergistic results* were identified as a significant factor in the success of the partnership. Trilogy Behavioral Healthcare and the State of Illinois collaborated to provide key resources such as social work, counseling, wellness, and recovery programs. These resources contributed to developing skills and achieving health goals during the transition from IMDs to a more independent community-based lifestyle. By utilizing these resources, the partnership is able to achieve yearly goals to move individuals out of the IMDs into the community for independent living.

EXEMPLAR 15.4 School-Based Clinics: Antagonistic Results

Rush University Medical Center has partnered with Chicago Public Schools to operate school-based health centers (SBHCs) for the provision of nurse-managed primary and mental health services to socially disadvantaged students. The SBHC model is designed to achieve health equity by providing safe and convenient access to quality, evidence-based healthcare to students experiencing health disparities. In these sites, nurse practitioners provide billable preventive and primary health-care services such as physical examinations, immunizations, and care for chronic conditions like asthma. Nurses partner with the school to provide schoolwide health education and programming. Comparing this partnership to the Bergen Model of Collaborative Functioning, Rush was able to identify both positive and negative outputs of partner processes. "Antagonistic results" were described as termination of established programs due to unpredictable school administration changes that resulted in decreased awareness of the SBHC services. This in turn resulted in decreased productivity and insurance reimbursements, jeopardizing SBHC financial sustainability. Rush was able to respond to this antagonistic result by recognizing the need to establish ongoing, structured communication between partners and increasing SBHC staff ability to adapt to the priorities of school administrators.

WHAT IS KNOWN ABOUT INTERSECTORAL COLLABORATION IN ACHIEVING BETTER HEALTH OUTCOMES?

Fundamentally, intersectoral collaboration becomes an option when the complex problem cannot be resolved by the work of a single sector such as healthcare (Bryson, Crosby, & Stone, 2006). Partnering with other groups outside of health sector is hypothesized to result in better health outcomes (Corbin, 2017). While the concept of intersectoral partnership has become an increasingly popular strategy, studies are limited regarding the impact of intersectoral action on addressing social determinants and on improving health and health equity (Ndumbe-Eyoh & Moffatt, 2013) or public policy (Chircop, Bassett, & Taylor, 2014). These initial conclusions were again confirmed in a review of 26 studies on the topic of what constitutes effective and influential partnerships (Corbin et al., 2018). While the authors identified nine key elements that can guide a positive partnership process (see Box 15.1), the authors still concluded that there was limited empirical evidence about different types of intersectoral partnerships in achieving health outcomes and that more process-focused and outcomes-oriented research was needed to truly understand the key features that enable the achievement of synergistic outcomes rather than additive or antagonistic outcomes (Corbin et al., 2018). However, intersectoral action is still seen as a key strategy in addressing health equity. The absence of strong documentation, especially for structural determinants of health interventions, does not necessarily mean that intersectoral partnerships cannot be effective (Ndumbe-Eyoh & Moffatt, 2013). Rather, the lack of resounding evidence may be due to the difficulty in measuring outcomes from complex and dynamic system changes that intersectoral partnerships attempt to create, especially as the interventions are more upstream to the access to healthcare delivery systems (Ndumbe-Eyoh & Moffatt, 2013).

> **Box 15.1: Core Properties of the Bergen Model for Collaborative Functioning**
>
> Develop a shared mission aligned to the partners' individual or institutional goals
>
> Include a broad range of participation from diverse partners and a balance of human and financial resources
>
> Incorporate leadership that inspires trust, confidence, and inclusiveness
>
> Monitor how communication is perceived by partners and adjust accordingly
>
> Balance formal and informal roles/structures depending on mission
>
> Build trust between partners from the beginning and for the duration of the partnership
>
> Ensure balance between maintenance and production activities
>
> Consider the impact of political, economic, cultural, social, and organizational contexts
>
> Evaluate partnerships for continuous improvement

■ Conclusion

The American Association of Colleges of Nursing includes healthcare policy and advocacy as essentials in nursing practice. As experts in health determinants, nurses are empowered to be creative in their practice in order to treat individuals holistically and reach wellness goals. Through comprehensive and critical assessments, nurses are leaders in determining factors that influence individuals' overall well-being and implement processes to alleviate harmful barriers. The knowledge, skills, and training nurses possess in assessing the needs of communities contribute to the nurse's role in implementing collaborative partnerships in achieving health equity. By working to change the underlying social conditions that lead to poor health outcomes, nursing is influential at many levels of policy. Nursing's knowledge and skills facilitate effective partnerships by collaborating across all sectors to provide education on healthy public policies.

Nursing collaboration within intersectoral partnerships can exert influence at multiple policy levels, including (a) structural, living, and working conditions; (b) community; and (c) individual interventions (Lathrop, 2013). By providing a scientific interpretation on how policies affect communities and contribute to poor health outcomes, nurses advocate for population groups on a national level. Nursing can promote policy changes by educating policy makers on health disparities seen across the socioeconomic gradient. Influencing sectors to implement economic strategies to promote health equity fits the nursing roles of being an educator and an advocate.

For example, nurses advocating for improved education policy also aid in the quest to achieve health equity. Providing knowledge and research surrounding health disparities between educational levels promotes sectors to consider restructuring policies that integrate an HiAP approach such as increasing access to college education for those who are experiencing poverty (Adler & Stewart, 2007).

Nursing must continue to educate legislators, policy makers, and those whose decisions impact greatly on communities. Additionally, nurses partnering with sectors such as the business sector can contribute to policies in favor of healthy working environments. Healthy workplaces decrease chronic stress, work injury, and/or environmental toxin exposure (Lathrop, 2013). Initiating health promotion strategies such as workplace wellness programs can also be implemented by nursing staff. Studies have shown employers save an average of $6 for every $1 spent on workplace wellness programs (RWJF, 2013). This proves that health and safety benefits both employee and business owners.

HOW CAN STUDENTS USE WHAT IS KNOWN TO DATE IN APPLYING INTERSECTORAL PARTNERSHIPS IN ACHIEVING HEALTH EQUITY IN THEIR CAREERS?

The nursing profession has been challenged to be a leader in achieving health equity. Nursing will need to move beyond direct care within hospital systems and focus on improving health collectively through collaboration, advocacy, political involvement, and education (Lathrop, 2013). In order to continue the quest to achieve health equity, nursing education will need to be restructured. Understanding and remaining updated on healthcare policy is fundamental for nursing leadership.

Health outcomes can be best understood through analyzing social, economic, and environmental relations. With focusing on a comprehensive approach to care, policy making that pertains to addressing social determinants of health to improve health equity should include the contribution of nurses.

Nurse educators must prepare nursing students for political participation. The nursing profession needs to restructure education to require a greater understanding of political competence. This training should include the influence of policy on community structures and social processes. As advocates for health equity, nursing students need to prepare for political involvement by developing policy analysis skills, and learning the processes of challenging the health system through political, social, economic, and environmental involvement (Association of State and Territorial Directors of Nursing, 2009). Many ways exist for the political development of nurses. One method is a staged approach where political development is achieved over time. The approach suggests health policy should be a stand-alone class in addition to greater discussion on the integration of health policy into other curriculum courses. Nurse faculty also must act as role models demonstrating the importance of health policy and engaging in activity. Nursing students will need to learn how to collaborate with sectors outside the health system in order to interpret the influence political, social, economic, and environmental factors have on health and healthcare (Box 15.2).

Box 15.2: Key Nursing Roles in Utilizing Intersectoral Partnerships for Health Equity

Key Points
- The nursing profession requires a greater understanding of the health implications of policies made by nonhealth sectors.
- Nursing contribution to intersectoral partnership requires improving health collectively through collaboration, advocacy, political involvement, and education.

WHAT ARE THE AVENUES OF FUTURE RESEARCH THAT NURSES CAN LEAD IN ACHIEVING HEALTH EQUITY THROUGH INTERSECTORAL PARTNERSHIPS TO ADDRESS CURRENT UNDERSTANDING GAPS?

Based on the available systematic reviews of the literature about intersectoral collaboration and health equity outcomes, much work remains in designing evaluation methods that capture the dynamics of complex interventions such as intersectoral collaboration. For intersectoral collaboration projects involving the nursing profession, more has to be done to document these projects in the scientific and general literature so that the entire community can learn about the design, implementation, and outcomes of these activities.

Improving health and health equity can be done through rigorous evaluation of what does and does not work in current policy and practice (Association of State and Territorial Directors of Nursing, 2009). Nurses must be aware of policies and opportunities to improve programs and health services for the populations served. Nurses must be trained and supported in using their knowledge and skills to lead the movement around researching effective ways to address health equity. Applying research findings to advocate for new health policies is fundamental in organizing health promotion initiatives (Mahony & Jones, 2013).

■ Critical Thinking Exercise

1. As a nurse working in the Chicago Department of Public Health on child lead exposure, you have been approached to participate with community organizations in developing the 5-year public health community health needs assessment and community health implementation plan to follow from the 2013 Healthy Chicago 2.0 plan (see www.cityofchicago.org/content/dam/city/depts/cdph/CDPH/Healthy%20Chicago/HC2.0Upd4152016.pdf). Since the plan was made, there have been studies of water in the schools and parks that have found elevated lead levels. The community is concerned and wants solutions. The public health department would like to continue the approach of achieving goals using a health equity lens. How would you build a strong intersectoral partnership to reduce the likelihood of children developing elevated lead levels through drinking water exposure in public areas such as schools and parks?

2. A recent community health needs assessment uncovered that life expectancy is 85 years in Chicago's downtown Loop but plummets to age 69 in West Garfield Park, located on the West Side of Chicago. This 16-year gap cannot be explained solely by a lack of access to healthcare, as academic health centers, safety-net hospitals, and federally qualified health centers are widespread across Chicago's West Side. Moreover, a growing body of scientific evidence shows that the fundamental causes of many illnesses that shorten life expectancy are rooted in social forces such as education, employment, food access, violence, and transportation. To address these social determinants of health, a new place-based, cross-sector collaborative is launched—West Side United (WSU; westsideunited.org). WSU focuses on the roles that education, economic vitality, healthcare, and the neighborhood or physical environment play on health outcomes. The collaborative includes six health institutions, community-based organizations, local government, residents, and other stakeholders. WSU has announced several initiatives to address disparities that

lead to poor life expectancy outcomes, including developing a community health strategy to identify gaps in care and access. WSU analyzed quantitative health outcomes data and interviewed 20 community health leaders from hospitals, federally qualified health centers, and social services organizations. Based on analysis of health outcomes on the West Side and the gaps identified through stakeholder interviews, the Steering Committee identified five priority morbidity disparities:

1. Maternal/child health
2. Childhood asthma
3. Behavioral health
4. Hypertension management
5. Healthy eating and active lifestyle

What role could nurses play to help build out the community health strategy with these priorities? Which priority would you address first and what intersectoral partnerships would you need to help develop and implement interventions for that priority?

■ Discussion Questions

1. Intersectoral partnerships have been hypothesized to be an important component for achieving health equity. Describe the evidence for or against this hypothesis.
2. Compare and contrast the Bergen Model of Collaborative Functioning for intersectoral partnerships with one other model. What are the strengths of the Bergen Model and what are the weaknesses?
3. Give one example of nursing involvement in community, intersectoral partnerships for achieving health equity.

■ Resources

Carnegie, E., & Kiger, A. (2009). Being and doing politics: An outdated model or 21st century reality. *Journal of Advanced Nursing, 65*(9), 1976–1984. doi:10.1111/j.1365 -2648.2009.05084.x

Corbin, J. H. (2017). Health promotion, partnership and intersectoral action. *Health Promotion International, 32,* 923–929. doi:10.1093/heapro/dax084

Corbin, J. H., Jones, J., & Barry, M. B. (2018). What makes intersectoral partnerships for health promotion work? A review of the international literature. *Health Promotion International, 33,* 4–26. doi:10.1093/heapro/daw061

Gilles, P. (1998). Effectiveness of alliances and partnerships for health promotion. *Health Promotion International, 13,* 99–120. doi:10.1093/heapro/13.2.99

Jones, J. M. (2011). Record 64% rate honesty, ethics of members of Congress low, ratings of nurses, pharmacists, and medical doctors most positive. *Gallup.* Retrieved from http://www.gallup.com/poll/151460/record-rate-honesty-ethics-members -congress-low.aspx

Kegler, M. C., & Swan, D. W. (2011). An initial attempt at operationalizing and testing the Community Coalition Action Theory. *Health Education & Behavior, 38*(3), 261–270. doi:10.1177/1090198110372875

Koelen, M. A., Vaandrager, L., & Wagemakers, A. (2012). The healthy alliances (HALL) framework: prerequisites for success. *Family Practice, 29*, i132–i138. doi:10.1093/fampra/cmr088

Lasker, R. D., Weiss, E. S., & Miller, R. (2001). Partnership synergy: A practical framework for studying and strengthening the collaborative advantage. *The Milbank Quarterly, 79*(2), 2001. doi:10.1111/1468-0009.00203

Lathrop, B. (2013). Nursing leadership in addressing the social determinants of health. *Policy, Politics, and Nursing Practice, 14*(1), 41–47. doi:10.1177/1527154413489887

■ Acknowledgments

The authors would like to thank Angela Moss, PhD, MSN, APN-BC, RN; Sally Lemke, DNP, APRN, WHNP-BC; and Susan Swider, PhD, PHNA-BC, FAAN, at the Rush University College of Nursing along with Alice Geis, DNP, APN, at the Rush University College of Nursing and Director of Integrated Health at Trilogy, Inc., for sharing real-world exemplars. They also thank Amber Miller, MPH, for providing feedback on improving initial versions of this chapter. The authors also wish to thank Darlene Hightower, JD, Associate Vice President of the Office of Community Engagement and Practice at Rush University Medical Center for sharing the second critical thinking exercise regarding West Side United.

■ Disclosures

Heather Miller is part of the Rush University College of Nursing Office of Faculty Practice Program and is assigned to work at Trilogy, Inc. Raj Shah has no disclosures pertinent to the material presented in this chapter.

■ References

Adler, N., & Stewart, J. (2007). *Reaching for a healthier life: Facts on socioeconomic status and health in the U.S.* Retrieved from https://macses.ucsf.edu/downloads/Reaching_for_a_Healthier_Life.pdf

Altman, S. H., Stith Butler, A., & Shern, L. (Eds.). (2016). *Assessing progress on the Institute of Medicine report* The Future of Nursing. Washington, DC: National Academies Press.

Association of State and Territorial Directors of Nursing. (2009). *The public health nurse's role in achieving health equity: Eliminating inequalities in health* [Position Paper]. Retrieved from http://archive.dialogue4health.org/phip/CHPHLI/PDFs12_13_10/ASTDN_health_equity.pdf

Braveman, P. A., Kumanyika, S., Fielding, J., LaVeist, T., Borrell, L. N., Manderscheid, R., & Troutman, A. (2011). Health disparities and health equity: The issue is justice. *American Journal of Public Health, 101*(Suppl. 1), S149–S155. doi:10.2105/AJPH.2010.300062

Bryson, J. M., Crosby, B. C., & Stone, M. M. (2006). The design and implementation of cross-sector collaborations: Propositions from the literature. *Public Administration Review, 66*, 44–55. doi:10.1111/j.1540-6210.2006.00665.x

Butterfoss, F. D., Goodman, R. M., & Wandersman, A. (1996). Community coalitions for prevention and health promotion: Factors predicting satisfaction, participation, and planning. *Health Education Quarterly, 23*(1), 65–79. doi:10.1177/109019819602300105

Chircop, A., Bassett, R., & Taylor, E. (2014). Evidence on how to practice intersectoral collaboration for health equity: A scoping review. *Critical Public Health, 25*(2), 178–191. doi:10.1080/09581596.2014.887831

Corbin, J. H., & Mittelmark, M. B. (2008). Partnership lessons from the Global Programme for Health Promotion Effectiveness: A case study. *Health Promotion International, 23*(4), 365–371. doi:10.1093/heapro/dan029

Dahlgren, G., & Whitehead, M. (1991). *Policies and strategies to promote social equity in health.* Stockholm, Sweden: Institute for Futures Studies.

Deatrick, J., Lipman, T., Gennaro, S., Sommer, M., de Leon Siantz, M., Mooney-Doyle, K., . . . Jemmott, L. (2009). Fostering health equity: Clinical and research training strategies from nursing education. *The Kouhsiung Journal of Medical Sciences, 25*(9), 479–485. doi:10.1016/S1607-551X(09)70554-6

Dobal, M. T., Wesley, Y., Gulstone, J., Archer, L. C., & Elias, M. (2017) African American nurse leaders and the American public: Do we really understand the healthcare law? *Diversity and Equality in Health and Care, 14*(1), 1–8. doi:10.21767/2049-5471.100085

Geller, L. (2014). Putting housing first. *Canadian Nurse.* Retrieved from https://www.canadian-nurse.com/en/articles/issues/2014/june-2014/putting-housing-first

Goering, P. N., Streiner, D. L., Adair, C., Aubry, T., Barker, J., Distasio, J., . . . Zabkiewicz, D. M. (2011). The At Home/Chez Soi trial protocol: A pragmatic, multisite, randomized controlled trial of a Housing First intervention for homeless individuals with mental illness in 5 Canadian cities. *BMJ Open, 1*(2), e000323. doi:10.1136/bmjopen-2011-000323

Institute of Medicine. (2011). *The future of nursing: Leading change, advancing health.* Washington, DC: National Academies Press.

Mahony, D., & Jones, E. J. (2013). Social determinants of health in nursing education, research, and health policy. *Nursing Science Quarterly, 26*(3), 280–284. doi:10.1177/0894318413489186

Mezibov, D. (2000). The American Association of Colleges of Nursing. *Policy, Politics & Nursing Practice, 1*(2), 139–143. doi:10.1177/152715440000100212

Ndumbe-Eyoh, S., & Moffatt, H. (2013). Intersectoral action for health equity: A rapid systematic review. *Biomedical Central Public Health, 13*, 1056. doi:10.1186/1471-2458-13-1056

Nelson, G., Caplan, R., MacLeod, T., Macnaughton, E., Cherner, R., Aubry, T., . . . Goering, P. (2017). What happens after the demonstration phase? The sustainability of Canada's at home/Chez Soi Housing First programs for homeless persons with mental illness. *American Journal of Community Psychology, 59*(1–2), 144–157. doi:10.1002/ajcp.12119

Newman, L., Baum, F., Javanparast, J., O'Rourke, K., & Carlon, L. (2015). Addressing social determinants of health inequities through settings: A rapid review. *Health Promotion International, 30*, 26–43. doi:10.1093/heapro/dav054

Office of Disease Prevention and Health Promotion. (n.d.-a). *Disparities.* Retrieved from https://www.healthypeople.gov/2020/about/foundation-health-measures/Disparities

Office of Disease Prevention and Health Promotion. (n.d.-b). *Social determinants of health.* Retrieved from https://www.healthypeople.gov/2020/topics-objectives/topic/social-determinants-of-health

Osypuk, T. L., Joshi, P., Geronimo, K., & Acevedo-Garcia, D. (2014). Do social and economic policies influence health? A review. *Current Epidemiology Reports, 1*(3), 149–164. doi:10.1007/s40471-014-0013-5

Public Health Agency of Canada and World Health Organizaton. (2008). *Health equity through intersectoral action: An analysis of 18 country case studies*. Geneva, Switzerland: World Heatlh Organization. Retrieved from http://www.who.int/social_determinants/resources/health_equity_isa_2008_en.pdf

Robert Wood Johnson Foundation. (2013). *How does employment, or unemployment, affect health?* Retrieved from https://www.rwjf.org/en/library/research/2012/12/how-does-employment--or-unemployment--affect-health-.html

Roussos, S. T., & Fawcett, S. B. (2000). A review of collaborative partnerships as a strategy for improving community health. *Annual Review of Public Health, 21*, 369–402. doi:10.1146/annurev.publhealth.21.1.369

Rudolph, L., Caplan, J., Ben-Moshe, K., & Dillon, L. (2013). *Health in all policies: A guide for state and local governments*. Washington, DC and Oakland, CA: American Public Health Association and Public Health Institute.

Sen, A. (2002). Why health equity? *Health Economics, 11*, 659–666. doi:10.1002/hec.762

Solar, O., & Irwin, A. (2010) A conceptual framework for action on the social determinants of health: Social determinants of health discussion paper 2 (Policy and Practice). Geneva, Switzerland: World Health Organization. Retrieved from https://www.who.int/sdhconference/resources/ConceptualframeworkforactiononSDH_eng.pdf

Stergiopoulos, V., Hwang, S. W., Gozdzik, A., Nisenbaum, R., Latimer, E., Rabouin, D., . . . At Home/Chez Soi Investigators. (2015). Effect of scattered-site housing using rent supplements and intensive case management on housing stability among homeless adults with mental illness: A randomized trial. *Journal of the American Medical Association, 313*(9), 905–915. doi:10.1001/jama.2015.1163

Tsemberis, S., Gulcur, L., & Nakae, M. (2004). Housing First, consumer choice, and harm reduction for homeless individuals with a dual diagnosis. *American Journal of Public Health, 94*(4), 651–656. doi:10.2105/AJPH.94.4.651

Weinstein, J. N., Geller, A., Negussie, Y., & Baciu, A. (Eds.). (2017). *Communities in action: Pathways to health equity*. Washington, DC: National Academies Press. doi:10.17226/24624

Wilkinson, R. G., & Marmot, M. G (Eds.). (2005). *Social determinants of health: The solid facts* (2nd ed.). Copenhagen, Denmark: World Health Organization. Retrieved from http://www.euro.who.int/__data/assets/pdf_file/0005/98438/e81384.pdf

World Health Organization. (n.d.). *Constitution*. Retrieved from https://www.who.int/about/who-we-are/constitution

World Health Organization. (2013). *Framework and statement: Consultation on the drafts of the "Health in All Policies Framework for Country Action" for the Conference Statement of 8th Global Conference on Health Promotion*. Retrieved from http://www.healthpromotion2013.org/conference-programme/framework-and-statement

Wyatt, R., Laderman, M., Botwinick, L., Mate, K., & Whittington, J. (2016). *Achieving Health Equity: A Guide for Health Care Organizations* [IHI White Paper]. Cambridge, MA: Institute for Healthcare Improvement. Retrieved from http://www.ihi.org/resources/Pages/IHIWhitePapers/Achieving-Health-Equity.aspx

16 Politics and Law at the Root of Health Equity

Daniel E. Dawes and Nelson J. Dunlap

CHAPTER OBJECTIVES

- ⊙ Expand understanding of health equity through an exploration of its historical context and prioritization via federal public policies
- ⊙ Explain the concept of the political determinants of health and the role of healthcare clinicians in advocating for policy change
- ⊙ Incorporate strategies to meaningfully address health inequities, foster greater interdisciplinary collaborations, and promote health equity by addressing the social and political determinants of health

KEY CONCEPTS

Health equity	Evidence-based
Cultural competency	Mental health equity
Social determinants of health	Immigration
Political determinants of health	Advocacy

KEY TERMS

Equity	Determinants
Disparities	Inequities

■ Introduction

Health equity (World Health Organization [WHO], n.d.-d) and the accompanying fight to ensure that every individual can achieve his or her optimal level of health is shaping up to be one of the defining challenges of our time. As healthcare clinicians, you will be on the proverbial "front lines" of this fight as you interact with a vast assortment of different types of patients on a daily basis. It is because of this direct and continued contact with individuals who actually suffer the ill effects of health inequities that you need to have a working knowledge of what health inequities look like on a practical level. As a nurse, caring for people is not just your job, but it is also a part of who you are as a person. Truly caring for patients goes beyond the four walls of the clinical setting and out into the community where the health issues begin, are perpetuated, and are exacerbated. Once you have a more solid understanding of what health inequities are and what causes them, you will be in a much better position to not only provide your patients with tailored and high-quality care, but you will also be able to ardently advocate on their behalf.

■ Historical Approaches

The U.S. health system is a complicated and sometimes convoluted system that is growing increasingly more complex as the country attempts to move away from a system of disparate parts to one that nudges consumers and clinicians alike toward better health outcomes. However, one of the major barriers to accomplishing this goal is the lingering presence of health disparities. Health disparities are the differences in health and healthcare between population groups (Orgera & Artiga, 2018). It is vital to keep in mind that disparities occur across the life course and in many dimensions, including race/ethnicity, socioeconomic status, age, location, gender, disability status, and sexual orientation. While the mere existence of health disparities has proven historically to be quite the effective barrier to effectuating a significant change in our healthcare system, healthcare clinicians have always played a pivotal role in the fight to address these disparities and will continue to do so for many years to come.

For more than 225 years, the United States has struggled with aligning the constitutional notions of equal protection and general welfare to our health policies, which has resulted in a chasm between researchers and the patients who need their discoveries (Dawes, 2016). Despite this struggle, there have been researchers, clinicians, policy makers, and advocates who have worked assiduously throughout the years to uphold the integrity of scientific research and build longer and stronger bridges to ensure that the discoveries made in a lab, a clinical setting, or in the field translated positively to all communities, including those that have historically been marginalized and underserved such as racial and ethnic minorities, women, children, Veterans, rural individuals, and most recently LGBTQ individuals (Dawes, 2016). The history of policy makers in the United States successfully attempting to address health inequities by legislative means goes back 150 years to after the Civil War, when the federal government attempted to give newly freed slaves access to essential resources such as employment, education, healthcare, and housing. Although that effort ultimately failed after 7 years of opposition in Congress, it set the stage for future attempts.

Most notably, during the 1980s, President Ronald Reagan and his administration were able to accomplish some significant success due in large part to the inclusion of clinicians and researchers. These individuals developed a report that highlighted the latest evidence at that time related to minority health and health disparities. Then Secretary of Health and Human Services, Margaret Heckler, recognized that while the overall health of the nation had been improving, the health status of African Americans and other racial and ethnical minorities was alarming (Heckler, n.d.). As a result of this report, a task force was convened that was charged with taking a closer look at the issue. This marks the first attempt by the federal government to take a comprehensive approach to addressing racial and ethnic disparities. What is most telling is that the groundswell of academic and clinical support that helped push the Reagan administration to take this step came from clinicians who understood the value of addressing health disparities.

Today, the division between those who develop and implement health policies and those whom the health policies impact is narrowing. This is due in large part to the inclusion of researchers, clinicians, and consumers in the policy-making process. Advancing health equity focused policies in America requires both a concerted effort by all involved parties as well as a sense of urgency. The fact of the matter is that in 25 years, racial and ethnic minorities are expected to comprise a majority of the U.S.

population (Colby & Ortman, 2014). This means that the health inequities that have historically been confined to minority populations will soon impact a broad swath of the American patient population. As the healthcare system slowly responds to these trends, it is vital that clinicians fully understand the root causes of inequities, the political determinants of health, as well as their role in addressing them.

■ Political Determinants of Health

Political determinants of health involve the systematic process of structuring relationships, distributing resources, and administering power, operating simultaneously in ways that mutually reinforce each other to shape opportunities that either advance health equity or exacerbate health inequities (Dawes, 2020). Today, we recognize that a variety of forces collectively impact our health and determine our life expectancy, including social, environmental, economic, behavioral health, healthcare, and genetic factors. Too often we stop at those drivers of inequities failing to dig even further to understand the bigger picture. As a result, we miss the link between all of these generally accepted determinants of health and the political determinants of health. These political determinants of health inequitably distribute social, medical, and other determinants, and create structural barriers to equity for population groups that lack power and privilege.

Researchers and clinicians have in recent years increasingly focused their attention on the generally broad social determinants of health, which are "the conditions in which people are born, grow, work, live, and age, and the wider set of forces and systems shaping the conditions of daily life" (WHO, n.d.-c, "What Are Social Determinants of Health?"). Often it is difficult to differentiate whether health inequities originate from political factors or whether the political factors are masked by social factors, but it can no longer be denied that political determinants are the greatest instigator among the "wider set of forces and systems" (WHO, n.d.-c, "What Are Social Determinants of Health?") that have created and exacerbated the inequities in our society.

■ Social Determinants of Health

The Centers for Disease Control and Prevention (CDC) defines social determinants of health as conditions in the places where people live, learn, work, and play that affect a wide range of health risks and outcomes (CDC, n.d.). What this means more practically is that all of the contributing factors that make up a person's life play an outsized role in both his or her health and why you ultimately will be caring for him or her in a clinical setting. It is a fact that poverty places limits on access to safe living communities and healthy foods and that more education is a predictor of better health. If you can improve individual and population health by addressing some of these social determinants of health, you can also advance health equity (Williams, Costa, Odunlami, & Mohammed, 2008). And if you can advance health equity, then you can make a positive and lasting impact on the lives of the patients you treat.

Health inequities present themselves in many various shades of insidious harm. There is behavioral and mental health equity, immigration, and housing mobility just to name a few. The common thread among them all, for the sake of this text, is that they can all be ameliorated by acknowledging and addressing the root causes directly.

■ Mental Health Equity

While we as a society have made significant gains in destigmatizing mental health, there is still a long way to go to elevating mental health to parity with other forms of physical health. Simply stated, mental health is not a fringe issue. Approximately one in five adults in the United States, or 46.6 million people, experiences mental illness in a given year (National Institute of Mental Health [NIMH], 2019). Further, roughly one in five youth aged 13 to 18 experiences a severe mental disorder at some point during his or her life (NIMH, 2019). What these numbers truly show is the prevalence with which any number of your future patients may present with mental health issues. More importantly, they show the increasing number of individuals in our country who struggle with mental health and are also willing to share their experiences with researchers and clinicians alike. This data operates to provide a more complete picture of the mental health landscape in our country, which can then be used to advocate for policy changes.

Communities of color often face significant shortages of behavioral and mental health clinicians, which in turn further exacerbates problems that are associated with seeking care for these mental health issues. A recent *Stress in America* survey released by the American Psychological Association documents the significant needs of many communities of color and highlights the need for both community-based primary prevention and strategies to improve access to mental and behavioral healthcare (American Psychological Association, 2018). There is great potential for partnerships to exist between clinicians and these communities to meet the dire needs of these communities, but in order for these partnerships to come to fruition, there has to be an open line of communication. As nurses, you will often develop a much more personal relationship with those for whom you care as opposed to other types of clinicians with whom they may interact. Understanding the social determinants of health that could be impacting or even exacerbating a patient's mental health disorder may be just the olive branch necessary to build a new bridge to the community.

■ Immigration and Health Equity

According to the Robert Wood Johnson Foundation, "[w]hen people in America are forced to live in fear because of their immigration status, their health and the health of our nation suffer" (Robert Wood Johnson Foundation, n.d., para. 1). The research firmly demonstrates that immigration can and does impact one's health status and bears out that families composed of immigrants often forgo vitally needed social services and healthcare because of fear of interaction with public agencies. This is in spite of the fact that immigrants are often identified as a "vulnerable population"—that is, a group at increased risk for poor physical, psychological, and social health outcomes and inadequate healthcare (Flaskerud & Winslow, 1998). Immigrants comprise a large, and ever-growing, portion of the population. In 2016, more than 43.7 million immigrants resided in the United States, accounting for 13.5% of the total U.S. population

(Zong, Zong, Batalova, & Burrows, 2019). Further, immigrants and their U.S.-born children accounted for approximately 86.5 million people or 27% of the U.S. population in 2017. Immigrants account for a non-insignificant portion of virtually every patient population and their fear-based reluctance to engage with the healthcare system makes them an especially vulnerable population.

What this means for clinicians is that when an immigrant does seek care, there are no safe assumptions to be made with regard to the last time that person sought care or when he or she will seek care again. Cultural competence is the ability to interact effectively with people of different cultures (Substance Abuse and Mental Health Services Administration, 2019). More importantly, cultural competence is a crucial aspect of interacting with immigrant patients. In order to truly provide high-quality care to any and all individuals, regardless of immigration status, you have to understand the background factors that may impact their health status. Being mindful of the hardships that immigrants face goes a long way to accomplish that.

■ Housing

When you think about where you live, do you also think about how that impacts your health? If you do not, you are not alone. It most likely just means that you have been fortunate enough to not be forced to consider the impact that housing, or lack thereof, may have on your health status. However, insufficient housing quality is associated with stress and mental health (WHO, n.d.-b). This reality is typically viewed through the prism of life expectancy and the effect that neighborhood choices can directly have on an individual's life span. However, that is not the full picture and most certainly does not illuminate the health equity issues.

Life expectancy rates continue to improve for the overall U.S. population, yet disparities persist and race remains a powerful predictor of them (White & Lipsitz, 2016). African Americans continue to have lower life expectancy rates than their White counterparts and higher morbidity and mortality from the leading causes of death. In fact, residential segregation—the degree to which two or more groups live separately from one another in a geographic region—is a characteristic of neighborhoods linked to persistent racial health disparities (White & Lipsitz, 2016). While housing inequity may, on its face, appear to be a policy issue with no significant impact on healthcare, that is simply not true. The social and political determinants of health begin at home and as such are heightened by housing choices. While communities across the country are attempting to be responsive to this reality and are making progress toward addressing the heavy concentration of health risks in low-income community and communities of color, health equity advocates have been slower to embrace this growing evidence (Dawes, 2016). While being cognizant of the impact that housing choices can have on individuals' health is indeed a vital first step toward addressing these inequities, it cannot be the only step.

■ Conclusion

The American Nurses Association has stated that nurses "instinctively advocate for their patients, in their workplaces, and in their communities, but legislative and political advocacy is no less important to advancing the profession and patient care" (n.d., para. 1). Policy makers are not inherently experts on every topic or subject they legislate or regulate. Rather, they rely on the knowledge of individuals who have spent their careers dedicated to mastering a specific topic. That is where you, as nurses, come in. In our society, when healthcare professionals speak up, people listen. When you answered the internal call to become a healthcare clinician, you also answered the call to advocate on behalf of those for whom you care. Use your skills and knowledge to inform policy that will effectuate positive changes in the communities you serve.

■ Critical Thinking Exercise

While you are, undoubtedly, fully versed in all of the clinical practices and techniques that you will need to be successful as a nurse, you may not be totally prepared to assess and handle cultural differences that can play an outsized role in providing quality care (Adler & Newman, 2002; Walker, Keane, & Burke, 2010).

Imagine, for a moment, that you are a new nurse who has just finished orientation at a hospital in Fort Lauderdale, Florida. It is your first overnight weekend shift on the floor and you are beginning to feel overwhelmed with an all too familiar problem with which many new nurses have to grapple: feeling understaffed. However, in the face of this adversity, you know that you are well prepared to rise to the occasion because you received stellar training and preparation during your many years of education. You can handle this.

A few hours in to your shift, two patients are admitted and assigned to your unit. Both patients are around the same age, both pregnant females, and both appear to be from the same area in Fort Lauderdale. Most importantly, both of the patients are presenting with similar health issues that they fear may be related to their pregnancy. *Begin to formulate the series of questions you might ask the patients, or their families if they are present, that you think would help fully inform you of the situation.*

As you begin to ask these two patients a series of questions to help fully understand their symptoms and what led to them coming to the hospital, *are you making any assumptions that could negatively impact the quality of care they will receive? Are you assuming that this is not their first prenatal visit? Did you assume that because they are from the same area in a bustling metropolis that they have not experienced any access to care issues?*

In Florida, as is the case with many places across the country, where you are born can and does play a major role in the quality of life you will most likely live. Across the state, the life expectancy of a newborn child can swing drastically from county to county. More alarmingly, in some neighborhoods in Broward County (where Fort Lauderdale is located), there can be upward of nearly a 15-year life expectancy difference depending on which side of the street a child grows up (National Center for Health Statistics, n.d.). Just being born on the wrong side of West Broward Boulevard can make all the difference when it comes to the social and political determinants of health a person will face.

You, as a nurse, will not always have access to the background of where your patients live or which determinants of health they face. But, you can always be mindful of the fact that there are most likely some inequities playing a role in the reason why your patient is in the hospital in the first place.

■ Discussion Questions

1. What role/responsibility do you think the nursing profession plays in addressing systemic health equity issues?
2. Given what you now know about health disparities and their impact on the health-care system, can you think of any examples of health inequities that you have over-looked in your community or clinical experiences?
3. When healthcare professionals speak up, lawmakers listen. What are some ways you would like to see the nursing profession, as a collective unit, speak up to tackle health disparities?

■ Resources

Health Affairs: https://www.healthaffairs.org

Health Equity Leadership & Exchange Network (HELEN): https://www.healthequity network.org

Hogg Foundation for Mental Health: https://hogg.utexas.edu

Kaiser J. Family Foundation: https://www.kff.org

National Conference of State Legislatures: http://www.ncsl.org

NursingWorld: https://www.nursingworld.org

Policies for Action: A Robert Wood Johnson Foundation Program: https://www.policies-foraction.org

Satcher Health Leadership Institute: http://www.satcherinstitute.org

The Commonwealth Fund: https://www.commonwealthfund.org

U.S. Department of Health and Human Services: https://www.hhs.gov

■ References

Adler, N. E., & Newman, K. (2002, March/April). *Socioeconomic disparities in health: Pathways and policies*. doi:10.1377/hlthaff.21.2.60

American Nurses Association. (n.d.). Nursing advocacy. Retrieved from https://www .nursingworld.org/practice-policy/advocacy

American Psychological Association. (2018). *Stress in America™: Generation Z.* Stress in America™ Survey. Washington, DC: Author. Retrieved from https://www.apa.org/ news/press/releases/stress/2018/stress-gen-z.pdf

Centers for Disease Control and Prevention. (n.d.). *Social determinants of health: Know what affects health*. Retrieved from https://www.cdc.gov/socialdeterminants/index .htm

Colby, S. L., & Ortman, J. M. (2014). *Projections of the size and composition of the U.S. population: 2014 to 2060* [Current Population Reports, P25-1143]. Washington, DC: U.S. Census Bureau. Retrieved from https://www.census.gov/content/dam/Census/ library/publications/2015/demo/p25-1143.pdf

Dawes, D. E. (2016). *150 years of Obamacare.* Baltimore, MD: Johns Hopkins University Press.

Dawes, D. E. (2020). *The political determinants of health.* Baltimore, MD: Johns Hopkins University Press.

Flaskerud, J. H., & Winslow, B. J. (1998). Conceptualizing vulnerable populations health-related research. *Nursing Research, 47*(2), 69–78. doi:10.1097/00006199-199803000-00005

Heckler, M. M. (n.d.). *Report of the Secretary's Task Force on black & minority health* (Vol. I). Washington, DC: U.S. Government Printing Office. Retrieved from https://minorityhealth.hhs.gov/assets/pdf/checked/1/ANDERSON.pdf

National Center for Health Statistics. (n.d.). National Vital Statistics System: U.S. Small-Area Life Expectancy Estimates Project—USALEEP. Retrieved from https://www.cdc.gov/nchs/nvss/usaleep/usaleep.html

National Institute of Mental Health. (2019). Mental illness. Retrieved from https://www.nimh.nih.gov/health/statistics/mental-illness.shtml

Orgera, K., & Artiga, S. (2018, August 08). *Disparities in health and health care: Five key questions and answers.* Retrieved from https://www.kff.org/disparities-policy/issue-brief/disparities-in-health-and-health-care-five-key-questions-and-answers

Robert Wood Johnson Foundation. (n.d.). Immigration, health care and health. Retrieved from https://www.rwjf.org/en/library/research/2017/09/immigration-status-and-health.html

Substance Abuse and Mental Health Services Administration. (2019). *A guide to SAMHSA's Strategic Prevention Framework.* Retrieved from https://www.samhsa.gov/sites/default/files/20190620-samhsa-strategic-prevention-framework-guide.pdf

Walker, R. E., Keane, C. R., & Burke, J. G. (2010). Disparities and access to healthy food in the United States: A review of food deserts literature. *Health & Place, 16*(5), 876–884. doi:10.1016/j.healthplace.2010.04.013

White, K., & Lipsitz, G. (2016). Using fair housing to achieve health equity. *Standford Social Innovation Review.* Retrieved from https://ssir.org/articles/entry/using_fair_housing_to_achieve_health_equity

Williams, D. R., Costa, M. V., Odunlami, A. O., & Mohammed, S. A. (2008). Moving Upstream. *Journal of Public Health Management and Practice, 14*(Suppl.), S8–S17. doi:10.1097/01.phh.0000338382.36695.42

World Health Organization. (n.d.-a). Health equity. Retrieved from https://www.who.int/topics/health_equity/en

World Health Organization. (n.d.-b). Housing and health equity. Retrieved from https://www.who.int/sustainable-development/housing/health-equity/en

World Health Organization. (n.d.-c). Social determinants of health. Retrieved from https://www.who.int/social_determinants/en

World Health Organization. (n.d.-d). *Glossary of terms used.* Retrieved from https://www.who.int/hia/about/glos/en/

Zong, J., Zong, J. B., Batalova, J., & Burrows, M. (2019, April 03). *Frequently requested statistics on immigrants and immigration in the United States.* Retrieved from https://www.migrationpolicy.org/article/frequently-requested-statistics-immigrants-and-immigration-united-states

17 The Intersection of Health Literacy, Health Equity, and Nursing Practice

Diana Peña Gonzalez, Rachel Roberts, and Kirby Johnson

CHAPTER OBJECTIVES

- ⊙ Identify demographic and social factors that can influence health literacy
- ⊙ Summarize the four steps of motivational interviewing
- ⊙ Describe how to use the teach-back technique to confirm patient understanding
- ⊙ Discuss the root causes of health disparities
- ⊙ Examine ways to achieve health equity through health literacy best practices
- ⊙ Evaluate the difference between plain language and medical jargon

KEY CONCEPTS

Health status disparities   Clinical competence
Effective communication   Causes for disparities
Narrative medicine

KEY TERMS

Health literacy   Plain language
Health equity   Shared decision-making
Health status disparities   Systemic racism
Social determinants of health

■ Introduction

For many patients, maintaining a healthy lifestyle requires them to be well versed in disease prevention, self-care, and disease management, all without a nursing or medical degree. When they do seek help from a healthcare provider, patients may be under duress from physical pain, medication side effects, or stress from caring for a loved one, making it more challenging to absorb, process, and understand information. Differences in culture, language, and health literacy skills can add considerable challenges to explaining difficult concepts such as discharge instructions or medication management, and an explanation that seems simple and straightforward to a clinician may be overly complicated for the patient. The result is that patients remember and understand less than half of what providers say, which has been linked to 98% of medical errors (American Medical Association Foundation, 2007).

This chapter provides a robust background on health equity and health literacy and then highlights key practices that can enhance patient understanding. The practical solutions discussed in this chapter include plain language, cultural considerations, teach-back, and motivational interviewing. By exploring the intersection of health equity and health literacy, you may begin to form new ideas on how to better serve your patients and move your community toward health equity.

■ Health Equity

WHAT IS HEALTH EQUITY?

Populations comprise diverse individuals who can be categorized into smaller groups; for example, by race, age, disability, sexual orientation, gender, geographic location, and so on. Differences in health status between these groups are referred to as "health disparities" (Brennan Ramirez, Baker, & Metzler, 2008). When these differences occur, it provides evidence that there are underlying "health inequities," or unjust limitations on access to conditions that support good health, otherwise known as the "social determinants of health" (Brennan Ramirez et al., 2008). For example, some groups have better access to healthy foods and safe housing, while other groups live in areas surrounded by liquor stores and violence. Achieving "health equity" means that everyone has a fair opportunity to achieve and maintain a healthy lifestyle, without being faced by undue obstacles to such a lifestyle (Braveman, Arkin, Orleans, Proctor, & Plough, 2017).

Achieving health equity has become a national priority in the United States through the Department of Health and Human Services *Healthy People 2030* framework. While previous iterations of *Healthy People* have included goals to reduce health disparities, it has evolved in *Healthy People 2030* to the most comprehensive approach to date: eliminate health disparities, achieve health equity, and attain health literacy to improve health and well-being for all (Office of Disease Prevention and Health Promotion, n.d.-a).

HISTORICAL HEALTH INEQUITIES

The prevalence of health inequities mirrors hidden injustices among minority populations. Individuals who feel discriminated against because of their race or ethnicity are more likely to suffer from illness and disease (Williams & Mohammed, 2009). To achieve health equity, barriers to health, such as poverty and discrimination, must be eliminated to ensure equal access to better health outcomes (Braveman et al., 2017). But how does discrimination manage to persist, even now, when individuals from disparaged populations hold decision-making positions in government?

The Iceberg Equity Model, illustrated in Figure 17.1, describes how health inequities and racism continue to exist in modern society (Gee, Ro, Shariff-Marco, & Chase, 2009). The tip of the iceberg, which is visible above water, represents *overt racism*, such as hate crimes. The larger portion of the iceberg that lies below the surface represents *systemic racism* or the social interactions, attitudes, and institutional policies that create inequities among different populations (Powell, 2008). Systemic racism provides the hidden infrastructure that enables overt racism to persist. It is

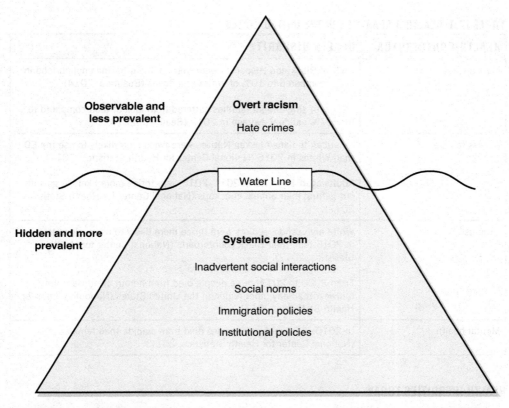

FIGURE 17.1 THE ICEBERG EQUITY MODEL. THE TIP OF THE ICEBERG REPRESENTS OVERT RACISM AND THE LARGER PORTION UNDER THE SURFACE REPRESENTS SYSTEMIC RACISM.

Source: Data from Gee, G. C., Ro, A., Shariff-Marco, S., & Chae, D. (2009). Racial discrimination and health among Asian Americans: Evidence, assessment, and directions for future research. *Epidemiologic Reviews,* *31*(1), 130–151. doi:10.1093/epirev/mxp009

also the most difficult to change as interventions often focus on correcting overt racism rather than the underlying system (Gee & Ford, 2011). To understand origins of systemic racism, consider past events and how they have influenced current social norms.

Recognizing and addressing historical events that built the infrastructure for systemic racism is essential to understanding the inequities that exist today. One example is a set of laws that enforced racial segregation between Blacks and Whites from the 1870s to the mid-1960s, known as the Jim Crow laws. These laws enforced unfair standards of etiquette, such as serving meals to Whites before Blacks, giving the right-of-way to White motorists, and requiring Whites to be spoken to with respectful language and tone (Pilgrim, 2012). More importantly, these laws impeded Black Americans from obtaining status that could influence their health, including property ownership, education, voting, and other civil liberties (Urofsky, 2018). Although the Civil Rights Movement was successful in dismantling Jim Crow laws that allowed for overt racism, it has proven to be more difficult to dismantle the negative social norms and attitudes that influence the systemic racism that persists today.

TABLE 17.1 HEALTH DISPARITIES IN THE UNITED STATES

HEALTH CONTRIBUTOR	HEALTH DISPARITY
Food access	25% of Black non-Hispanics were worried about having enough food in 2012 compared to 10% of White Americans (Beaulieu, 2014). 12.7% of single-mom families suffered from lack of food compared to the 5.7% national average in 2012 (Beaulieu, 2014).
Access to care	American Indians/Alaskan Natives were twice more likely to use the ED than Whites in 2016 (National Center for Health Statistics, 2017). Adults aged 19 to 25 in 2015–2016 were thrice more likely to go without getting their annual checkups (National Center for Health Statistics, 2017).
Drug use	White high school seniors were thrice more likely to use e-cigarettes in 2016 than their Black counterparts (National Center for Health Statistics, 2017). From 2000 to 2013, more people died from heroin overdose in the Midwest than any other region in the United States (National Center for Health Statistics, 2017).
Mental health	In 2016, 3.5 times more males died from suicide than females (National Center for Health Statistics, 2017).

HEALTH INEQUITIES TODAY

In addition to racism, people continue to experience overt and subtle discrimination based on gender, age, income, immigration status, marital status, and more; see Table 17.1 for some examples. For many, this creates unnecessary barriers to quality healthcare. Environmental and social challenges can also directly affect an individual's ability to achieve positive health outcomes. Those facing poor social and physical conditions often experience the worst health outcomes, while populations with better circumstances fare better (Brennan Ramirez et al., 2008). Unfortunately, access to healthy environments and other resources is not equally distributed (Braveman et al., 2017). Despite a forward progression toward health equity, some groups continue to face higher morbidity and mortality rates when compared with others.

■ Health Literacy

A POPULAR DEFINITION

Although the term "health literacy" has been in use since the 1970s, there has been a general lack of consensus about the precise definition. As of 2012, scholars have offered 17 different definitions (Sørensen et al., 2012). The most widely used in the United States defines health literacy as "the degree to which individuals can obtain, process, and understand the basic health information and services they need to make appropriate health decisions" (Ratzan, Parker, Selden, & Zorn, 2000, pp. v–vi). Though *literacy* has often been used as a proxy for *health literacy*, they are not the same. "Literacy" refers to an individual's ability to read and write and "health literacy" generally refers to an individual's ability to obtain, process, understand, and apply health information. To efficiently promote health literacy among populations of patients, clients, and consumers, it is helpful to be able to gauge the effectiveness of the efforts to do so. Determining what works, and what may not work, requires measurement. Over the past 30 years, the body of research on health literacy has grown substantially.

HEALTH LITERACY: A BRIEF HISTORY

The work of Doak, Doak, and Root in the late 1980s launched the health literacy movement by combining theories of adult education and health education. *Teaching Patients with Low Literacy Skills*, written by Doak, Doak, and Root in 1988, "became the major resource book available to health providers who knew that their patients weren't getting the message" (Doak, Doak, & Root, 1996, p. v). The second edition of the book, like the first, was the only book on the topic, and it "pays careful attention to both theory and application and offers us teaching skills always respectful to client, practical, and cost-effective" (Doak et al., 1996, p. v).

In conjunction with this movement, the results of two large-scale studies of literacy skills in the United States (the National Adult Literacy Study [NALS] and the National Assessment of Adult Literacy [NAAL]) conducted by the U.S. Department of Education were presented in 1993 and 2003, respectively [Kirsch, Jungeblut, Jenkins, & Kolstad, 2002; Kutner, Greenberg, Jin, & Paulsen, 2006]). To date, the NALS and NAAL studies have not been replicated. However, it is important to note the results from these studies indicated that nearly half of the U.S. adult population (47% in 1993 and 43% in 1992) were reading at marginal levels and below. Until that time, many people felt that marginal literacy was an issue for only a very small part of the population. Physicians spoke to patients in medical terms, and print materials, though often glossy and attractive, were visually dense and conceptually complex. Only a limited number of "easy-to-read" materials were available for "the unfortunate few" who struggled with reading.

Realizing that much greater percentages of adults were struggling to read basic information, medical researchers began to wonder what impact this might have on health outcomes (Rudd, 2017). A flurry of health literacy research ensued, yielding valuable insights into the effects of inadequate literacy on healthcare access and health outcomes. As a result, much has been revealed about this complex topic and the populations at risk for low health literacy.

POPULATIONS AT RISK FOR LOW HEALTH LITERACY

Although low health literacy affects persons of all demographics, certain populations experience higher rates of low health literacy. Data from the 2003 NAAL (Kutner et al., 2006) indicate that the following populations are at risk for low health literacy:

- Members of certain racial/ethnic groups (Black, Hispanic, American Indian/Alaska Native, and multiracial adults) with Hispanic adults having lower average health literacy than adults in any other racial/ethnic group
- Adults who spoke other languages alone or other languages and English
- Adults who were aged 65 or older

TABLE 17.2 FACTORS THAT CAN HAVE AN IMPACT ON OR CONTRIBUTE TO THE LEVEL OF PEOPLE'S HEALTH LITERACY

DEMOGRAPHIC AND SOCIAL FACTORS		
■ Socioeconomic status ■ Occupation ■ Employment ■ Income ■ Social support ■ Language ■ Environmental forces	■ Peer influence ■ Parental and family influence ■ Health promotion activities ■ Political forces ■ Media use	■ Education ■ The verbal communication skills of providers of service and care ■ The written communication skills of information providers
PERSONAL CHARACTERISTICS		
■ Age ■ Race ■ Gender ■ Cultural background ■ Vision	■ Hearing ■ Verbal ability ■ Memory ■ Reasoning ■ Physical abilities	■ Social skills ■ Fundamental literacy ■ Science literacy ■ Civic literacy

Source: Data from Sørensen, K., Van den Broucke, S., Fullam, J., Doyle, G., Pelikan, J., Slonska, Z., . . . HLS-EU Consortium. (2012). Health literacy and public health: A systematic review and integration of definitions and models. *BMC Public Health, 12*(80). doi:10.1186/1471-2458-12-80

- Adults who had never attended or did not complete high school
- Adults living below the poverty level

   People within these groups often report lower levels of satisfaction with the relationship they have with their provider, leading to a higher risk of decreased access to healthcare and other services (Berkman et al., 2011).

   In 2012, Kristine Sørensen and her team from the European Health Literacy Project conducted a study to explore contributing factors and consequences of health literacy. The results illustrate some of the factors that can affect health literacy skills, as listed in Table 17.2.

THE HEALTH IMPACT OF LOW HEALTH LITERACY

Only 12% of the U.S. population has proficient health literacy, which means the majority of Americans are unable to make important healthcare decisions or navigate the healthcare system.

   Due to a complex healthcare system and low health literacy rates, it is not surprising that low health literacy affects a patient's health and proper use of care. In the most recent comprehensive systematic literature review on health literacy, impact was categorized into two domains: (a) health outcomes and (b) use of healthcare services.

   With respect to health outcomes, the authors found strong evidence to suggest that lower literacy levels are associated with a higher risk of mortality for seniors, poorer overall health status among seniors, poorer ability to demonstrate taking medications appropriately, and poorer ability to interpret labels and health messages (Berkman et al., 2011).

With respect to health services, Berkman and colleagues found moderate evidence to suggest that lower literacy levels are associated with increased hospitalization, greater emergency care use, less use of preventive services such as mammograms, and lower receipt of immunizations including the influenza vaccine (2011).

The rationale for these results is due to many factors that can include culture, ability to share personal health information, and high emotional demands of the healthcare system. Individuals may feel uncomfortable in unfamiliar health situations and become overwhelmed with health information. Other individuals may have difficulty with math, which makes it challenging to measure medication, understand nutrition labels, or calculate their share of cost from the hospital visit. In addition, individuals with limited health literacy skills lack knowledge to understand the pathology of diseases or the anatomy of the human body. This can pose a challenge considering they may not understand how one might affect the other (Office of Disease Prevention and Health Promotion, n.d.-b).

BENEFITS OF IMPROVING HEALTH LITERACY

Kristine Sørensen and her team in the 2012 study also explored the possible benefits of improved health literacy skills, described in Table 17.3. These include demographic, psychological, cultural, and individual factors that may contribute to or result from a person's level of health literacy (Sørensen et al., 2012).

Although delving deeper into the variables presented in Table 17.3 cannot be achieved in this brief chapter, we can summarize by noting that improving health literacy can decrease the burden on the healthcare system and yield positive personal outcomes, which in turn impacts the community.

TABLE 17.3 POSSIBLE BENEFITS THAT MAY RESULT FROM HIGHER LEVELS OF PEOPLE'S HEALTH LITERACY

POSSIBLE PERSONAL BENEFITS	
■ Improved self-reported health status ■ Lower healthcare costs ■ Shorter hospitalization ■ Longer life ■ Less frequent use of healthcare services ■ Compliance with prescribed actions ■ Stronger incentive to develop their own knowledge and skills	■ Stronger incentive to develop their children's health knowledge and skills ■ Improved capacity to act independently ■ Improved motivation ■ More self-confidence ■ Improved resilience to social and economic adversity
POSSIBLE COMMUNITY BENEFITS	
■ Increased participation in population health programs ■ Increased capacity to influence social norms ■ Higher labor market productivity, contributing to rather than withdrawing from pension schemes	■ A lower demand for health services ■ Increased capacity to interact with social groups ■ Enhanced capacity to act on social and economic determinants of health

Source: Data from Sørensen, K., Van den Broucke, S., Fullam, J., Doyle, G., Pelikan, J., Slonska, Z., . . . HLS-EU Consortium. (2012). Health literacy and public health: A systematic review and integration of definitions and models. *BMC Public Health*, 12(80). doi:10.1186/1471-2458-12-80.

MAKING CHANGES TO IMPROVE HEALTH LITERACY

From the late 1990s into the early 21st century, the Pfizer Clear Health Communication Initiative provided grants for both health literacy researchers and practitioners (Pfizer, 2004). This encouraged multidisciplinary collaboration, adding to the growing diversity of professionals involved in addressing the problem of low health literacy. Over the years, state-based health literacy projects formed, as did partnerships with adult education organizations. According to the Centers for Disease Control and Prevention (n.d.), 20 states in the United States implemented formal initiatives to promote interdisciplinary collaboration and improve health literacy. In addition, several national organizations have called for action, including the U.S. Department of Health and Human Services, Institute of Medicine, American Medical Association, and National Institutes of Health (Berkman et al., 2011). Guidelines are available to help organizations and government agencies respond to the needs of the patients, clients, consumers, and citizens they serve. The guidelines offer best practice recommendations for developing print and online patient education materials, verbal communication, and creating a health literate environment.

Health literacy researchers around the world are increasingly collaborating on tackling the tasks of defining, assessing, and promoting people's health literacy. There is an effort currently under way to form and grow an International Health Literacy Association composed of professionals committed to "unite people around the world to promote health literacy." It will be of interest to see the extent to which researchers, healthcare providers, and health educators will collaborate and share results of their efforts to meet the health literacy needs of all people, and especially those with lower incomes, lower levels of educational attainment, and lower social status.

◼ Practical Solutions for Patient Teaching

In addition to direct patient care responsibilities, healthcare providers play a critical role in helping patients achieve positive health outcomes through patient teaching. Historically, the patient–provider relationship was unidirectional, meaning the provider made decisions for the patient. In 1956, Szasz and Hollander recommended shifting the patient–provider relationship from one where the patient is a passive listener to one where there is "mutual participation." This relationship became known as "shared decision-making" and is defined as "an approach where clinicians and patients share the best available evidence when faced with the task of making decisions, and where patients are supported to consider options, to achieve informed preferences" (Elwyn et al., 2010, p. 1361).

Inviting patients to be active partners in their healthcare and treatment plan is widely accepted as the new patient–provider communication norm. However, successful shared decision-making requires clinicians to communicate the information in plain language, or define complex medical terminology where no plain language substitute exists, and to select appropriate tools to enhance instruction.

PLAIN LANGUAGE

For many years, patients were labeled as "noncompliant" if they did not adhere to provider recommendations. However, the American Medical Association Foundation's video, *Health Literacy and Patient Safety: Help Patients Understand*, helped raise awareness about how well clinicians communicated with their patients (Weiss, 2007). This documentary showed clinicians explaining treatment options, chronic disease, and medication management using medical terminology and verbiage unfamiliar to the layperson.

According to 2014 results from the Program for the International Assessment of Adult Competencies (PIAAC), 18% of Americans read at or below the basic reading level; certain populations are at greater risk for low health literacy, especially those who suffer from limited literacy. Nevertheless, all patients have the potential to suffer from low health literacy to a certain degree. An assumption is that patients who have higher socioeconomic status or education level can understand medical instructions and effectively manage their condition or disease. However, the reality is that even if a patient has a doctorate in engineering, the patient may benefit from a plain language description of the diagnosis to effectively manage his or her disease or condition. Keep this in mind when continuing on to Case Study 17.1.

Routinely using plain language during patient interactions helps ensure patients succeed in areas including managing their health status, reducing disease-related complications, and maintaining lower healthcare costs. Some typical everyday terms used by clinicians are "persistent cough," "profound fatigue," and "injection." But these terms may not be common in a patient's everyday language. Choosing simpler terms such as "cough that won't go away," "new fatigue (feeling very tired)," and "shot" can

CASE STUDY 17.1 Assessing Language Used in Patient Interactions

A 14-year-old male patient presents with flu-like symptoms and fever of 105°F in the ED. The patient and his mother wait 5 hours in a crowded waiting room. Exhausted from the wait, they are relieved when they hear their names called. The nurse takes them to their assessment room, only to wait another 4 hours. After waiting 9 hours and finally being seen by the doctor, the following conversation takes place between the doctor and patient's mother upon discharge from the ED.

Doctor: Your son has influenza A. I'm prescribing Tamiflu. Give him one pill BID. I'm also prescribing Zofran for the nausea. He needs to take one pill sublingually as needed. Do you have any questions?

Mother: No.

Most healthcare professionals understand medical jargon since it is part of their everyday vocabulary. Care should be taken to ensure that these words are translated into plain language when explaining critical instructions to the patient. There may be many reasons the mother replies "no" when asked if she understands.

Discussion Questions

- What words or phrases did the doctor use that might be difficult for the mother to understand? Brainstorm plain language alternatives.
- What internal or external factors may have caused the mother to have difficulty understanding the information?

achieve the same outcomes while reducing confusion (Warde et al., 2018). The *Plain Language Medical Dictionary* is a useful tool used by clinicians to search for easy-to-understand alternatives to medical jargon (University of Michigan, Taubman Health Sciences Library, 2014).

In cases where there is no plain language substitute, such as hemoglobin A1c (HbA1c), use the medical term but follow up with a plain language definition. This allows patients to not only become familiar with the terminology commonly used by their healthcare team but also provides them with a "translation" of the term. For example, a provider may say,

> Mrs. Garcia, I'd like you to have a blood test called hemoglobin A1c (HbA1c). Some people call it A1c test. It tracks how much glucose or sugar has been in your blood over the past 3 months. This helps us understand if your diabetes plan is working or if we need to make changes.

WRITTEN MATERIALS

Clinicians rely on written materials to supplement education during a medical appointment or upon discharge from the hospital or outpatient facility. Many clinicians do not have the luxury or resources to write and design their own print media. However, they are often tasked with identifying patient education materials. The *Federal Plain Language Guidelines* (Plain Language Action and Information Network, 2011) offers comprehensive instructions on how to write and design consumer-friendly materials. It also serves as a useful tool to help identify low literacy resources when creating new materials is not an option. Here is a quick, albeit not comprehensive, checklist to identify if the patient material follows some of the guidelines:

- *Plain language*: Content is written in layperson terms or medical terminology is defined as needed.
- *Chunking*: Messages are grouped into logical sections.
- *White space*: The page is not filled with text; there are sections with no text or images (commonly referred to as "white space") to provide eye rest and make the page seem less difficult to navigate.
- *Type size*: Type size is 12 or 14 point. Use a larger type size, 14 to 16 point, for older adults to accommodate vision problems.
- *Images*: Culturally appropriate images are used to illustrate important points.

TEACH-BACK

Teach-back is a technique that providers can use to evaluate how effectively they conveyed information to the patient. It is not a test of *patients'* comprehension; rather, it is a test for the clinicians to see how well *they* have conveyed the information. It provides an opportunity for the clinician to explain things more clearly if their explanations were too complex at first.

To facilitate teach-back, the provider first instructs the patient using simple terms and materials. Then the clinician asks the patient to explain, in his or her own words, the information that was just discussed or presented. If the patient does not correctly "teach back" the information to the clinician, this is an opportunity for the provider to correct

CASE STUDY 17.2 Using Teach-Back to Further Patient Understanding

Doctor: Your son has influenza A. I'm prescribing Tamiflu. Give him one pill BID. I'm also prescribing Zofran for the nausea. He needs to take one pill sublingually as needed. Mrs. Smith, you've been here a long time and it's very late. I would like to be sure I explained everything correctly, so you can leave feeling confident you can take care of your son at home. Would you please explain to me what I just told you?

Mother: Well, I've heard of influenza. But I don't know what the A means. Is that the flu?

Doctor: Yes, that's correct. Influenza A and B are common during flu season and can be treated with antivirals or medicine.

Mother: So my son needs to take the medicine you're giving him. I know he needs one pill but you said something about B and D. Then you're giving him something that starts with a Z. Is he supposed to drink that too?

Doctor: Let me explain the medicines again. I did not explain well the first time. The flu medicine is called Tamiflu. Give your son one pill two times a day. Give him one in the morning and one at night before he goes to bed. Zofran is for the upset stomach. If your son feels nauseous like he might throw up, he needs to put one pill under his tongue. The pill will slowly melt to make his stomach feels better. Can you explain how to give him his medicine?

Mother: My son needs to take two Tamiflu pills every day. If he feels like he's going to throw up, he needs to put one Zofran pill under his tongue.

Doctor: Yes, that is correct.

Discussion Questions

- How is this interaction different when compared with the previous scenario? Did you notice how the provider acknowledged the mistake and corrected it? Although teach-back takes a few minutes longer, it helps to reduce the possibility of medical errors, ensuring patient safety.

misinformation and confusion, using a different approach, thereby reducing self-management errors. Let us look again at the scenario presented in Case Study 17.1, but this time, consider how things might unfold if teach-back is utilized as shown in Case Study 17.2.

MOTIVATIONAL INTERVIEWING

Along with providing clinical care, nurses also elicit behavior al change related to lifestyle choices and habits, medication management, and self-care. Several studies show that patients respond positively when the information is delivered using plain language and motivational interviewing techniques (Hettema, Steele, & Miller, 2005). Motivational interviewing is defined as "a directive, client-centered approach for eliciting behavior change by helping clients explore and resolve ambivalence" (Hettema et al., 2005, p. 91). While the goal of motivational interviewing is to help patients identify and modify behaviors that place them at risk for developing health-related complications, their success is dependent on their readiness to change and how the information is delivered (American College of Obstetricians and Gynecologists, 2009). Case Study 17.3 provides a good example of both.

Motivational interviewing is a useful technique to help patients achieve behavioral change, based on where they are in their stage of change, and to ultimately achieve their goal. The following are the four steps in motivational interviewing:

1. *Express empathy*: Communicate understanding about the patient's hesitancy to change behaviors and their experiences. For example, patients with diabetes may feel discouraged with high glucose levels and overwhelmed with their attempt to manage diabetes. They may be hesitant to try a different medication or make further changes out of fear their health will remain unchanged.

2. *Develop discrepancy*: Help patients become aware of and identify behaviors that may hinder them from achieving their goals. For example, a patient who self-reports smoking a pack of cigarettes a day is being discharged from the hospital after suffering a heart attack. The patient is motivated to change behaviors. The nurse may want to review risk factors for heart disease and then ask the patient what, if any, behaviors may prevent him or her from having a healthy heart.

3. *Roll with resistance*: Recognize behavioral change can be a difficult process and may be met with resistance. Help the patient find solutions to barriers getting in the way of making changes. For example, if patients are not meeting their weight

---

CASE STUDY 17.3 Motivational Interviewing to Encourage Positive Health Changes

A 53-year-old male Latino patient is seeing his healthcare provider to review his blood test results.

Doctor: The results of your fasting plasma glucose test remains elevated again at 215. Considering this is the second fasting plasma glucose test that yielded results 126 or higher, you definitely have diabetes. I'd like you to schedule a follow-up appointment to discuss your dietary habits and needs. I am also prescribing oral medication to bring your glucose levels down. You need to start exercising and quit smoking. I would like to see you again in 1 month. Do you have any questions?

Patient: No. My mom has diabetes, so I know all about it. In my culture, when a man is sick it means he's weak so I can't tell anyone, especially my wife. Don't give me anything to take home that says diabetes on it because my wife might find it.

Discussion Questions

- Rewrite the provider's instructions using plain language and the *Plain Language Dictionary* as needed. Remember to include teach-back techniques.
- Discuss talking points for each of the four motivational interviewing steps.

loss goals, acknowledge their busy schedule and ask them how they can incorporate additional activity into their busy day. Suggest getting off the elevator one floor earlier and using the stairs to climb one flight.

4. *Support self-efficacy*: Increase patients' self-confidence by stating you believe they are capable of making changes and achieving their goals. For example, ask patients what they feel *they* can do to reach their health goals (Levensky, Forcehimes, O'Donohue, & Beitz, 2007).

■ Conclusion

Despite our best efforts, health inequities continue to exist. While some people experience discrimination because of the color of their skin or sexual orientation, others face barriers due to the physical environment in which they live. All of this directly or indirectly influences one's health. While the health status of individuals today may be attributed to a number of factors including historical events, past laws, and present-day legislation, each person deserves to have the opportunity to make informed choices about his or her health.

Taking simple precautions such as communicating in simple terms, using teach-back, and incorporating techniques such as motivational interviewing can help patients make difficult health decisions and access better health outcomes. Increasing individual health literacy levels is one step toward increasing fair access to health for all.

Many opportunities exist to advance health literacy efforts and improve health equity. In 2017, the National Center for Education Statistics launched the International Survey of Adult Skills (ISAS), which measures math, reading, computer, and Internet skills. The results will provide updated adult literacy measures initially reported in the 1993 NAAL and 2003 NALS studies. This is an opportunity for health literacy professionals to gauge their success with past efforts and improve on ways to reduce poor patient outcomes through new methods.

Assessing the environment in which you work to determine whether it meets the criteria for a health literate environment is another chance to impact health literacy and health equity. From the person answering the phone to visible signage throughout the workplace, you can measure whether each interaction is geared toward helping a patient make informed decisions or acting as a barrier to understanding.

And last, scan the forms you ask patients to read, understand, and sign, such as consent and new patient forms, and discharge instructions. Ask yourself if the terminology used throughout is plain language or terms you find in a legal document. Every patient education material or informed consent document can be modified to retain the legal integrity and help patients make informed healthcare choices.

■ Critical Thinking Exercise

- How did Jim Crow laws affect social determinants of health?
- What, if any, are other past events that have dismantled overt racism but traces of systemic racism can still be seen in its wake?
- What are some examples of health disparities that exist between populations?

- What governmental policies contribute to or help decrease healthy disparities?
- What can you do to improve health equity?
- What words, acronyms, or jargon are commonly used in nursing? How can you put these into plain language or translate into simpler terms?

Resources

Always Use Teach-back! training toolkit: http://www.teachbacktraining.org

Brega, A. G., Barnard, J., Mabachi, N. M., Weiss, B. D., DeWalt, D. A., Brach, C., . . . West, D. R. (2015). *Health literacy universal precautions toolkit* (2nd ed., Tool #10). Rockville, MD: Agency for Healthcare Research and Quality. Retrieved from http://www.ahrq.gov/professionals/quality-patient-safety/quality-resources/tools/literacy-toolkit/healthlittoolkit2-tool10.html

Centers for Disease Control and Prevention. (n.d.). *Health literacy.* Retrieved from https://www.cdc.gov/healthliteracy/index.html

Droppa, M., & Lee, H. (2014). Motivational interviewing. *Nursing, 44*(3), 40–45. doi:10.1097/01.nurse.0000443312.58360.82

Glanz, K., Rimer, B. K., & Viswanath, K. (2015). *Health behavior: Theory, research, and practice.* San Francisco, CA: Jossey-Bass.

Hansan, J. E. (2011). Jim Crow laws and racial segregation. *Social Welfare History Project.* Retrieved from http://socialwelfare.library.vcu.edu/eras/civil-war-reconstruction/jim-crow-laws-andracial-segregation

Harvard T. H. Chan School of Public Health. (2019). Health literacy studies. Retrieved from http://www.hsph.harvard.edu/healthliteracy

Meadows, G. (2017). Shared decision making: A consideration of historical and political contexts. *World Psychiatry, 16*(2), 154–155. doi:10.1002/wps.20413

National Center for Education Statistics. (2014). Program for the International Assessment of Adult Competencies (PIAAC), U.S. PIAAC 2012/2014. Retrieved from https://nces.ed.gov/surveys/piaac/results/summary.aspx

Nielsen, L., Panzer, A. M., & Kindig, D. A. (Eds.). (2004). *Health literacy: A prescription to end confusion.* Washington, DC: National Academies Press. doi:10.17226/10883

Pleasant, A., McKinney, J., & Rikard, R. V. (2011). Health literacy measurement: A proposed research agenda. *Journal of Health Communication, 16*(Suppl. 3), 11–21. doi:10.1080/10810730.2011.604392

Rost, K., & Roter, D. (1987). Predictors of recall of medication regimens and recommendations for lifestyle change in elderly patients. *The Gerontologist, 27*(4), 510–515. doi:10.1093/geront/27.4.510

Sørensen, K., Pelikan, J. M., Röthlin, F., Ganahl, K., Slonska, Z., Doyle, G., . . . Brand, H. (2015). Health literacy in Europe: Comparative results of the European health literacy survey (HLS-EU). *The European Journal of Public Health, 25*(6), 1053–1058. doi:10.1093/eurpub/ckv043

Sørensen, K., Van den Broucke, S., Pelikan, J. M., Fullam, J., Doyle, G., Slonska, Z., . . . Brand, H. (2013). Measuring health literacy in populations: Illuminating the design and development process of the European Health Literacy Survey Questionnaire (HLS-EU-Q). *BMC Public Health, 13*(1). doi:10.1186/1471-2458-13-948

The Center for Plain Language: http://www.centerforplainlanguage.org

U.S. Department of Health and Human Services, Office of Disease Prevention and Health Promotion. (2018). *Plain language: A promising strategy for clearly communicating health information and improving health literacy.* Retrieved from http://www.health.gov/communication/literacy/plainlanguage/PlainLanguage.htm

Welch, J. (2014). Building a foundation for brief motivational interviewing: Communication to promote health literacy and behavior change. *The Journal of Continuing Education in Nursing, 45*(12), 566–572. doi:10.3928/00220124-20141120-03

Zarcadoolas, C., Pleasant, A., & Greer, D. S. (2005). Understanding health literacy: An expanded model. *Health Promotion International, 20*(2), 195–203. doi:10.1093/heapro/dah609

■ References

American College of Obstetricians and Gynecologists. (2009). Motivational interviewing: A tool for behavior change. Retrieved from https://www.acog.org/Clinical-Guidance-and-Publications/Committee-Opinions/Committee-on-Health-Care-for-Underserved-Women/Motivational-Interviewing-A-Tool-for-Behavior-Change

American Medical Association Foundation. (2007). *Health literacy and patient safety: Help patients understand* [Video]. Retrieved from https://www.youtube.com/watch?v=cGtTZ_vxjyA&t=16s

Beaulieu, S. M. (2014). *Current and prospective scope of hunger and food security in America: A review of current research.* Research Triangle Park, NC: RTI International.

Berkman, N. D., Sheridan, S. L., Donahue, K. E., Halpern, D. J., Viera, A., Crotty K., . . . Viswanathan M. (2011). *Health literacy interventions and outcomes: An updated systematic review* (Evidence Report/Technology Assessment No. 199). Rockville, MD: Agency for Healthcare Research and Quality.

Braveman, P., Arkin, E., Orleans, T., Proctor, D., & Plough, A. (2017). *What is health equity? And what difference does a definition make?* Princeton, NJ: Robert Wood Johnson Foundation.

Brennan Ramirez, L. K., Baker, E. A., & Metzler, M. (2008). *Promoting health equity: A resource to help communities address social determinants of health.* Atlanta, GA: U.S. Department of Health and Human Services, Centers for Disease Control and Prevention.

Centers for Disease Control and Prevention. (n.d.). *Health literacy activities by state.* Retrieved from https://www.cdc.gov/healthliteracy/statedata/index.html

Doak, C. C., Doak, L. G., & Root, J. H. (1996). *Teaching patients with low literacy skills* (2nd ed.). Philadelphia, PA: J.B. Lippincott.

Elwyn, G., Coulter, A., Laitner, S., Walker, E., Watson, P., & Thomson, R. (2010). Implementing shared decision making in the NHS. *BMJ, 341,* c5146. doi:10.1136/bmj.c5146

Gee, G. C., & Ford, C. L. (2011). Structural racism and health inequities. *Du Bois Review: Social Science Research on Race, 8*(1), 115–132. doi:10.1017/s1742058x11000130

Gee, G. C., Ro, A., Shariff-Marco, S., & Chae, D. (2009). Racial discrimination and health among Asian Americans: Evidence, assessment, and directions for future research. *Epidemiologic Reviews, 31*(1), 130–151. doi:10.1093/epirev/mxp009

Hettema, J., Steele, J., & Miller, W., (2005). Motivational interviewing. *Annual Review of Clinical Psychology, 1,* 91–111. doi:10.1146/annurev.clinpsy.1.102803.143833

Kirsch, I. S., Jungeblut, A., Jenkins, L., & Kolstad, A. (2002). *Adult literacy in America: A first look at the findings of the National Adult Literacy Survey* (3rd ed.). Washington, DC: National Center for Education Statistics.

Kutner, M., Greenberg, E., Jin, Y., & Paulsen, C. (2006). *The health literacy of America's adults: Results from the 2003 National Assessment of Adult Literacy (NCES 2006-483).* Washington, DC: National Center for Education Statistics.

Levensky, E. R., Forcehimes, A., O'Donohue, W. T., & Beitz, K. (2007). Motivational interviewing. *American Journal of Nursing, 107*(10), 50–58. doi:10.1097/01.naj.0000292202.06571.24

National Center for Health Statistics. (2017). *Emergency department visits within the past 12 months among adults aged 18 and over, by selected characteristics: United States, selected years 1997–2016* [Data file]. Retrieved from http://www.cdc.gov/nchs/hus/contents2017.htm#074

U.S. Department of Health and Human Services. (2019). *Healthy People 2030* framework. (n.d.). Retrieved from http://www.healthypeople.gov/2020/About-Healthy-People/Development-Healthy-People-2030/Framework

Office of Disease Prevention and Health Promotion. (n.d.-b). *Quick guide to health literacy.* Retrieved from https://health.gov/communication/literacy/quickguide/factsbasic.htm

Pfizer. (2004). *Pfizer principles for clear communication* (2nd ed.). Retrieved from http://www.pfizer.com/files/health/PfizerPrinciples.pdf

Pilgrim, D. (2012). *What was Jim Crow.* Retrieved from http://www.ferris.edu/jimcrow/what.htm

Plain Language Action and Information Network. (2011). Federal plain language guidelines. Retrieved from https://www.plainlanguage.gov/media/FederalPLGuidelines.pdf

Powell, J. A. (2008). Structural racism: Building upon the insights of John Calmore. *North Carolina Law Review, 86,* 791–816. Retrieved from https://scholarship.law.berkeley.edu/cgi/viewcontent.cgi?article=2637&context=facpubs

Ratzan, C. S., Parker, R., Selden, R. C., & Zorn, M. (2000). *National Library of Medicine current bibliographies in medicine: Health literacy.* Bethesda, MD: National Institutes of Health.

Rudd, R. (2017). Health literacy: Insight and issues. In R. A. Logan & E. R. Siegel (Eds.), *Health literacy: New directions in research, theory, and practice* (pp. 60–78). Clifton, VA: IOS Press.

Sørensen, K., Van den Broucke, S., Fullam, J., Doyle, G., Pelikan, J., Slonska, Z., . . . HLS-EU Consortium. (2012). Health literacy and public health: A systematic review and integration of definitions and models. *BMC Public Health, 12*(80). doi:10.1186/1471-2458-12-80

Szasz, T. S., & Hollander, M. H. A. (1956). A contribution to the philosophy of medicine: The basic models of the doctor-patient relationship. *American Medical Association Archives of Internal Medicine, 97.* 585–592. doi:10.1001/archinte.1956.00250230079008

University of Michigan, Taubman Health Sciences Library. (2014). *Plain language medical dictionary.* Retrieved from http://www.lib.umich.edu/taubman-health-sciences-library/plain-language-medical-dictionary

Urofsky, M. I. (2018, August 20). *Jim Crow law.* Retrieved from http://www.britannica.com/event/Jim-Crow-law

Warde, F., Papadakos, J., Papadakos, T., Rodin, D., Salhia, M., & Giuliani, M. (2018). Plain language communication as a priority competency for medical professionals in a globalized world. *Canadian Medical Education Journal, 9*(2), e52–e59. Retrieved from https://www.ncbi.nlm.nih.gov/pmc/articles/PMC6044302

Weiss, B. D. (2007). *Health literacy and patient safety: Help patients understand.* Chicago, IL: American Medical Association Foundation.

Williams, D. R., & Mohammed, S. A. (2009). Discrimination and racial disparities in health: Evidence and needed research. *Journal of Behavioral Medicine, 32*(1), 20–47. doi:10.1007/s10865-008-9185-0

The Role of Community Health Centers in Health Equity

Kevin C. Lo and Thomas Tsang

CHAPTER OBJECTIVES

- ⊙ Define a Federally Qualified Health Center (FQHC)
- ⊙ Describe the history and evolution of the FQHC movement
- ⊙ Describe the role of nurses in FQHCs
- ⊙ Highlight the development of several community health centers (CHCs)
- ⊙ Showcase the impact and explain the continued challenges for CHCs

KEY CONCEPTS

Health disparities	Comprehensive care
Social determinants of health	Patient-centered care
Integrated healthcare	Enabling services
Cultural competency	Underserved communities
Linguistic competency	Health outcomes
Community governance	

KEY TERMS

Paternalism	Displacement
Uninsured	Sustainability
Underinsured	Outreach
Service	Multicultural
Advocacy	Workforce
Gentrification	

■ Introduction

FQHCs number nearly 1,400 to date, serving 28 million people (National Association of Community Health Centers [NACHC], 2018a) and providing 110 million patient visits annually. FQHC's pioneered integrated care is based on the social determinants of health, the idea that health outcomes are a result of much more than illness and healthcare. Throughout its 50-year history, the FQHC movement has survived elastic waves of support and opposition from public officials (Lefkowitz, 2007).

As health disparities persist and shift, integrated care has persevered to become the model for healthcare delivery.

In the following pages, we describe the history of the CHC movement, define the CHC integrated model of care, showcase several CHCs, discuss their impact, and the continued challenges they face.

The CHC was born out of the Civil Rights Movement and President Lyndon B. Johnson's "War on Poverty." In a major departure, the federal government moved away for the paternalism of public welfare and heeded local community leaders wanting programs that were developed *with* them and not *for* them. Fifty years later, the Affordable Care Act (ACA) would recognize the importance of CHCs and make a major investment in the nation's healthcare safety net.

In the early 1960s, the Office of Economic Opportunity (OEO), which would become part of the Department of Health and Human Services, was tasked to research, develop, and implement new social welfare programs. In another departure, the office would bypass city and state governments that had previously not responded to the needs of the poor. The federal government worked directly with educational institutions, nonprofit organizations, and disenfranchised community members. Early OEO staffers also sought nontraditional sources such as activists, protestors, and even youth gangs. These early meetings helped officials fully realize that health was essential to fighting poverty.

Until this point, health services for the low-income and poor were far away, impersonal, episodic, expensive, or did not exist at all. Activist physician Jack Geiger, who is largely credited for the early health center model, advocated for more personalized care from a team of physicians and other health professionals in convenient locations. The model would have a community focus, be family-centered, and account for economic and environmental factors that contribute to poor health. By 1965, the OEO granted funding to the first health centers that used this full-scale model for care. In the years that followed, a struggle would ensue for greater community involvement and input because a majority of funding and control had gone to medical schools and teaching hospitals. So, in 1970, specific guidelines were created to provide job training and career advancement to neighborhood residents, create advisory boards with half of its members eligible for services, and create governing boards with one-third eligible for services.

■ Medicaid

FQHCs would continue to experience varying levels of support from government officials throughout the years, but the relationship between Medicaid and health centers played an enormous role in their growth. In 1967, the OEO committed to creating 1,000 health centers by 1973 and 80% of the operational financing would be provided by Medicaid. The growth would continue in the 1980s and 1990s when special payment rules were established to: expand eligibility to children, pregnant women, and low-income parents in some states; increase the scope of services; and increase the number of sites. This era also saw the creation of the 340B Drug Pricing Program, which provided CHCs with select pharmaceuticals at reduced prices. Under the George H. W. Bush administration, Congress enacted legislation that would create the designation known as Federally Qualified Health Centers. This legislation integrated the health center model with Medicaid and Medicare, which effectively pay closer to its full share of coverage per patient and replace federal grants as the highest source of CHC revenue. Additionally, the legislation defined the health center as an entity, the services covered, the patient's method of payment, and cost-related reimbursements for FQHCs and "look-alikes" (organizations that did not receive federal grants but otherwise met federal requirements). As a distinct benefit class, FQHCs would establish rules regarding clinical care from physicians, nurse practitioners (NPs), physician assistants (PAs), psychologists, social workers, dental, preventive care, and other ambulatory care services.

Medicaid revenues would increase from 15% in 1985 to nearly 38% in 2011 prior to ACA enactment (Shin, Sharac, & Rosenbaum, 2015) and grew to 44% by 2016 after Medicaid expansion and inclusion of the Children's Health Insurance Program (CHIP; see Kaiser, 2017). Yet this 50-year relationship has its tensions as Medicaid and health centers differ in structure and reach. For example, patients with inconsistent coverage do not fall under the scope of Medicaid, whereas health centers serve patients regardless of their ability to pay. Additionally, Medicaid beneficiaries do not necessarily live in an area with health centers whose community is largely geographically based. Still, Medicaid reimbursement remains one of the largest and much needed sources of FQHC revenue.

■ What Is a Federally Qualified Health Center?

In 2018, nearly 1,400 FQHCs served 28 million people (NACHC, 2018a) and provided 110 million patient visits annually. Health center patients are disproportionately poor with 13 million in poverty and 91% being low-income. Most are uninsured or publicly insured with 49% on Medicaid, 9% on Medicare, 23% uninsured, and 1% on other public insurance. Racial and ethnic minority groups make up 63% of health center patients, the two largest being Hispanics at 35% and Black/African Americans at 23% (NACHC, 2018b).

The guiding principles behind the health center model are today known as the "social determinants of health." This is the idea that health is affected by many more factors than medical care. According to the NACHC, social and economic factors account for 40% of life expectancy, health behaviors for 30%, physical environment for 10%, while clinical care accounts for 20%.

Ignoring social and economic, environmental, and accessibility issues can create barriers to care. This in turn can impact identifying, assessing, and treating a health problem. The health center model is built on making multiple and simultaneous interventions accessible while remaining culturally competent.

Responding to community needs requires building programs and infrastructure through community partnerships, input, and collaboration. This has resulted in the provision of multiple nonclinical services that include health education, eligibility assistance, social support, and outreach (NACHC, 2018c).

Understanding these social determinants of health, FQHCs must deliver comprehensive culturally competent, patient-centered clinical care and enabling services. To do so, health centers must be colocated in the community they serve and have a patient-majority governing board. Care delivery must be open to everyone, regardless of their ability to pay, and charge for services on a sliding fee scale. Additionally, they must meet administrative, clinical, and financial requirements under the oversight of the Health Resources and Services Administration (HRSA) Bureau of Primary Health Care (BPHC). In turn, FQHCs and look-alikes receive reimbursement for services delivered through Medicare, Medicaid, and the 340B Drug Pricing Program and the Vaccines for Children Program.

■ National Health Service Corps (NHSC)

FQHCs also receive assistance in the recruitment and retention of primary care providers through the federally funded NHSC. In 1972, NHSC was created in response to an increase in young physicians choosing to specialize rather than pursue general practice. This trend created a workforce gap in high-need areas around the country. A program was created that would provide scholarships for primary care practitioners and dentists willing to practice in underserved rural communities. As the program developed, FQHCs in urban areas found that workforce recruitment was difficult particularly in competition with large hospitals and private practices. Several health centers acquired data to fight and change legislation to include underserved urban communities, and their demands were heard. Today, the program offers scholarships and loan repayment to multiple disciplines including physicians (MDs or DOs), dentists, NPs, certified nurse-midwives (CNMs), and PAs. Members must commit to 2 years of service at an approved healthcare site in an urban, rural, or tribal area.

In 2018, NHSC has nearly 11,000 members, with 5,000 members serving at approved sites and 13,000 scholars enrolled in school or residency. Since its inception, more than 50,000 primary care medical, dental, and mental and behavioral health professionals have served across the country. More than 60% of NHSC CNMs, NPs, and physicians are working at a health center. More than half of the members who completed their service obligations continue to practice in underserved communities 10 years later (NACHC, 2018d).

■ National Association of Community Health Centers

Another advent of the CHC movement was the formation of the NACHC in 1971. Early community health leaders came together to provide education, training, and technical assistance to health center staff and board members. It has grown to serve as a national advocacy organization for the medically underserved and uninsured, and the growth of health centers that serve them. To achieve this, the NACHC conducts independent and collaborative research to advance healthcare knowledge and develops strategic public and private sector partnership to support health centers and communities.

■ The Role of Nurses

Staffing NPs, PAs, and certified nurse-midwives (CNMs) are an important component to improving access to care, improving patient outcomes, and reducing health disparities. In fact, health centers are 88% more likely to use NPs, PAs, and CNMs, which is twice as likely than other primary care practices (Hing, Hooker, & Ashman, 2011). Between 2007 and 2016, NPs, PAs, and CNMs increased by 131% at health centers (NACHC, 2018b) and account for 9 out of every 10 full-time doctors.

> *As of 2017, one-third of health center clinical visits are by NPs, PAs, and CNMs (HRSA, 2018c) and are the main sources of health education, counseling services as compared to those by physicians (NACHC, 2018c).*

In the following section, the importance of nurses at FQHCs will become particularly clear in the development and sustainability of health centers.

■ Case Study: Asian American Health

Health disparities persist across the spectrum of underserved communities, and each group has worked to respond to the needs of its community. For example, as compared to their White counterparts, American Indian and Alaskan Natives are 39% more likely to smoke, and obesity is higher among African Americans (39%) and Hispanics (32%; see Kaiser, 2019). Health gaps remain and new challenges continue to emerge across all underserved communities. In this chapter, we take a special look at the Asian American community, a group encompassing a broad range of ethnic groups, with an even broader range of languages and varying healthcare needs.

The story of Asian American health is one that is deeply rooted in a sense of pooling community resources to affect change. Many were started with simply a notion and grew to be important hubs for not only healthcare but also as a point of connectivity for community members. In the following, we look specifically at Asian and Pacific Islander (API) health organizations. APIs are tasked with addressing the needs of a community that encompasses a wide section of cultures and language and is a historically overlooked community in the American social fabric. The following profiles show how communities around the country mobilized to address their own needs and continue to serve them even as new waves of immigration bring new health concerns and challenges.

ASSOCIATION OF ASIAN PACIFIC COMMUNITY HEALTH ORGANIZATIONS (AAPCHO)

In 1985, several Asian American–serving CHCs came together at a national conference to express their frustration over the lack of API representation in advocacy and discuss ways to raise a collective voice for a growing and diverse population. This frustration was also prompted by a report of the Secretary's Task Force on Black and Minority Health by the U.S. Department of Health and Human Services that neglected to include data on the health status of API communities (USDHHS, 1985–1986). In 1987, the groups officially came together to form the AAPCHO.

The AAPCHO's mission is to be a leading national and critical voice to promoting advocacy, collaboration, and leadership that improves the health and access to health resources through its member Asian American, Native Hawaiian, and Pacific Islander (AA and NHPI) CHCs. To this end, they ensure that the community would have better access to affordable, high-quality, and culturally and linguistically proficient healthcare. The AAPCHO also develops, tests, and evaluates health education and promotion programs, offers technical assistance and training to the expansion of services, and shares the collective knowledge and experience of its membership with policy makers at the national, state, and local levels.

The AAPCHO's early advocacy initiatives included advocating for the inclusion of AA and NHPIs in the Disadvantaged Minority Health Improvement Act of 1990 and advocating for patients with limited English proficiency to have an interpreter under Title VI of the Civil Rights Act. Today their advocacy efforts fall under five major policy initiatives: promoting the patient-centered medical home (PCMH) model, implementing the ACA, eliminating health disparities, advocating for health professional shortage areas and medically underserved areas/populations, and supporting the White House Initiative on Asian Americans and Pacific Islanders. The AAPCHO works continuously and collaboratively to promote policies and legislation that support the protection of CHCs and eliminate health disparities for the underserved in their community.

The collective accomplishment of the member organizations is formidable. A 2017 analysis of the AAPCHO's 29 member organizations showed that across 12 states and one freely associated state, over 500,000 patients were served. Between 2005 and 2015, membership jumped from 16 to 29 members and the total number of patients served rose by 115%. In the same time period, patients on Medicaid increased by 173% (likely due to ACA implementation). Nineteen percent of patients were uninsured, 56% had Medicaid, and at some member CHCs 100% of patients were uninsured. The AAPCHO members serve patients in over 15 languages and dialects with 52% of patients best served in a language other than English as compared to 23% nationally. The AAPCHO FQHCs also provide more than twice the national average number of enabling service encounters at 10,642 as compared to 4,825 nationally (AAPCHO, 2017). In the following profiles, we showcase three member organizations in urban communities of the continental United States to illustrate their individual stories of struggle, sustainability, and the wide-reaching effect on their communities.

ASIAN HEALTH SERVICES (AHS; OAKLAND)

In 1973, East Bay Asians for Community Action, a group of students from an Oakland Chinatown-based advocacy group and alternative school, created a committee to assess the health needs of Oakland's Chinatown and Manilatown (AHS, 2018). They decided to conduct a door-to-door survey and found that residents used healthcare services half as often as the general U.S. population due mostly to the lack of linguistically competent and affordable healthcare. During this time, Oakland's API population was rapidly growing in both size and diversity with a large influx of immigrants. Armed with this knowledge, 11 community organizations met to discuss the need for adequate healthcare and they decided on hosting the first Asian Health Day. The huge turnout emphasized the need for affordable multilingual healthcare, and in 1974, the county awarded a grant to incorporate AHS. In the first year, the one-room clinic on 10th and Harrison Streets was staffed by young students and volunteers and provided 1,500 medical visits.

AHS continues to hold fast to its roots in the community and provide services that are informed by the community. Each year the General Membership Meeting is convened to inform patients about the healthcare policies that affect them. The feedback and inquiry from patients guide the priorities and strategic planning of the subsequent year. Additionally, the Patient Leadership Council (PLC) trains patients to become health advocates in their community. Over 100 council members participate in seven councils that represent a subset of the community including: Cantonese, Korean, Khmer, Mandarin, Tagalog, Vietnamese, and Young Adults. PLCs engage in an array of activities such as distributing patient satisfaction surveys, voter registration outreach, and supporting the review of health education materials.

As with AHS's inception, advocacy is a cornerstone of their work. In 1978, Proposition 13 was a state initiative to reduce property taxes resulting in funding cuts that would eliminate community-based contracts in Alameda County. AHS mobilized patients and staff to testify at a public hearing and on television with the use of interpreters. Along with a coalition of community organizations, protest marches were organized to send home the message that sustaining language-appropriate and affordable care was a priority. To the relief of the coalition, AHS did not lose funding and only a handful of community-based organizations experienced funding cuts. Another coup came in 1981 when AHS and other local community clinics negotiated with the Office of Civil Rights to establish a core unit of interpreters at the local Highland Hospital.

AHS's advocacy would take on a national role when it participated in the formation of the AAPCHO and Asian & Pacific Islander American Health Forum (APIAHF), an advocacy organization that provides policy and political analysis, research and data support, and effective communications strategies to mobilize communities and influence local, state, and national legislation. In 1999, the APIAHF and the AAPCHO's advocacy resulted in Presidential Executive Order 13125, a federal initiative that would recognize and improve the needs of APIs in health, education, housing, and economic and community development. Most recently, AHS has worked on the California Healthy Nail Salon Bill, Workers Rights Education in Barbering and Cosmetology Establishments, the Data Disaggregation Bill, and an initiative to address commercially sexually exploited children and human trafficking.

AHS also has outreach initiatives such as: the Community Liaison Unit for raising awareness on healthcare services; youth programs that foster the next generation of community leaders; Banteay Srei that provides a safe haven and enabling services to Southeast Asian Women at risk of or engaged in sexual exploitation; and Revive Chinatown!, a community initiative to make Oakland Chinatown safer, more pedestrian-friendly, attractive, and economically viable. To emphasize the importance of nursing at AHS, the Nurse Practitioner Fellowship was established as a comprehensive training program for recent NP graduates focusing on developing skills imperative to the community health setting and who have a commitment to working with the underserved. The salaried 1-year program with benefits provides practical, didactic, and mentored training.

Since AHS's inception, Alameda County has seen an exponential growth in the API population, having grown from 3% in 1970 to 31% in 2017 (Census, 2018). To support this burgeoning community, AHS sees more than 28,000 patients with over 115,000 visits per year providing comprehensive adult and pediatric medical, dental, behavioral, and enabling services. Patients on public insurance including Medi-Cal (California's Medicaid program), Medi-Medi (dual eligibles), or are uninsured account for 94% of patients. Services are offered in 14 languages to patients, 73% of whom experience linguistic isolation. Overall, 93% of patients are Asian, 67% are Chinese, 10% Vietnamese, and another 23% represent over eight more Asian cultures (Chinese, Vietnamese, Cambodian, Filipino, Korean, Mongolian, Burmese, Mien; see AHS, 2016).

As gentrification and economic development changes the face of Oakland and displaces longtime residents, new challenges will emerge for AHS. Yet the reach of their work beyond healthcare is what will sustain their presence. Their advocacy and outreach has provided affordable and culturally competent healthcare to the API community of Oakland.

INTERNATIONAL COMMUNITY HEALTH SERVICES (ICHS; SEATTLE)

The healthcare landscape for APIs in Seattle's Chinatown-International District of the late 1960s was plagued by several environmental factors. Seattle's Harborview Hospital scaled back services to low-income patients, and a recession caused thousands of layoffs from the Boeing Company, Seattle's largest employer of the time. Additionally, the construction of the King County Domed Stadium and Interstate 5 was believed by activists to displace longtime residents and generations of family-run businesses. These factors spurred young activists to rally against the development, and they put forth a list of demands to the King County Executive. One of these demands was to meet the healthcare needs of the community.

During this time, a concurrent movement was taking place with Sister Heide Parreno, a Catholic nun and recent immigrant from the Philippines, who volunteered to bring blood pressure screenings to elderly Filipino residents of the Chinatown-International District. At the time, the only available community health clinic was in an adjacent neighborhood too far and unsafe for elderly residents to access. Sister Heide, as she was affectionately known, saw that the International District—a historic home to APIs including Chinese, Filipino, Japanese, and Vietnamese—needed a clinic with affordable linguistically and culturally proficient healthcare.

In 1973, the student activists, Sister Heide, medical students, nurses, and many others came together to develop the Asian Community Health Clinic. Dr. Eugene Ko, a physician in Beacon Hill, invited the founding group to create a free "walk-in" clinic on Tuesday evenings. By 1975, a small storefront was secured at 416 Maynard Avenue South in the International District. The space was across the street from the newly constructed Hing Hay Park, a recreational space frequented by the elderly Filipino and Chinese residents who would become its first group of patients. Securing the storefront had been precarious as it was home to a Filipino gambling operation run by a menacing looking "proprietor" with a cigar and gun. With some negotiating, the outfit was moved upstairs and immediately volunteers from the Beacon Hill clinic moved in to set up the space.

This triumph was not a guarantee of sustainability for the newly renamed International District Community Health Clinic (IDCHC). On a shoestring budget, the clinic relied heavily on volunteers and ingenuity to offset operational costs. Soon they obtained the first of a few funding opportunities that would allow them to hire a new director and the first full-time desk receptionist. Before long, lobbying efforts on the city, county, and state levels secured $90,000 to renovate the space. Additionally, Sister Heide wrote a grant for a "nurses demonstration project" that would create a full-time nursing position for much needed outreach. Rather than wait for patients to come to the clinic, staff and volunteers visited elderly residents where they congregated including social clubs, pool halls, and in the deteriorated hotel apartments where they lived. Clearly in need for more staff, IDCHC joined the fight in the late 1970s to expand NHSC eligibility and was among the first to receive funding for a doctor and an NP.

Still, continued challenges came at the end of the Vietnam War when waves of refugees from Southeast Asia flooded the International District and the clinic. Unexpectedly, the influx of new patients resulted in Washington State funding support to recruit interpreters. Relative financial stability would come in the early 1990s when CHCs collaborated to create the Community Health Plan of Washington. The program provided a stable source of health insurance coverage for community members and a steady stream of clinic reimbursement. Another coup came in 1996 when the clinic acquired a South Seattle satellite site in Holly Park. This growth would expand services to a wider spectrum of the API diaspora and so the clinic decided to change its name to International Community Health Services. Finally, a permanent home would come in 1998 in a former Metro "bus barn." This was part of the "Village Square" initiative bringing together the ICHS, Asian Counseling and Referral Service, and the Denise Louie Education Center.

Through the many ups and downs of financial stability, ICHS is today a multi-award-winning community healthcare facility that serves nearly 31,000 patients with over 420,000 health encounters at eight clinic locations. Patients are served in over 50 languages with 55% of total patients requiring interpretation services. Three out of four patients have low income and 76% of patients are on Medicaid or Medicare, or are uninsured. ICHS continues to meet the challenges of an ever-shifting community. The influx of immigrants, refugees, and the imminent effect of gentrification threatens to displace the communities they serve. Yet it is the commitment to multiculturalism, agility, openness to change, and a welcoming presence that will continue to be the hallmark of care at ICHS.

CHARLES B. WANG COMMUNITY HEALTH CENTER (CBWCHC; NEW YORK CITY)

In 1971, a group of young community volunteers and organizers saw the need for healthcare services in New York City's Chinatown. The group wanted to bring the examining room to the community and simultaneously develop an advocacy effort for the community. The result was the first Chinatown Health Fair, which would have three main purposes: health screenings, health education, and raising community awareness of minority employment issues at the new Gouverneur Hospital east of Chinatown. The night before the weeklong fair, New York City had experienced one of the worst thunderstorms in years. Undeterred, the fair was set up and opened with a Chinese dragon dancing through the street to ensure the success of the event.

The Chinatown Health Fair provided many bilingual medical services and educational materials to the Chinatown community. Statistics gathered from the fair—that was extended for 3 additional days—showed that nearly 2,492 people had registered for at least one test, 90% of them had been Chinese, and of those 69% lived in Chinatown. The success of the fair, public demonstrations, and community meetings was finally enough pressure for the city to agree to hire 19 Chinese-speaking nurses' aides when Gouverneur Hospital opened.

The success of the fair also proved that health services were needed in the community. By the end of the same year, a group of the health fair volunteers opened the Chinatown Health Clinic in a donated space at the Episcopal Church of Our Savior. The youthful idealism of the volunteers, much influenced by the social activism of the 1960s, had no experience or license to run a clinic. Yet for 6 years, doctors, nurses, social workers, students, and others volunteered to provide two evenings and a Sunday afternoon of free health services at the church. Their work reached beyond the clinic hours when volunteers would provide interpretation services at local hospitals that were not sympathetic to the needs of racial and ethnic minorities, particularly those requiring translation.

The dedication to patients in the early days helped to increase the number of appointments and walk-in patients. By 1972, the clinic was able to incorporate as a nonprofit, began applying to public and private grant funding, and moved to a new location on Catherine Street. In the continued spirit of encouraging community youth to pursue careers in healthcare, Project AHEAD (Project Asian Health Education and Development) was started as an 8-week summer program providing college students with a field placement, workshops, and mentorship. A mark of success for this program is shown by the many former participants who returned to work for and with the clinic.

As the 1970s came to a close, the clinic had taken major steps toward obtaining a New York State operating license and federal funding. An important moment came in 1977 when the clinic was awarded $249,000 in federal funds, allowing it to hire a full-time medical director, a nurse through the NHSC program, and additional clinical and operational staff. Further funding would allow the clinic to offer a sliding fee scale based on income to qualified uninsured patients. Yet in a catch-22, the Catherine Street site did not meet the requirements necessary for state licensure and the clinic would not be able to receive the federal funds. Soon the clinic would acquire and renovate a former seafood warehouse on Baxter Street.

The clinic survived the tempestuous funding climate of the 1980s and in 1995 established the Chinatown Health Clinic Foundation to provide more financial stability for the organization. Fundraising efforts soon led to the renovation of the Canal Street site in 1999 and, in recognition of a major donor, the clinic would be renamed the Charles B. Wang Community Health Center (Hoobler & Hoobler, 2011). Today, the CBWCHC serves over 52,000 patients through over 280,000 visits operating out of five sites in Lower Manhattan and Flushing, Queens. Of these, 88% are at or below the 200% federal poverty level, 88% are better served in a language other than English, and 18% of adult patients are uninsured.

One such service is the Bridge Program, an innovation designed in response to Asian Americans being the least likely of any American ethnic group to seek mental healthcare. The program improves access to mental health services in a primary care environment, trains providers to recognize mental health symptoms, and raises

CBWCHC has achieved the highest status as a patient-centered medical home, a designation that ensures high-quality coordinated care across the spectrum of clinical and enabling services.

community awareness of mental health issues. The CBWCHC is also a recognized leader in screening and treatment of hepatitis B. The Centers for Disease Control and Prevention (CDC) reports that Asian Americans account for 50% of the nearly 1 million people living with chronic hepatitis B (CDC, 2018). In response, the health center has participated in citywide advocacy, research, and care coordination efforts. The CBWCHC has also responded during times of crisis such as the attacks of September 11, 2001. A mere 5 miles from Ground Zero, the health center and its patients were directly affected by the attack. Despite the devastation around them, the CBWCHC pushed to keep their doors open and collaborated with several organizations to participate in assistance programs through the September 11th Fund. The staff not only forged ahead to inform patients of their eligibility for benefits but also took care to reinforce mental healthcare through the Bridge Program. Additionally, concern about the environmental impact of the collapse of the Twin Towers prompted a community-based study that helped identify the need to address pediatric asthma. Although many of the youthful idealists from the early years have come and gone, it is clear that that spirit lives on in the CBWCHC's ability to identify issues affecting the community and evolve to continue serving this ever-changing population.

◼ Impact

CHCs have provided comprehensive, affordable, and culturally competent healthcare to some of the hardest to reach populations in the country. They provide care that is more cost-effective with patient outcomes that meet or exceed other primary care providers. CHCs have been able to increase both the breadth of services to 35% between 2010 and 2016. These include enabling services, medical, dental, behavioral health, and vision; the latter two experienced the largest growth of 83% and 96%, respectively. Health centers also have higher rates of accepting new patients compared to other primary care providers. Not only are CHCs cost-effective, but they also save the healthcare system $24 billion annually. This is predominantly achieved by lowering the average daily cost per patient and saving 24% per Medicaid patient. CHCs also employ over 220,000 people and create $45.6 billion in total economic activity annually within the country's most underserved communities (NACHC, 2018b).

Health centers lead the nation in achieving PCMH designations and account for 68% of all healthcare providers to be awarded this distinction. PCMH is a model of care that has been shown to relate to better clinical performance (NACHC, 2018e). The development of this standard is owed to the experimental beginnings of the early health clinics that rose out of the Civil Rights Movement. To this day, CHC patient care recognizes cultural and linguistic differences while understanding that socioeconomic factors and environment all contribute to health outcomes. No matter what changes in the healthcare landscape, it is clear that care must be accessible and coordinated beyond the primary care setting and be in tune with the ideal that community health-care treats the whole person.

The CHC model for care in addressing the social determinants of health has even permeated the private sector. Technologically driven healthcare startups and inno-vators are seeing the value in addressing social determinants of health by providing linkages to social services, mental health providers, care management, Medicaid and Medicare enrollment, and transportation to providers (MedCity News, 2019; Modern Healthcare, 2019). In fact, it is now more widely understood that addressing change-able behaviors that negatively impact health outcomes can reduce health costs. Many of the ideals and time-tested CHC methodology of integrated healthcare are now the model of care that is guiding the healthcare landscape.

■ Challenges

The sustainability of CHCs has historically been subject to the politics of the day. Over the years, legislation or the lack thereof has threatened funding and support of CHCs. For example, while the ACA made a significant investment in the growth of CHCs, a funding cliff regularly threatens it at the end of each funding cycle. The ACA estab-lished a 5-year, $11 billion Health Center Trust Fund and $1.5 billion in the NHSC. The investment allowed for discretionary funds for basic operations, expanded Med-icaid to low-income adults, established subsidized health insurance through new state exchanges, continued special payment rules under Medicaid and CHIP, and extended payment rules to Qualified Health Plans sold through the exchanges (Kaiser, 2018b). The funding was extended in 2015 and 2018 but with severe cuts to discretionary funds. Policy makers also threaten FQHC's long beneficial relationship with Medic-aid, Federal Section 330 grants, and the prospective payment system that requires a defined bundle of comprehensive services that is then reimbursed in a sustainable regular way. As each renewal period approaches, there is much concern of the funding cliff, which would have huge ramifications on adherence to Federal Section 330 com-pliance regulations, employment of thousands of clinical and nonclinical staff, and most importantly the millions of patients they serve (NACHC, 2018e). Funding cuts would also affect workforce recruitment and retention, a continued issue for health centers that are faced with more competitive salaries at private healthcare organiza-tions. Additionally, the NHSC and the Teaching Health Centers Graduate Medical Education program (places residency programs in community-based settings) rou-tinely face funding cuts.

CHCs must also keep up with the fast-paced and costly technological changes in health information technology (HIT) that is vital for recording patient data and com-munity-based research. In 2009, the Health Information Technology for Economic and Clinical Health (HITECH) Act created incentive, training, and services, for electronic health record (EHR) adoption referred to as "meaningful use." Adoption grew rapidly, and in 2017, HRSA reported that 99% of health centers have EHR programs installed (HRSA, 2018a). In recognition of the shift in EHR needs, the Centers for Medicare and Medicaid Services (2019) changed the focus and created the Promoting Interoperability program. This initiative seeks to give patients better access to their health records and more fluid, confidential, and efficient exchange of healthcare data. Other technologies such as telehealth, video interpretation, and patient portals are also costly to maintain. Staying up to date with these technologies, training staff, and analyzing data are important to identifying population-level health trends and serving individual patient needs.

Gentrification, real estate development projects, and increased costs have impacted CHCs across the country and threatened to displace disenfranchised communities. Yet the number of people who need affordable healthcare continues to increase and will require CHCs to expand and renovate their facilities through capital projects. A vast majority of health centers have planned capital projects that would result in millions of square feet of new space, but nearly all these projects have large funding gaps.

Health centers have long proven that they can survive and vocalize the needs of their communities. However, the support of all levels of government is essential to the existence and growth of CHCs. As we continue to debate healthcare reform, hopefully these and other needs will be addressed so that CHCs can sustain comprehensive high-quality care and preserve the country's healthcare safety net.

■ Conclusion

The early activist and experimental years of the CHC model faced many hurdles, but continues to adhere to the original model of providing holistic, comprehensive, personalized, and accessible healthcare. Struggles remain as populations and community boundaries shift, competition for funding and patients increase, and the uncertain political climate of healthcare reform continues. Whether they are clinical or nonclinical staff, each of these health professionals has taken on bigger roles that are beyond his or her scope of work and training. The accomplishments of CHCs and their dedication to underserved communities truly honor their reputation as the nation's healthcare safety net.

■ Critical Thinking Exercises

- You notice a new wave of immigration in your area but you neither have the workforce nor language capacity to serve these patients; some have even refused care. What should the administration at your CHC do?
- Major real estate developments are reported to be coming to the community you serve and residents are threatened with displacement. What are some steps you can take to address this issue?

■ Discussion Questions

- What is integrated healthcare?
- What is the importance of community involvement in healthcare?
- What role does gentrification and displacement play in health outcomes?

■ Resources

Association of Asian Pacific Community Health Organizations: https://www.aapcho.org

Charles B. Wang Community Health Center. (2018). *2016 Annual Report*. Retrieved from https://issuu.com/cbwchc1971/docs/annual_report_2017_final

Health Resources and Service Administration. (2018a). *Health information technology capabilities and quality recognition*. Retrieved from https://bphc.hrsa.gov/uds/datacenter.aspx?q=tehr&year=2018&state=

Health Resources and Service Administration. (2018b). *National Health Service Corps*. Retrieved from https://bhw.hrsa.gov/loansscholarships/nhsc

Health Resources and Service Administration. (2018c). *Table 5 – Staffing and utilization*. Retrieved from https://bphc.hrsa.gov/uds/datacenter.aspx?q=t5&state=

Health Resources and Service Administration. (2018d). *What is a health center?* Retrieved from https://bphc.hrsa.gov/about/what-is-a-health-center/index.html

The Henry J. Kaiser Family Foundation. (2018a). *Community health center revenues by payer source*. Retrieved from https://www.kff.org/other/state-indicator/distribution -of-revenue-by-source-for-community-health-centers/?currentTimeframe=0&sort Model=%7B%22colId%22:%22Location%22,%22sort%22:%22asc%22%7D

The Henry J. Kaiser Family Foundation. (2018b). *Issue paper: Medicaid and the uninsured March 2013*. Retrieved from https://www.kff.org/issue-paper-community-health -centers-in-an-era-of-health-reform/

The Henry J. Kaiser Family Foundation. (2019). *Key facts on health and health care by race and ethnicity*. Retrieved from https://www.kff.org/report-section/key-facts -on-health-and-health-care-by-race-and-ethnicity-section-3-health-status-and -outcomes

International Community Health Services. (2018a). *2017 annual report*. Retrieved from https://www.ichs.com/wp-content/uploads/2018/05/2017-annual-report-final2_ reduced.pdf

International Community Health Services. (2018b). *International Community Health Services: A documentary history 1973–2008*. Retrieved from http://chewcommunications .com/docs/ICHSHistory.pdf

National Association of Community Health Centers: http://www.nachc.org

National Association of Community Health Centers. (2018). *Community health centers past, present, and future: Building on 50 years of success March 2015*. Retrieved from http://www.nachc.org/wp-content/uploads/2016/12/NACHC_50th-Report.pdf

National Association of Community Health Centers. (2018). *Mission*. Retrieved from http://www.nachc.org/about/about-nachc/

National Health Service Corps: https://nhsc.hrsa.gov/scholarships/index.html

Trinh-Shevrin, C., Islam, N. S., & Rey, M. J. (2009). *Asian American communities and health: Context, research, policy and action*. San Francisco, CA: Jossey-Bass.

U.S. Census Bureau. (2018). QuickFacts: Alameda County, California. Retrieved from https://www.census.gov/quickfacts/fact/table/alamedacountycalifornia,US/PST045217

■ References

Asian Health Services. (2018). *The history of Asian Health Services*. Retrieved from http://www.chcchronicles.org/sites/default/files/4818FAB9-7E93-EE10-E006D D4FAFB03D37.pdf

Association of Asian Pacific Community Health Organizations. (2017). *An analysis of AAPCHO health centers: UDS 2015*. Retrieved from http://www.aapcho.org/wp/wp -content/uploads/2016/05/2017-UDS-Fact-Sheet_2015-Data_052217.pdf

Centers for Disease Control and Prevention. (2018). *Asian Americans and Pacific Islanders and chronic hepatitis B*. Retrieved from https://www.cdc.gov/hepatitis/populations/api.htm

Centers for Medicare and Medicaid Services. (2019). *Promoting Interoperability (PI)*. Retrieved from https://www.cms.gov/Regulations-and-Guidance/Legislation/EHRIncentivePrograms/index.html

The Henry J. Kaiser Family Foundation. (2017). *Community health centers: Growth and the role of the ACA*. Retrieved from https://www.kff.org/report-section/community-health-centers-recent-growth-and-the-role-of-the-aca-issue-brief/

Hing, E., Hooker, R., & Ashman, J. (2011). Primary health care in community health centers and compensation with office-based practice. *Journal of Community Health, 36*(3), 406–413.

Hoobler, D., & Hoobler, T. (2011). *From street fair to medical home*. China: Charles B. Wang Community Health Center.

Lefkowitz, B. (2007). *Community health centers: A movement and the people who made it happen*. New Brunswick, NJ: Rutgers University Press.

MedCity News. (2019). *Solera Health partners with Blue Cross Blue Shield Institute to tackle social determinants nationwide*. Retrieved from https://medcitynews.com/2019/03/solera-health-partners-with-blue-cross-blue-shield-institute-to-tackle-social-determinants-nationwide

Modern Healthcare. (2019). *Tending to social determinants of health with software*. Retrieved from https://www.modernhealthcare.com/article/20190126/TRANSFORMATION03/190129973/tending-to-social-determinants-of-health-with-software

National Association of Community Health Centers. (2018a). *America's Health Centers August 2018*. Retrieved from http://www.nachc.org/wp-content/uploads/2018/08/AmericasHealthCenters_FINAL_8.12.18.pdf

National Association of Community Health Centers. (2018b). *Community Health Center Chart Book June 2018*. Retrieved from http://www.nachc.org/wp-content/uploads/2018/06/Chartbook_FINAL_6.20.18.pdf

National Association of Community Health Centers. (2018c). *Powering healthier communities: Community health centers address the social determinants of health. August 2012*. Retrieved from http://www.nachc.org/wp-content/uploads/2016/07/SDH_Brief_2012.pdf

National Association of Community Health Centers. (2018d). *Staffing the safety net: Building the primary care workforce at American's health centers. March 2016*. Retrieved from http://www.nachc.org/wp-content/uploads/2015/10/NACHC_Workforce_Report_2016.pdf

National Association of Community Health Centers. (2018e). *Strengthening the safety net: Community health centers on the front lines of American health care. March 2017*. Retrieved from http://www.nachc.org/wp-content/uploads/2017/03/Strengthening-the-Safety-Net_NACHC_2017.pdf

Shin, P., Sharac, J., & Rosenbaum, S. (2015). Community health centers and Medicaid at 50: An enduring relationship essential for health system transformation. *Health Affairs, 34*(7), 1096–1104. doi:10.1377/hlthaff.2015.0099

United States Department of Health and Human Services. Secretary's Task Force on Black and Minority Health. http://resource.nlm.nih.gov/8602912

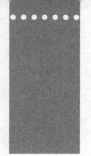

Epilogue

The previous chapters underscore the tremendous role nurses must play in achieving health equity. As nursing continues to advance as a profession, we must assume progressive levels of leadership and influence engaging in critical discussions related to improving the health profile of all populations. The goal of achieving health equity where everyone has "a fair opportunity to be as healthy as possible" will require sustained and deliberate efforts on the part of many individuals, communities, disciplines, sectors, and other entities. Achieving this goal, while daunting at times, resonates with nursing's social mandate to society and requires that nursing remain committed to integrating the principles of social justice, health equity, and a culture of health into its daily nursing endeavors. As we push forward in this regard, we must move further upstream advocating for social policies that advance the health equity agenda. When social injustices and structural inequities lead to poor health outcomes, we must move swiftly to lend our voices to causes that support better health and longevity. This commitment is particularly important for marginalized, underserved, and socially disadvantaged populations across all segments within our society. As nurses we are well positioned to help institutionalize the principles of health equity regardless of specialty or practice setting. This expanded focus on health equity is central to building a culture of health now and well into the future. Achieving health equity is a professional imperative for nursing and those we serve. Moving forward we must continue to build strong interprofessional partnerships to help leverage the expertise and resources that are needed to achieve this goal. Such attention to achieving health equity has the potential to change the health and well-being of populations worldwide. Anything less is counter to our duty as nurses.

"Of all the forms of inequality, injustice in health care is the most shocking and inhumane." —Dr. Martin Luther King Jr.

Janice M. Phillips, PhD, RN, FAAN, CENP

Index